MW00909838

PLANS OF CARE FOR SPECIALTY PRACTICE

Medical Nursing

PLANS OF CARE FOR
SPECIALTY PRACTICE

Medical Nursing

BONNIE ALLBAUGH, RN, MS, CDE
Clinical Nurse Manager
University of Wisconsin Hospitals and Clinics
Madison, Wisconsin

KATHY V. GETTRUST, RN, BSN ~ *Series Editor*
Case Manager
Midwest Medical Home Care
Milwaukee, Wisconsin

Delmar Publishers Inc.™

I(T)P™

NOTICE TO THE READER

Publisher does not warrant or guarantee any of the products described herein or perform any independent analysis in connection with any of the product information contained herein. Publisher does not assume, and expressly disclaims, any obligation to obtain and include information other than that provided to it by the manufacturer.

The reader is expressly warned to consider and adopt all safety precautions that might be indicated by the activities described herein and to avoid all potential hazards. By following the instructions contained herein, the reader willingly assumes all risks in connection with such instructions.

The publisher makes no representations or warranties of any kind, including but not limited to, the warranties of fitness for particular purpose or merchantability, nor are any such representations implied with respect to the material set forth herein, and the publisher takes no responsibility with respect to such material. The publisher shall not be liable for any special, consequential or exemplary damages resulting, in whole or in part, from the readers' use of, or reliance upon, this material.

Delmar publishing team:
Publisher: David C. Gordon
Administrative Editor: Patricia Casey
Associate Editor: Elisabeth F. Williams
Project Editor: Danya M. Plotsky
Production Coordinator: Mary Ellen Black
Art and Design Coordinator: Megan K. DeSantis
Timothy J. Conners

For information, address

Delmar Publishers Inc.
3 Columbia Circle, Box 15015
Albany, NY 12212-5015

Printed in the United States of America
Published simultaneously in Canada
by Nelson Canada,
a division of The Thomson Corporation

1 2 3 4 5 6 7 8 9 10 XXX 00 99 98 97 96 95 94

Library of Congress Cataloging-in-Publication Data

Medical nursing / (edited by) Bonnie Allbaugh.
p. cm.—(Plans of care for specialty practice)
Includes index.
ISBN 0-8273-5947-0
1. Nursing. 2. Nursing care plans. I. Allbaugh, Bonnie. II. Series.
[DNLM: 1. Nursing Care. 2. Patient Care Planning. WY 100 M4874 1994]
RT41.M478 1994
610.73—dc20
DNLM/DLC
for Library of Congress 93-9030
CIP

TABLE OF CONTENTS

COMMON RESPIRATORY CONDITIONS AND PROCEDURES

COMMON NEUROLOGICAL CONDITIONS AND PROCEDURES

COMMON RENAL AND UROLOGICAL CONDITIONS AND PROCEDURES

COMMON INFECTIOUS DISEASE AND SKIN CONDITIONS

CONTRIBUTORS

Bonnie Allbaugh, RN, MS, CDE
Clinical Nurse Manager, Diabetes, Renal and Geriatric Clinics
University of Wisconsin Hospitals and Clinics
Madison, WI

- Diabetes Mellitus: Effects of Hospitalization and Surgery
- Diabetes Mellitus: Initiating Insulin
- Diabetic Ketoacidosis and Hyperosmolar Nonketotic Syndrome

Maureen R. Anderson, RN, BSN, CRRN
Nurse Clinician III, Rehabilitation Clinic
University of Wisconsin Hospitals and Clinics
Madison, WI

- Parkinson's Disease
- Spinal Cord Injury

Penny M. Bernards, RN, MS, GNP
Clinical Nurse Specialist, Peripheral Vascular Nursing
University of Wisconsin Hospitals and Clinics
Madison, WI

- Arteriography (Arteriogram)
- Peripheral Arterial Occlusive Disease
- Thrombophlebitis/Deep-Vein Thrombosis

Linda A. Briggs, RN, MS, CCRN
Clinical Nurse Specialist, Cardiovascular Nursing
Rural Wisconsin Hospital Cooperative
Sauk City, WI

- Angina Pectoris
- Cardiomyopathy
- Congestive Heart Failure
- Digitalis Toxicity
- Endocarditis
- Hypertension
- Myocardial Infarction
- Pericarditis

Elizabeth A. Bruckbauer, RN, MS
Nurse Practitioner, Wingra Family Practice Clinic
University of Wisconsin Department of Family Practice
Madison, WI

- Multiple Sclerosis

Rochelle M. Carlson, RN, MS, CRRN
Clinical Nurse Specialist, Geriatrics and Rehabilitation
William S. Middleton Memorial Veterans Hospital
Madison, WI

- Lumbar Puncture
- Spinal Cord Injury
- Stroke/Cerebral Vascular Accident
- Traumatic Brain Injury

Mercy Galacia, RN, BSN
Nurse Manager, Orthopedic, Gynecology, Urology, Plastic and Oral Surgery
St. Vincent Hospital and Medical Center
Portland, OR
- Nephrostomy

Gail Gaustad, RN, MS
Director, Project Access
Sauk Prairie Memorial Hospital
Prairie du Sac, WI
(previously, Manager, General Surgery Unit, Meriter Hospital, Madison, WI)
- Nephrostomy

LuAnn Greiner, RN, BSN
Assistant Clinical Nurse Manager, General Medicine Unit
University of Wisconsin Hospitals and Clinics
Madison, WI
- Acquired Immunodeficiency Syndrome

Deborah R. Johnson, RN, MS, CNSN
Clinical Nurse Specialist, Medical/Surgical Nursing
Meriter Hospital
Madison, WI
- Cholecystitis/cholelithiasis
- Diverticular Disease
- Hiatal Hernia: Medical Management
- Inflammatory Bowel Disease: Crohn's Disease and Ulcerative Colitis
- Nutrition Support: Enteral Nutrition
- Nutrition Support: Total Parenteral Nutrition
- Pain Management: Patient-Controlled Analgesia
- Pancreatitis
- Peptic Ulcer Disease

Ellen M. Jovle, RN, MS
Clinical Nurse Specialist, Chronic Illness
Meriter Hospital
Madison, WI
- Asthma
- Chronic Obstructivc Pulmonary Disease: Acute Exacerbation
- Corticosteroid Therapy
- Pleural Effusion
- Pneumonia

Barbara King, RN, MS, CCRN, ANP
Geriatric Nurse Practitioner
University of Wisconsin Hospitals and Clinics Regional Services
Madison, WI
- Prevention and Care of Pressure Ulcers
- Venous Stasis Ulcers

Susan Murray, RN, MS
Clinical Nurse Manager, General Surgery/Enterostomal Therapy
University of Wisconsin Hospitals and Clinics
Madison, WI
- Prevention and Care of Pressure Ulcers
- Venous Stasis Ulcers

Lynn Schoengrund, RN, MS
Director of Nursing
Meriter Hospital
Madison, WI
- Cirrhosis and Esophageal Varices
- Hemodialysis
- Hepatitis
- Peritoneal Dialysis
- Renal Failure

Andrea Strayer, RN, MS, CNRN
Clinical Nurse Specialist,
Neuroscience and Epilepsy
William S. Middleton Memorial
Veterans Hospital
Madison, WI

- Altered Consciousness
- Amyotrophic Lateral Sclerosis
- Brain Tumors
- Central Nervous System Infections: Meningitis and Encephalitis
- Guillain-Barré Syndrome
- Seizure Disorders

Mary A. Vassalotti, RN, MS
Clinical Nurse Specialist, Oncology
Meriter Hospital
Madison, WI

- Long-Term Venous Access Devices

Linda Wonoski, RN, MSN
Manager, Intermediate Care Unit
Meriter Hospital
Madison, WI

- Cardiac Catheterization
- Chest Tubes

PREFACE

Medical-surgical nursing is one of the largest specialties within the nursing profession. Medical or surgical nursing is most often selected by nurses as they begin their nursing career. The body of knowledge required to practice medical nursing is growing constantly. The skilled nurse faces a multiplicity of medical diagnoses and problems requiring familiarity with extensive pathophysiology, human psychosocial needs, and current nursing diagnoses and treatments. While the roles and responsibilities of the nurse are expanding, the time to carry these out is decreasing. Care must be planned and coordinated to be accomplished efficiently. The plans of care in this book are designed to assist the experienced nurse with prioritizing care, to give direction, and to provide continuity of care during hospitalization and after discharge.

In medical nursing, the professions of nursing and medicine are closely interrelated. Recognizing this fact, this book is organized by medical diagnosis and/or procedure. The most common hospital admitting diagnoses and procedures have been included. The plans are comprised of background information on the medical problem: etiologies or indications, clinical manifestations, and clinical diagnostic findings; nursing diagnoses, expected patient outcomes, and nursing interventions and rationales; and discharge planning/continuity of care strategies.

Practicing nurse experts from all areas of medical-surgical nursing have contributed to this project. Their knowledge, practical experience, and high standards of care are reflected in the content of each plan of care.

ACKNOWLEDGMENTS

This book could not have been written without the willingness and interest of the contributors to share their expertise and time in writing the plans of care. Much can be learned from each. I would like to thank Trish Casey, Administrative Editor, Health Sciences, Beth Williams, Health Sciences Editor, and Elena Mauceri, Project Editor, for their support and assistance and Delmar Publishers for this opportunity. For assistance with typing and manuscript development, I want to thank Trisha Borgrud, who cheerfully gave up many evenings and weekends. I especially want to thank my husband, Stu, for his encouragement, patience, and willingness to take over house and dog responsibilities during the long hours of preparing this book, and my daughter, Gaylin, for her moral support from afar.

SERIES INTRODUCTION

Scientific and technological developments over the past several decades have revolutionized health care and care of the sick. These rapid and extensive advancements of knowledge have occurred in all fields, necessitating an ever-increasing specialization of practice. For nurses to be effective and meet the challenge in today's specialty settings, the body of clinical knowledge and skill needs to continually expand. *Plans of Care for Specialty Practice* has been written to aid the practicing nurse in meeting this challenge. The purpose of this series is to provide comprehensive, state-of-the-art plans of care and associated resource information for patient situations most commonly seen within a specialty that will serve as a standard from which care can be individualized. These plans of care are based on the profession's scientific approach to problem solving—the nursing process. Though the books are written primarily as a guide for frontline staff nurses and clinical nurse specialists practicing in specialty settings, they have application for student nurses as well.

DOCUMENTATION OF CARE

The Joint Commission on Accreditation of Healthcare Organizations (JCAHO) assumes authority for evaluating the quality and effectiveness of the practice of nursing. In 1991, the JCAHO developed its first new nursing care standards in more than a decade. One of the changes brought about by these new standards was the elimination of need for every patient to have a handwritten or computer-generated care plan in his or her chart detailing all or most of the care to be provided. The Joint Commission's standard that describes the documentation requirements stipulates that nursing assessments, identification of nursing diagnoses and/or patient care needs, interventions, outcomes of care, and discharge planning be permanently integrated into the clinical record. In other words, the nursing process needs to be documented. A separate care plan is no longer needed; however, planning and implementing care must continue as always, but using whatever form of documentation that has been approved by an institution. *Plans of Care for Specialty Practice* can be easily used with a wide variety of approaches to documentation of care.

ELEMENTS OF THE PLANS OF CARE

The chapter title is the presenting situation, which represents the most commonly seen conditions/disorders treated within the specialty setting. It may be a medical diagnosis (e.g., diabetes mellitus), a syndrome (e.g., acquired immunodeficiency syndrome), a surgical procedure (e.g., mastectomy), or a diagnostic/therapeutic procedure (e.g., thrombolytic therapy).

An opening paragraph provides a definition or concise overview of the presenting situation. It describes the condition and may contain pertinent physiological/psychological bases for the disorder. It is brief and not intended to replace further investigation for comprehensive understanding of the condition.

Etiologies

A listing of causative factors responsible for or contributing to the presenting situation is provided. This may include predisposing diseases, injuries or trauma, surgeries, microorganisms, genetic factors, environmental hazards, drugs, or psychosocial disorders. In presenting situations where no clear causal relationship can be established, current theories regarding the etiology may be included.

Clinical Manifestations

Objective and subjective signs and symptoms which describe the particular presenting situation are included. This information is revealed as a result of a health history and physical assessment and becomes part of the data base.

Clinical/Diagnostic Findings

This component contains possible diagnostic tests and procedures which might be done to determine abnormalities associated with a particular presenting situation. The name of the diagnostic procedure and the usual abnormal findings are listed.

Nursing Diagnosis

The nursing management of the health problem commences with the planning care phase of the nursing process. This includes obtaining a comprehensive history and physical assessment, identification of the nursing diagnoses, expected outcomes, interventions, and discharge planning needs.

Diagnostic labels identified by NANDA through the Tenth National Conference in April 1992 are being used throughout this series. (Based on North American Nursing Diagnosis Association, 1992. *NANDA Nursing Diagnoses: Definitions and Classification 1992.*) We have also identified new diagnoses not yet on the official NANDA list. We endorse NANDA's recommendation for nurses to develop new nursing diagnoses as the need arises and we encourage nurses using this series to do the same.

"Related to" Statements

Related to statements suggest a link or connection to the nursing diagnosis and provide direction for identifying appropriate nursing interventions. They are termed contributing factors, causes, or etiologies. There is frequently more than one related to statement for a given diagnosis. For example, change in job, marital difficulties, and impending surgery may all be "related to" the patient's nursing diagnosis of anxiety.

There is disagreement at present regarding inclusion of pathophysiological/medical diagnoses in the list of related to statements. Frequently, a medical diagnosis does not provide adequate direction for nursing care. For example, the nursing diagnosis of chronic pain related to rheumatoid arthritis does not readily suggest specific nursing interventions. It is more useful for the nurse to identify specific causes of the chronic pain such as inflammation, swelling, and fatigue; these in turn suggest more specific interventions. In cases where the medical diagnosis provides the best available information, as occurs with the more medically oriented diagnoses such as decreased cardiac output or impaired gas exchange, the medical terminology is included.

Defining Characteristics

Data collection is frequently the source for identifying defining characteristics, sometimes called signs and symptoms or patient behaviors. These data, both subjective and objective, are organized into meaningful patterns and used to verify the nursing diagnosis. The most commonly seen defining characteristics for a given diagnosis are included and should not be viewed as an all-inclusive listing.

Risk Factors

Nursing diagnoses designated as high risk are supported by risk factors that direct nursing actions to reduce or prevent the problem from developing. Since these nursing diagnoses have not yet occurred, risk factors replace the listing of actual defining characteristics and related to statements.

Patient Outcomes

Patient outcomes, sometimes termed patient goals, are observable behaviors or data which measure changes in the condition of the patient after nursing treatment. They are objective indicators of progress toward prevention of the development of high-risk nursing diagnoses or resolution/modification of actual diagnoses. Like other elements of the plan of care, patient outcome statements are dynamic and must be reviewed and modified periodically as the patient progresses. Assigning realistic "target or evaluation dates" for evaluation of progress toward outcome achievement is crucial. Since there are so many considerations involved in when the outcome could be achieved (e.g., varying lengths of stay, individual patient condition), these plans of care do not include evaluation dates; the date needs to be individualized and assigned using the professional judgment and discretion of the nurse caring for the patient.

Nursing Interventions

Nursing interventions are the treatment options/actions the nurse employs to prevent, modify, or resolve the nursing diagnosis. They are driven by the related to statements and risk factors and are selected based on the outcomes to be achieved. Treatment options should be chosen only if they apply realistically to a specific patient condition. The nurse also needs to determine frequencies for each intervention based on professional judgment and individual patient need.

We have included independent, interdependent, and dependent nursing interventions as they reflect current practice. We have not made a distinction between these kinds of interventions because of institutional differences and increasing independence in nursing practice. The interventions that are interdependent or dependent will require collaboration with other professionals. The nurse will need to determine when this is necessary and take appropriate action. The interventions include assessment, therapeutic, and teaching actions.

Rationales

The rationales provide scientific explanation or theoretical bases for the interventions; interventions can then be selected more intelligently and actions can be tailored to each individual's needs.

The rationales provided may be used as a quick reference for the nurse unfamiliar with the reason for a given intervention and as a tool for patient education. These rationales may include principles, theory, and/or research findings from current literature. The rationales are intended as reference information and, as such, should not be transcribed into the permanent patient record. A rationale is not provided when the intervention is self-explanatory.

Discharge Planning/Continuity of Care

Because stays in acute care hospitals are becoming shorter due to cost containment efforts, patients are frequently discharged still needing care; discharge planning is the process of anticipating and planning for needs after discharge. Effective discharge planning begins with admission and continues with ongoing assessment of the patient and family needs. Included in the discharge planning/continuity of care section are suggestions for follow-up measures, such as skilled nursing care; physical, occupational, speech, or psychiatric therapy; spiritual counseling, social service assistance; follow-up appointments, and equipment/supplies.

References

A listing of references appears at the conclusion of each plan of care or related group of plans. The purpose of the references is to cite specific work used and to specify background information or suggestions for further reading. Citings provided represent the most current nursing theory and/or research bases for inclusion in the plans of care.

Clinical Clips

Interspersed throughout the books are brief pieces of information related to the particular specialty. The intent is to blend some concept or theory tidbits with the practical nature of the books. This information not only may enrich the nurse's knowledge base but also may be used in the dissemination of patient education information.

A Word About Family

The authors and editors of this series recognize the vital role that family and/or other significant people play in the recovery of a patient. Isolation from the family unit during hospitalization may disrupt self-concept and feelings of security. Family members, or persons involved in the patient's care, must be included in the teaching to ensure that it is appropriate and will be followed. In an effort to constrain the books' size, the patient outcome, nursing intervention, and discharge planning sections usually do not include reference to the family or other significant people; however, the reader can assume that they are to be included along with the patient whenever appropriate.

Any undertaking of the magnitude of this series becomes the concern of many people. I specifically thank all of the very capable nursing specialists who authored or edited the individual books. Their attention to providing state-of-the-art information in a quick, usable form will provide the reader with current reference information for providing excellent patient care.

The editorial staff, particularly Patricia E. Casey and Elisabeth F. Williams, and production people at Delmar Publishers have been outstanding. Their frank criticism, comments, and encouragement have improved the quality of the series.

Finally, but most importantly, I thank my husband, John, and children, Katrina and Allison, for their sacrifices and patience during yet another publishing project.

Kathy V. Gettrust
Series Editor

LIST OF TABLES

Special Needs and Procedures

LONG-TERM VENOUS ACCESS DEVICES

Mary A. Vassalotti, RN, MS

Long-term venous access devices are used to administer intravenous (IV) antibiotics, chemotherapy, hydration fluids, and total parenteral nutrition in either the home or the hospital setting. They may be inserted peripherally, centrally through the chest or implanted in a pocket on the chest. These devices are either external catheters or implanted ports accessed through the skin with a noncoring needle. There are two types of catheters: closed end (Groshong) and open end (Hickman). Placement of either an external catheter or implanted port can be performed as an outpatient procedure under local anesthetic. This plan encompasses centrally placed access devices.

ETIOLOGIES

None

CLINICAL MANIFESTATIONS

- Poor peripheral access for short-term IV catheters
- Receiving vesicant/irritating medication
- Potential for prolonged therapy (months)
- Fear of repetitive needle sticks
- Need for frequent blood draws/blood products

CLINICAL/DIAGNOSTIC FINDINGS

None

▼

NURSING DIAGNOSIS: KNOWLEDGE DEFICIT—PROCEDURE AND POSTOPERATIVE CARE

Related To

- New experience
- No previous exposure to information

Patient Outcomes

The patient will

- state reasons for and process of placement of device.
- state immediate postoperative complications: bleeding, pneumothorax.
- demonstrate site care, dressing change, inspection of the site, cap changes, and flushing technique appropriate for the type of catheter.
- state who and when to call for assistance.
- define comfort measures to relieve pain and discomfort after placement of the line.

Nursing Interventions	Rationales
Discuss reason(s) for device being placed (see Clinical Manifestations and Table 1.1).	
Explain process for placement: 1. sterile procedure 2. IV placed prior to procedure 3. potential IV sedation with placement 4. use of local anesthetic 5. actual procedure time as little as 30 min 6. chest x-ray taken to confirm placement	Implanted ports are placed in the right infraclavicular fossa (see Figure 1.1). The catheter is threaded through the subclavian vein and terminates at the junction of the superior vena cava and the right atrium. Incision will be approximately 3 in. long with internal stitches. External catheters are threaded through the subclavian vein and terminate at the junction of the superior vena cava just above the right atrium (see Figure 1.2). The proximal end is tunnelled from the entrance site in the subclavian vein through the subcutaneous fascia of the chest wall and brought out through an exit site on the chest. The catheter will have a Dacron polyester fiber cuff placed about 2 mm from the exit site. This cuff promotes fibrin growth, which helps anchor the catheter in place.The cuff will also prevent bacteria from migrating up the catheter.

Nursing Interventions	Rationales
Instruct patient to expect shoulder stiffness and soreness for 24–72 hr after placement of the line. Comfort measures could include 1. nonsteroidal analgesics (NSAIDs) Tylenol, or mild narcotics 2. heat to shoulder area 3. ice to exit site if bleeding occurs	
Discuss the potential for pneumothorax induced with placement of the line, signs and symptoms, and how treated.	
Teach site care, dressing change. See steps under High Risk for Infection and Table 1.2.	
Review care of healed site. When site is healed, exit site may be cleansed in the shower.	
Teach patient cap changes. See steps under High Risk for Infection.	
Teach patient flushing solution/technique appropriate for type of catheter.	
Instruct to observe for signs of complications daily while device is present and appropriate resource persons to call if problems occur. The following problems and/or their symptoms should be reported immediately: 1. infection: locally at site—redness, drainage, erythema, tenderness; systemically—fever and chills 2. catheter malfunction: leakage, breakage of line 3. catheter thrombosis: swelling of arm, discomfort in chest and arm catheter displacement: cuff becomes visible, catheter falls out, unable to draw or infuse	These complications need immediate attention to prevent increasing problems. None are life threatening, but they could lead to major problems.

Table 1.1 • General Comparison of Venous Access Device

External Silastic Catheter	Implantable Ports
May remain in place as long as trouble free.	Silicone septum good for 1000–2000 punctures (varies per manufacturer).
Open-system catheter capped with injection cap.	Completely closed system.
Barrier against infection: tunnelled Dacron cuff.	Barrier against infection: skin.
Surgically inserted, may be removed in office setting.	Surgically inserted and removed.
Features: single, double, and triple lumens available.	Features: single and double lumens/septums available.
Maintenance: requires daily to weekly flush with normal saline or heparin, 10 U/mL). Regular dressing change and injection cap change. Care is done by patient, family, or home health agency. Maintenance costs include heparin or saline, syringes, needles, alcohol wipes, dressing supplies, injection caps, etc.	Maintenance: requires heparin or normal saline flush every 4 weeks. Usually done by nurse or trained phlebotomist. Maintenance cost minimal.
Appearance: tube outside of body and limits to physical freedom. Four to 5 inches of external catheter present.	Appearance: minimal alteration in body image because port is totally under the skin. Minimal limits on physical freedom.
Access: catheter accessed directly into catheter or through needle into injection cap.	Access: special needle (Huber non-coring) required to puncture skin and septum of catheter.
Placement: exit site of catheter will vary depending on surgical technique.	Placement: placed over bony prominence to allow stability during accessing. Potential areas of placement are limited, especially in overweight patients.
Complications: 1. Catheter-related infections. 2. Occluding thrombosis. 3. Infuses, but cannot draw. 4. Catheter damage, leakage, or dislodgment. 5. Spontaneous blood backflow (open-ended catheters).	*Complications*: 1. Port-related infections. 2. Occluding thrombosis. 3. Infuses but cannot draw. 4. Catheter, migration, damage, or leakage. 5. Catheter-needle dislodgment.

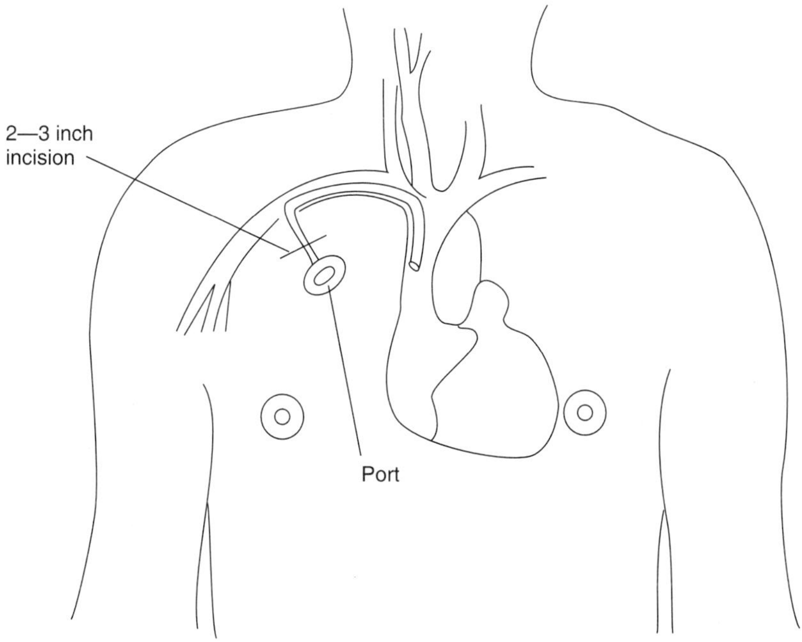

Figure 1-1. Implanted Port

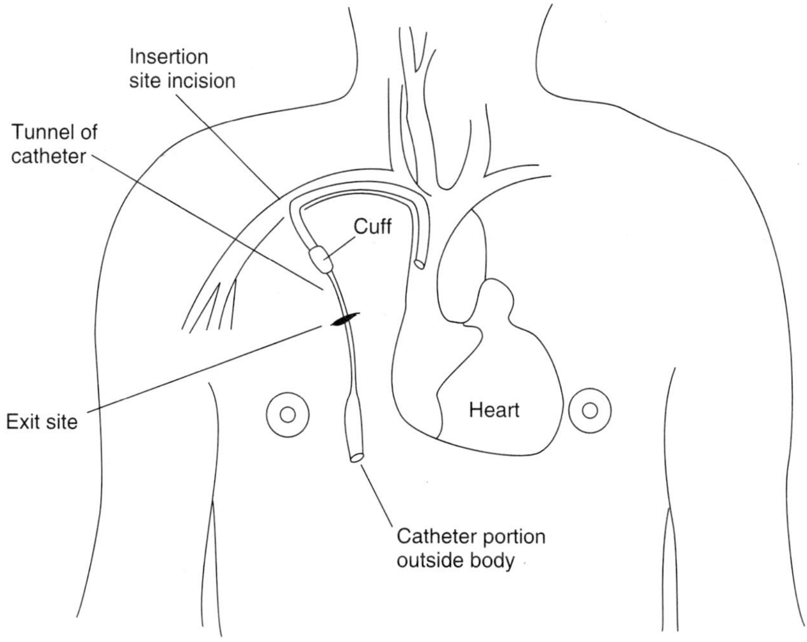

Figure 1-2. Central Catheter Placement:
Insertion and Exit Site

Table 1.2 • Postoperative Care of Long-Term Venous Access Devices

	External	Implanted Port
Dressing change exit site	Change initial dressing after 24–48 hr. Dressing may need reinforcement if bleeding present after placement.	Anticipate 3-inch incision with absorbable sutures. Dressing removed after 24–48 hr. Usually requires no further dressing.
Dressing change entrance site	Remove initial dressing after 24–48 hr. Observe for redness or drainage. Cover with Band-Aid, clear dressing, or no dressing.	No entrance site.

▼

NURSING DIAGNOSIS: HIGH RISK FOR IMPAIRED GAS EXCHANGE

Risk Factors

- Potential for pneumothorax with surgical procedure
- Difficulty placing line

Patient Outcomes

The patient will not exhibit symptoms of pneumothorax, as evidenced by an absence of pain with inspiration, shortness of breath, and anxiety.

Nursing Interventions	Rationales
Assess patient for signs and symptoms of pneumothorax; assess for pain with inspiration, shortness of breath, or anxiety frequently after catheter placement.	
If patient is discharged on the same day as placement, instruct on the symptoms to assess at home.	If symptoms occur, patient should call physician immediately.

▼

NURSING DIAGNOSIS: HIGH RISK FOR INFECTION

Risk Factors

- Traumatized tissue with placement
- Altered immune system/chronic disease
- Poor personal hygiene

Patient Outcomes

The patient and/or caregiver will

- demonstrate site care, dressing change, inspection of the site, cap changes, and flushing technique appropriate for the type of catheter.
- identify resources to call with questions/problems.

Nursing Interventions	Rationales
Protect insertion and exit site (see Figure 1.2).	
1. Remove initial dressing on *insertion site* after 24 hr. Keep site clean and observe for signs of infection.Remove sutures (if present) once healing occurs (2–3 weeks).	
2. Leave the initial, occlusive, pressure dressing on the *exit site* intact for 2–3 days after surgery. Then change the dressing every 2–3 days until the exit site is healed (2–3 weeks). At this time, the sutures anchoring the catheter in place should be removed. Once healed, the site may be washed daily in the shower and a Band-Aid placed. Some patients may want to continue to use a transparent dressing. Depending on the patient situation and institution policy, the healed site may require no dressing.	The initial dressing is left in place to permit surgical healing and lessen the risk of bacteria being introduced.
3. Change dressing immediately when soiled, wet, or no longer intact.	

Nursing Interventions	Rationales
Aseptically change dressing wearing nonsterile gloves (universal precautions).	
1. Remove old dressing and discard. Never use scissors to remove dressing as the catheter could be inadvertently severed or damaged.	
2. Remove gloves and wash hands.	
3. Inspect catheter *exit site* for leaking fluid, bloody or purulent drainage, redness, swelling, or induration.	
4. Palpate along tunnel route for swelling or tenderness. Notify appropriate personnel if these problems occur.	
5. Organize supplies on work area. Put on sterile examination gloves and maintain aseptic technique.	
6. Cleanse *exit site* if bloody or crusty drainage is present with hydrogen peroxide. Then cleanse with povidone-iodine swabs as for the exit site.	
7. Clean exit site with 2 povidone-iodine swabsticks. Cleansing must begin at the *exit site* and move away from the catheter. Clean in a circular motion covering an area of 3 in. in every direction. Never return to the *exit site* with the same swabstick. Let dry for at least 60 s.	The antimicrobial activity of povidone-iodine occurs as the solution dries on the skin.
8. With the swabstick, clean the catheter from the *exit site* distally. Allow the povidone-iodine to dry.	
9. Antimicrobial ointment may be applied to the *exit site* with sterile cotton tip applicators.	The efficacy of using antimicrobial ointment to decrease exit site colonization remains controversial.

Nursing Interventions	Rationales
10. A skin protective preparation (i.e., Skin Prep) may be applied to the area around the catheter and allowed to dry.	Use of Skin Prep may decrease skin irritation and create better adhesion of dressing.
11. Apply dressing of choice (see Table 1.3).Ensure dressing is occlusive.	Randomized studies have found no statistical difference between use of transparent gauze or no dressing.
12. Secure the catheter and its tubing to the dressing or skin with tape.	If catheter is inadvertently pulled on, the tape will help prevent the initial tug from the catheter from being pulled out.
13. Label dressing with date and initials.	
Change the cap of external catheters weekly and as needed. Each manufacturer has recommendations for frequency of cap changes.	
1. Use only short luer-lock injection caps.	Short luer-lock injection caps will not require injection of flushing solution into cap before flushing entire line.
2. Clamp catheter (Hickman).	
3. Clean the junction between the catheter or extension tubing and old injection cap with disinfectant. Allow to dry.	
4. Put on nonsterile gloves (universal precautions).	
5. Remove old injection cap and attach the new injection cap.	
6. Secure external catheter to chest with tape.	
Flush catheter using aseptic technique (see Table 1.4).	
If unable to flush catheter, consider using antithrombolytic agent such as urokinase 5000 IU (1 mL) per physician and manufacturer's recommendation.	

Nursing Interventions	Rationales
For implanted ports, aseptically a insert noncoring needle (straight or 90° bent) into implanted port to flush or use the port. 1. Locate the portal septum by palpating it under the skin. 2. Cleanse the injection site with povidone-iodine (or alcohol). Allow to dry.	Noncoring needles are available in straight or right-angle configurations in various lengths and gauges. The noncoring needle has a deflected point that helps avoid damage to the septum.
3. While the port is held firmly between two fingers of the nondominant hand, grasp the wings of the noncoring needle with the dominant hand and insert needle, perpendicular to the septum, through the skin and septum until it reaches the bottom of the portal system. 4. If the needle is to be left in, place a 2 x 2 gauze under the wings of the extension tubing; use a 3 x 5 clear dressing over the entire site to anchor.	Care should be taken when inserting a noncoring needle into an implanted port. Excessive insertion pressure or "grinding" of the needle against the portal base may damage the needle point. A "barbed" needle point may damage the resealing septum.

▼

NURSING DIAGNOSIS: HIGH RISK FOR BODY IMAGE DISTURBANCE

Risk Factors

- Tube hanging outside the body (Groshong, Hickman)
- Bulge present in the body (port)
- Required physical restrictions

Patient Outcomes

The patient will

- be involved in choice (if treatment plan allows) of type of line to be used preoperatively.
- express feelings/concern over having the catheter present in the body.
- identify coping mechanisms that will be of assistance.

Table 1.3 • Catheter Exit Site Dressings

Type	Advantages	Disadvantages
Transparent	Permeable membrane allows oxygen, moisture out; impermeable to bacteria. Allows visualization of site. Can remain in place 3–7 days. Greater patient comfort. Provides barrier for catheter dislodgment.	Expense. Allows cleansing of site with dressing change only. May increase colonization of bacteria. Poor adhesion with diaphoresis or bleeding at site.
Gauze	Absorbs moisture or drainage. Less expensive. Provides barrier for catheter dislodgment.	No visualization of site. Risk of irritation from tape. Increased frequency of dressing change: daily to every 3 days.
No dressing	Daily cleansing of site. Allows visualization of site. No irritation related to adhesive. No expense.	Greater risk of catheter dislodgment. No barrier to contamination.

▼

Table 1.4 • Flushing Solutions

Catheter Type	Frequency	Solution/Amount
Groshong (closed end) with two-way valve	Brisk flush after each use, or every 7 days	5 mL normal saline (*do not flush with heparin*) 20 mL normal saline following viscous solutions such as lipids.
Hickman (open end)	Before and after each use Above followed by heparin (10 U/mL) after each use or every 12–24 hr	3–5 mL normal saline 3–5 mL 10 U/mL heparin solution

▼

Nursing Interventions	Rationales
Assure patient understanding of care and maintenance and the effect the required restrictions will have on his or her lifestyle.	Patient may not be clear about the care and maintenance of a particular line.
Allow patient to express any concerns over the existence of a line. Provide strategies on how to incorporate the addition of the line into patient's lifestyle, i.e., types of clothing to wear, dealing with small children.	

▼

DISCHARGE PLANNING/CONTINUITY OF CARE

- Assure understanding of and ability to perform care and maintenance of line.
- Provide patient with needed supplies (usually 1 month's supply) and establish a plan for obtaining refills as needed.
- Assure follow-up with physician/nurse for questions and continued management.
- Refer to a home care agency if further assistance is needed for teaching or ongoing follow-up.

REFERENCES

Access Device Guidelines Module I—Recommendations for Nursing Education and Practice. Module I—Catheters. (1989). Pittsburgh, PA: Oncology Nursing Society.

Burke, M., Berg, W., Ingwersen, B. et al. (1991). *Cancer chemotherapy: A nursing process approach.* Boston: Jones and Bartlett.

Lucas, A.(1992). A critical review of venous access devices: The nursing perspective. *Current Issues in Cancer Nursing Practice*, *1*(7), 1–10.

Tillman, K. R. (1991). Venous access devices: Guidelines for home healthcare nurses. *Home Healthcare Nurse*, *9*(5), 13–17.

▼

NUTRITION SUPPORT: ENTERAL NUTRITION

Deborah R. Johnson, RN, MS, CNSN

Enteral nutrition is the delivery of nutrients directly into a functioning gastrointestinal (GI) tract. Total enteral nutrition is delivered by a tube when normal GI motility and absorption are present but caloric needs are unmet by usual oral intake because of some underlying illness or deficit. Malnourished patients requiring tube feeding may or may not outwardly appear clinically starved. Patients may present in a simple starvation state and appear cachetic; the body's adaptive mechanism (decreased metabolic rate and gradual wasting of body fat and skeletal muscle) operates to preserve protein stores. The patient with sepsis or trauma or one requiring an extensive surgical procedure may not appear malnourished or starved on physical exam but is significantly metabolically stressed. The metabolically stressed patient also requires enteral nutritional support to meet his or her needs because of limited body adaptive mechanisms, accelerated protein catabolism, and increased energy expenditure. See Decision Tree for Enteral vs. Parenteral Nutrition Support Delivery System (Figure 2.1).

ETIOLOGIES

- Neuromuscular impairments (usually permanent enteral access is needed with feeding into stomach or past the pylorus):
  - impaired gag or swallow reflexes
  - head trauma, cerebral vascular accidents, multiple sclerosis, or comatose state
- The lack of desire or incapability to ingest adequate oral intake to meet metabolic needs
  - chemo- or radiation therapy with mucositis, stomatitis
  - obstructive lesions of the esophagus, pharynx
  - the transition time during weaning from total parenteral nutrition and introducing oral feedings
- Inability to eat as a result of underlying illness (access temporary or permanent with feeding tube placed past the pylorus)
  - trauma

- burns
- sepsis

CLINICAL MANIFESTATIONS

- Muscle weakness, fatigue
- Anorexia, poor oral intake
- Aversion to food
- Weight loss, lack of interest in food
- Aspiration of food/fluids

Signs of severe malnutrition
- Subcutaneous fat loss, generalized muscle wasting
- Scaly dermatitis
- Dilated veins
- Petechia
- Poor skin turgor
- Dry mucous membranes
- Extremity edema
- Brittle thin nails
- Lack of hair luster, thinning hair
- Blepharitis
- Bitot's spots (grey triangular spots related to vitamin A deficiency)
- Lethargy, irritability, confusion
- Glossitis, cheilosis, angular stomatitis
- Parotid or thyroid enlargement

CLINICAL/DIAGNOSTIC FINDINGS

- Inadequate calorie counts or a dietary history assessment that indicates food intolerances, aversions, poor oral intake, or underlying clinical conditions causing decreased nutrient intake
- Somatic protein compartment assessment
  - weight less than normal for height
  - abnormal skin fold anthropometric measurements
- Visceral protein compartment assessment
  - decreased serum albumin
  - decreased serum transferrin
  - decreased hemoglobin and hematocrit levels.
- Immunocompetence assessment
  - delayed cutaneous hypersensitivity (anergic response)
  - decreased total lymphocytic count
- Abnormal swallow study

  NOTE: The above diagnostic findings may not be absolute indicators to diagnose the need for enteral nutrition. Certain diagnostic findings can be influenced by nonnutritional factors such as general anesthesia, steroid use, and fluid resuscitation. The decision to tube feed a patient with a functioning GI tract should be made only after examining the patient holistically.

NURSING DIAGNOSIS: ALTERED NUTRITION—LESS THAN BODY REQUIREMENTS

Related To

- Inability to ingest nutrients orally
- Inability to ingest adequate nutrient amounts
- Increased metabolic demand for nutrients

Defining Characteristics

Demonstrated protein/calorie malnutrition for more than 5–7 days
Inability to take over 50% of necessary calories by mouth
Greater than 10% unintentional weight loss despite oral intake
Altered level of consciousness
Impaired swallowing
Muscle weakness, anorexia, depression
Inability to meet increased nutritional needs by oral intake due to accelerated metabolic demands caused by sepsis, major trauma, or illness

Patient Outcomes

Patient will progress toward an improved nutritional state, as evidenced by

- weight increases towards normal range for age, sex, height, and activity level
- serum albumin, transferrin, hemoglobin, hematocrit, lymphocyte count, blood sugar, and electrolytes within normal range or improved
- urine area nitrogen balanced or positive
- improved strength, energy, and activity tolerance
- healing wounds or improved tissue integrity/skin turgor
- predictable bowel elimination patterns
- anthropometric measurements progressing toward normal

Nursing Interventions	Rationales
Consult dietitian or nutrition support team, if available, for recommended calorie, protein, carbohydrate, fat requirements, assistance with enteral formula selection and enteral access route (nasogastric, nasoduodenal, percutaneous endoscopic gastrostomy (PEG), or jejunostomy tube. See Decision Tree for Enteral vs. Parenteral Nutrition Support Delivery System (Figure 2.1).	

Nursing Interventions	Rationales
Weigh patient every other day at same time with the same amount of clothing and equipment using the same scale.	Accurate serial measurements are important to establish patient response to therapy.
Maintain accurate intake and output measurement. Intake includes colloid, crystalloid, and enteral feeding formula. Output includes all urine, loose stool, gastric losses, wound drainage, and presence of febrile episodes.	Attention to insensible losses is important to assure additional free water requirements are being met to prevent dehydration.
Implement techniques to maintain feeding tube patency:	
1. Flush feeding tube with at least 20–30 mL of water every 4 hr during continuous feeding, before and after giving medications, and after each intermittent gravity feeding or gastric residual check.	Tubes that are routinely and prophylactically irrigated with water have a lower incidence of obstruction. Tubes irrigated with cranberry juice have a higher rate of tube obstruction and shorter duration of use than tubes irrigated with water.
2. Insert a feeding tube made of a polyurethane material if available.	Formula flows more quickly through tubes made of polyurethane than silicone.
3. Administer medications in elixir form if available. Consult with the pharmacist.	Pill fragments from inadequately crushed medications are a frequent cause of tube obstruction.
4. Use an infusion pump when viscous enteral formulas are being used or if feedings are given at a slow rate.	A slow, low-pressure formula flow can promote feeding formula to adhere to the feeding tube lumen and cause obstruction.
5. If feeding tube becomes obstructed, attempt to irrigate it with water or cola. Avoid using meat tenderizer or pancreatic enzyme slurry mixtures.	Although meat tenderizer solutions can dissolve protein coagulated materials and pancreatic enzyme materials are often superior to meat tenderizer solutions, in dissolving some obstructions, use of these materials is discouraged because they can cause severe lung damage if given through a feeding tube that is accidently malpositioned in the respiratory tract.

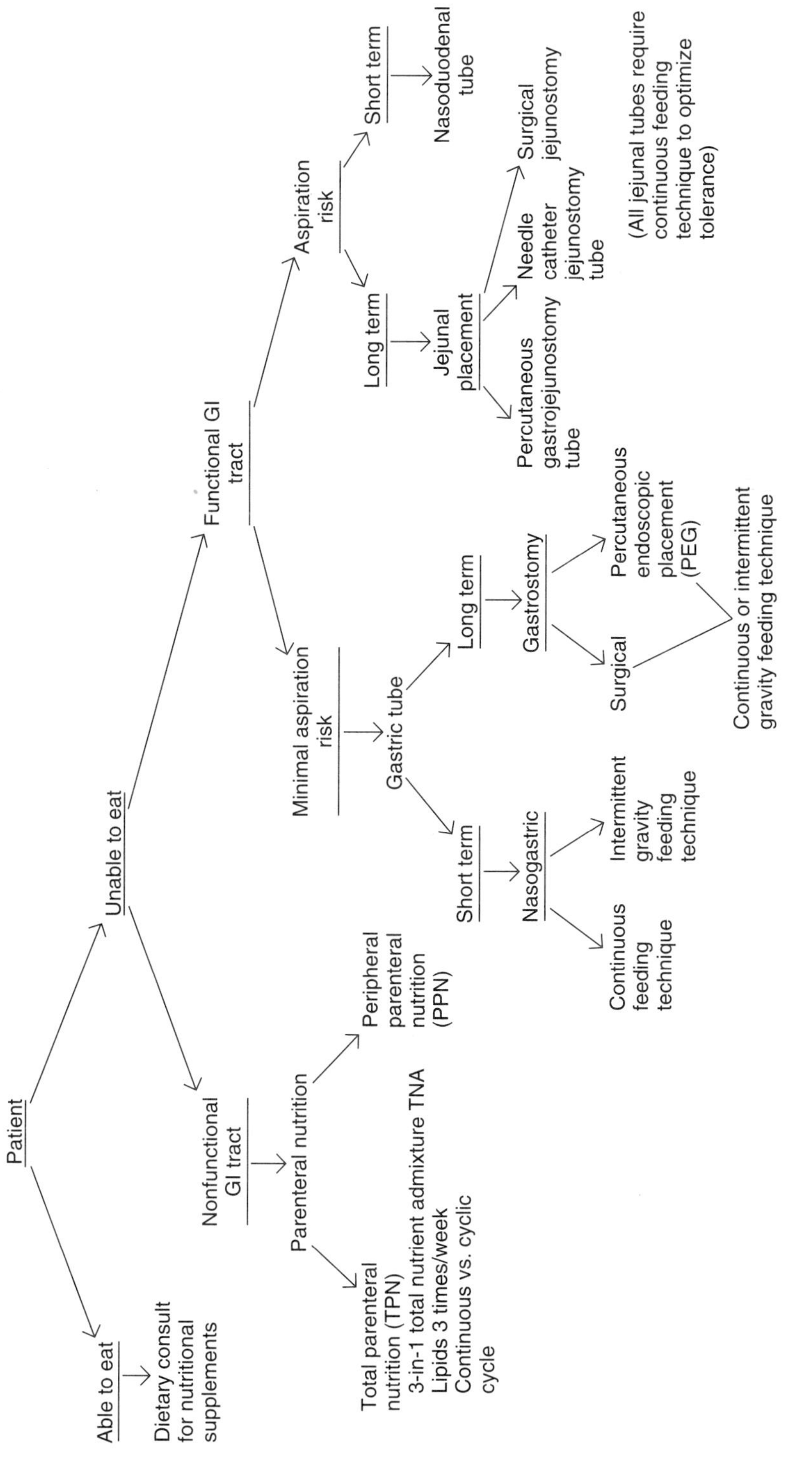

Figure 2–1. Decision Tree for Enteral vs. Parenteral Nutrition Support Delivery System

NURSING DIAGNOSIS: HIGH RISK FOR ASPIRATION

Risk Factors

- Malpositioned feeding tube
- Inability to maintain airway
- Impaired cough and gag reflexes
- Altered level of consciousness
- Incompetent esophageal sphincter (history of reflux or hiatal hernia)
- Delayed gastric emptying (gastroparesis associated with diabetes)
- Demonstrated GI intolerance to feeding with nausea, vomiting, abdominal fullness, and gastric residuals > 100–150 mL
- Inability to elevate head of bed 30°–45° at all times during continuous feeding or 1 hr before, during, and after intermittent gravity feeding

Patient Outcomes

Patient will demonstrate no aspiration, as evidenced by

- unlabored respirations
- normal complete blood cell count and differential
- adequate aeration in all lung fields via auscultation
- warm, dry, pink skin
- clear chest x-ray
- no unexplained fever

Nursing Interventions	Rationales
Insert a small-bore (7–8 French size) nasal enteral feeding tube to deliver formula.	Small-bore tubes are less likely to disrupt the esophageal sphincter and cause reflux compared to larger bore (14–16 French size) nasal tubes.
Assure proper enteral tube placement:	Pulmonary complications are generally caused by improper tube placement during insertion or from formula aspiration.
1. Measure tube for insertion landmarks and place tube as instructed on manufacturer's recommendation.	
2. After tube is placed, attempt to aspirate gastric contents to confirm gastric placement.	It may be impossible to aspirate gastric contents from a small-bore feeding tube because the tube may collapse during attempts to aspirate. Be aware that fluid can be aspirated from pleural space and mistaken for gastric contents.

Nursing Interventions	Rationales
3. Auscultate air insufflation over abdomen to confirm gastric placement.	This may also be misleading. The tube could be in the pleural space and sounds transmitted below the diaphragm can be mistaken for proper gastric placement.
4. Verify placement with x-ray.	This is the most accurate and reliable way to verify proper placement of a small-bore enteral feeding tube.
Tape nasal tube securely, after x-ray verification, and measure tube from nose to a predetermined point. Check this measurement at least once a shift.	Prevents migration of the tube and provides clues if the tube is migrating out of position.
If patient is at very high risk for aspiration, anticipate the need to place a weighted transpyloric feeding tube (jejunal or duodenal).	Placing a transpyloric tube minimizes incidence of gastric reflux and subsequent aspiration.
Elevate head of bed to 30°–45° while on continuous tube feeding or 1 hr before, during, and after each intermittent gravity feeding, if possible.	Optimizes stomach emptying and prevents reflux.
Encourage ambulation if not clinically contraindicated.	Optimizes stomach emptying and prevents reflux.
Add a small amount of vegetable-based food coloring to tube feeding in all patients at risk for aspiration.	Color will indicate presence or absence of tube feeding in sputum when coughing or suctioning.
Assure presence of bowel sounds by auscultating abdomen at least once a shift.	

Nursing Interventions	Rationales
Check gastric residuals every 4 hr and as needed when patient is on a continuous tube feeding or before each intermittent gravity feeding. Stop tube feeding or hold scheduled intermittent gravity feeding if residuals are above 100–150 mL. Slowly refeed the residual. Recheck residuals after 1 hr and resume feeding if residuals are below 100–150 mL.	Stomach may not be emptying well and distention and vomiting could occur. It may be difficult to check residuals with a small-bore (7–8 French size) nasal tube, hence assess patient for feeling of fullness, nausea, or increased abdominal girth. NOTE: There will be no residuals when a jejunostomy tube is placed because unlike the stomach, the jejunum is not a reservoir for food. The enteral formula should be delivered continuously via an enteral pump to maximize GI tolerance when a jejunostomy tube is used.

▼

NURSING DIAGNOSIS: HIGH RISK FOR IMPAIRED SKIN INTEGRITY

Risk Factors

- Enteral tube pressure on skin
- Enteral tube shearing motion on skin
- Drainage from enteral tube site
- Existing alteration in nutritional state

Patient Outcomes

Area at enteral tube site is clean and dry without redness, swelling, pain or drainage.

Nursing Interventions	Rationales
Assess skin around enteral tube for redness, swelling, tenderness, and drainage daily, and more frequently as needed.	
If nasal feeding is indicated, attempt to place a small (7–8 French size) soft polyurethane nasal enteral tube.	It is less irritating to nares and throat than the larger (14–18 French size) polyvinyl nasal gastric tubes.

Nursing Interventions	Rationales
If a nasal enteral tube is in use:	
1. Assess security of tape at nose regularly. Secure and position feeding tube to patient's gown/clothing to prevent shearing, friction, and unnecessary motion.	A secured tube without shearing motion minimizes tissue breakdown or areas of pressure necrosis.
2. Lubricate nares regularly; cleanse nose if crusting; provide mouth care every 2–4 hr.	
If a surgically and percutaneously placed gastric or jejunal tube is used:	
1. Cleanse tube site regularly with soap and water; apply split gauze or a sterile transparent dressing.	
2. Apply half-strength hydrogen peroxide to tube site if area is crusted and make sure to rinse peroxide from the skin.	
3. Tape the tube securely to minimize any shear, drag, and/or tension on tube.	
4. Apply abdominal binder over the tube if the patient is confused or agitated and pulling at tube.	
5. Avoid application of any topical ointments to the tube site unless specifically preserved.	Betadine ointment applied to a tube site for any length of time can destroy healthy granulation tissue. Chronic use of antibiotic ointment can foster a yeast infection.

▼

NURSING DIAGNOSIS: HIGH RISK FOR DIARRHEA

Risk Factors

- Non-tube-feeding related
  - low serum albumin levels
  - antibiotic administration
  - antacid administration

  - medications in elixir form (sorbital based)
- Tube-feeding related
  - bacterial contamination
  - improper feeding formula composition, hyperosmolar solution, absence/presence of fiber, solution high in fat
  - Formula infusion rate is too fast.

Patient Outcomes

Patient tolerates tube feeding volume, concentration, rate, and formula type, as evidenced by

- soft, formed, stools evacuated on a regular predictable schedule
- no more than 3 stools a day
- improved serum albumin

Nursing Interventions	Rationales
Assess for all non-tube-feeding related causes of diarrhea, including	
1. low serum albumin	Hypoalbuminemia disrupts intestinal cell osmotic pressure, hence compromising tube-feeding formula absorption.
2. drug therapy that may cause diarrhea, such as antibiotics, histamine 2 (H_2) blockers, oral medications in elixir form, and magnesium antacid	Antibiotics alter normal intestinal flora and bacterial overgrowth occurs; may need to administer a lactobacillus acidophilus preparation to restore GI flora. Histamine 2 blockers alter gastric pH, which causes bacterial overgrowth and diarrhea. Elixirs can contain sorbitol or another hypertonic base, which if given undiluted, may increase diarrhea. Alternating magnesium antacids with calcium- or aluminum-containing antacids may decrease diarrhea.

Nursing Interventions	Rationales
3. bacterial contamination	Prevent bacterial contamination by: using good hand washing technique when handling tubes, formula, or other equipment; avoid touching the inside of the tube-feeding delivery set during refilling and decanting; use only enough formula for 4–6 hr of tube feeding at one time; rinse tube-feeding delivery set with water before adding new formula; change tube-feeding delivery sets every 24 hr; when possible use full-strength, commercially prepared, ready-to-use formula.
4. presence of fecal impaction if not clinically contraindicated.	May be stooling around fecal impaction.
Assess for causes of diarrhea related to the tube-feeding formula. 1. Consult dietitian for assistance. 2. Examine enteral formula composition, including • fat content • fiber content • osmolality • lactose content	A fat content greater than 20 g fat/L can induce diarrhea. Dietary fiber and bulking agents may prevent or help control diarrhea in tube-fed patients. Hyperosmolar solutions greater than 280 mOsm/L may be poorly tolerated by the GI tract of a severely malnourished patient. The patient with a malabsorption problem may produce a "dumping syndrome" characterized by cold sweats, dizziness, distention, weakness, tachycardia, nausea, and diarrhea; the nurse may need to dilute this hyperosmolar formula to a more isotonic formula. Lactose intolerance is rarely a problem, as most commercially prepared enteral formulas do not contain lactose.

▼

DISCHARGE PLANNING/CONTINUITY OF CARE

- Assure patient/family understands self-care management plan:
  - feeding tube site care, assessments, and dressing changes
  - medication administration
  - tube-feeding formula storage
  - proper administration of formula by intermittent gravity feeding or continuous feeding technique
  - troubleshooting equipment
  - troubleshooting signs/symptoms of GI distress or feeding intolerance
  - when to call the physician
- Refer patient to a home health care agency if continued nursing care, teaching, or assistance with a self-care management plan is needed.
- Arrange follow-up with nurse and/or physician for continued management after discharge.
- Assist patient with obtaining prescriptions and establish a plan of refilling prescriptions.
- Assure that the financial arrangements (cost and reimbursement) for the enteral nutrition supplies be reviewed, discussed, and accepted by the patient prior to discharge.
- Establish a workable plan with the patient to deliver additional enteral supplies when materials need replenishing.

REFERENCES

Eisenberg, P. (1989). Enteral nutrition—indications, formulas and delivery techniques. *Nursing Clinics of North America*, *24*, 315–338.

Keithley, J. K. & Kohn, C. L. (1992). Advances in nutritional care of medical-surgical patient. *Medical Surgical Nursing*, *1*, 13–21, 67.

Kennedy-Caldwell, C., & Guenter, P. A. (1988). *Nutrition support nursing core curriculum* (2nd ed). Silver Spring, MD: American Society for Parenteral and Enteral Nutrition.

Kohn, C. L. & Keithley, J. K. (1989). Enteral nutrition: Potential complications and patient monitoring. *Nursing Clinics Of North America*, *24*, 339–353.

Rombeau, J. L. & Caldwell, M. D. (1990). *Clinical nutrition enteral and tube feeding* (2nd ed). Philadelphia, PA: Saunders.

▼

NUTRITION SUPPORT: PARENTERAL NUTRITION

Deborah R. Johnson, RN, MS, CNSN

Patients who cannot meet their caloric needs by the usual oral route or through a tube feeding because of abnormal gastrointestinal (GI) absorption or motility may be candidates for total parenteral nutrition (TPN). Total parenteral nutrition, also called hyperalimentation, is the administration of intravenous (IV) nutrients directly into the peripheral or central venous circulation. Peripheral parenteral nutrition (PPN) is administered through a large peripheral vein when nutrition support may only be needed for a short time, protein and calorie requirements are not high, or the placement of a central venous catheter (CVC) would be dangerous or technically difficult. Parenteral solutions that contain glucose as the primary energy source have a high osmolality, which can be *very irritating* to peripheral veins; hence PPN solutions rely on isotonic lipid emulsions for the main source of nonprotein calories. Phlebitis is frequently reported with PPN, and there are often times it is not possible to meet an adult's total nutritional needs with PPN. Central parenteral nutrition is most often given through a catheter inserted into the subclavian vein and threaded into the superior vena cava; the jugular or femoral vein may be used if the subclavian is inaccessible. A CVC enables the administration of hypertonic dextrose solutions to meet the nutritional needs of severely stressed or hypermetabolic patients. Central parenteral solutions may be compounded as a dual mixture of carbohydrates and amino acids (protein) or with a lipid (fat) source which is infused, *separately*, two to three times a week, or the lipids may be combined *with* the carbohydrate and amino acids in one large bag. This latter option is referred to as a "3-in-1" solution or a total nutrient admixture (TNA). All 3-in-1 solutions, including bags and tubing, must be changed every 24 hr.

ETIOLOGIES

- Conditions requiring complete bowel rest:
  - pancreatitis, enteric fistulas
  - inflammatory bowel disease
- Conditions that interfere with GI nutrient absorption
  - Short bowel syndrome
  - radiation enteritis
  - bowel obstruction/ileus
  - Congenital malformations
- Persistent uncontrollable vomiting or diarrhea related to
  - chemotherapy/radiation therapy
  - hyperemesis gravidarum
  - pseudomembranous colitis

CLINICAL MANIFESTATIONS

- Weight loss
- Persistent vomiting/diarrhea
- Documented intolerance to oral intake
- Documented intolerance to tube feeding

CLINICAL/DIAGNOSTIC FINDINGS

- Fluid and electrolyte imbalances
- Abnormal abdominal x-ray: obstruction or motility disturbance
- Elevated serum amylase/lipase
- Decreased serum albumin
- Decreased serum transferrin
- Weight outside of referenced normal for recorded height

OTHER PLANS OF CARE TO REFERENCE

- Nutrition Support: Enteral Nutrition
- Long-Term Venous Access Devices

▼

NURSING DIAGNOSIS: ALTERED NUTRITION–LESS THAN BODY REQUIREMENTS

Related To

- Inability to ingest foods orally
- Inability to absorb nutrients in adequate amounts
- Increased metabolic demand for nutrients

Defining Characteristics

Weight loss
Reported inadequate food intake less than recommended daily allowance
Aversion to eating
Abdominal pain with associated pathology
Satiety immediately after ingesting food
Abdominal cramping
Diarrhea
Vomiting
Weakness, fatigue
Poor muscle tone

Patient Outcomes

Patient will progress toward an improved nutritional state, as evidenced by

- weight increases toward normal range for age, sex, height, and activity level
- serum albumin, transferrin, hemoglobin, hematocrit, electrolytes, blood sugar, and chemistries within normal range or improved
- urine urea nitrogen balanced or positive
- improved strength, energy, and activity tolerance
- healing wounds or improved tissue integrity/skin turgor
- predictable bowel elimination patterns
- anthropometric measurements progressing toward a normal range

Nursing Interventions	Rationales
Consult dietitian, pharmacist, or nutrition support team, if available.	These resource people can provide recommendations for caloric needs, fat, carbohydrate, and protein requirements. They can also assist with monitoring blood chemistries and fluid and electrolyte balance as well as compounding the TPN solution.
Administer TPN at a constant rate using an infusion pump: 1. Do not interrupt the flow of TPN. 2. Do not increase or decrease the TPN rate to accommodate total IV fluids that could have fallen behind or infused too quickly. 3. If TPN catheter clots and TPN cannot be infused, notify physician, start a peripheral IV with at least a 5% dextrose solution at same rate as TPN.	An infusion pump regulates the flow rate more accurately than gravity and decreases the likelihood of fluid, metabolic, and electrolyte imbalances. Hyperglycemia or hypoglycemic reactions can occur if TPN solutions are not given at a steady rate or if the TPN is suddenly discontinued.

Nursing Interventions	Rationales
Monitor serum or capillary glucose levels as needed (e.g., every 6–8 hr when TPN is at a final rate and more frequently when TPN is initiated) to establish patients' baseline serum glucose levels and their tolerance to the infused glucose load. Serum glucose levels should stay between 100–200 mg/dL.	Blood glucose levels above 200 mg/dL may indicate the following: the need for supplemental insulin to increase tolerance to the infused glucose load; an expected short-term postoperative surgical stress response; and impending infection or sepsis. Blood glucose monitoring is more sensitive and allows tighter control/titration than urine glucose testing because urine is only positive for glucose when levels exceed renal threshold at approximately 240 mg/dL.
Infuse IV fat (lipid) emulsions as prescribed: 1. If lipids are given separately, infuse through an additional peripheral IV line or through a Y connector attached to the TPN catheter: • Infuse each fat emulsion over 4–8 hr two to three times per week. • Administer separate fat emulsion slowly over the first 15–30 min (60 mL/hr 10% lipid emulsion, and 30 mL/hr, 20% lipid emulsion); if tolerated increase to maximum of 125 mL/hr (10% lipid emulsion) or 160 mL/hr (20% lipid emulsion). • Observe for dyspnea, chest or back pain, and pain at IV site during infusions.	Lipids prevent essential fatty acid deficiency and provide caloric source: Infusion of fats separately prevents breakdown of fat emulsions and decreases risk of fat emboli. Slower rates allow body to assimilate the fat and prevent hyperlipidemia. Allergic reactions to fat emulsions may be local or systemic.

Nursing Interventions	Rationales
2. Infuse lipids in the specially prepared TPN, 3–in-1/TNA solution.	There is better normalization of blood glucoses when all nutrients are combined. Fat sources may be better tolerated when combined together with carbohydrates and amino acids and not given separately. There may be reduced infection rates because no additional breaks in IV tubing are done to hang fat emulsions separately. The TNA solutions may be more cost effective and time saving for Pharmacy and Nursing when compared to hanging separate bags of solution throughout the patient's course of TPN therapy.
3. Do not hang the TNA solution if there is any fat separation observed, as evidenced by a yellow-colored ring around the edges of the bag. Notify the pharmacy.	These solutions can separate if not correctly mixed by pharmacist. This may cause fat emboli.
4. Do not use IV filters with any fat emulsion infusions.	Fat particle size exceeds filter pore size and solution will not infuse.
Weigh patient daily or every other day at the same time with the same amount of clothing and equipment utilizing the same scale.	Accurate serial measurements are important to establish patient response to therapy.
Monitor and record accurate intake and output. Assess for signs and symptoms of fluid imbalances.	Overhydration or underhydration may occur with TPN and TPN solutions need to be reformulated accordingly.
Monitor serum electrolytes and blood chemistries.	Chemical and metabolic imbalances may occur in patients receiving TPN.
Assess for continued improvement in GI function, e.g., improved tolerance to oral intake, decreased nausea, vomiting, and diarrhea. Collaborate with physician and/or dietitian to follow progress.	Patients receiving TPN should be transitioned to enteral feeding when appropriate as the enteral route is the preferred method to provide nutrition support to patients with a functioning GI tract.

Nursing Interventions	Rationales
Collaborate with nutrition support team, physician, pharmacist, and/or dietitian when TPN is to be discontinued for assistance with weaning or tapering parameters. Total parenteral nutrition can usually be discontinued within 4–6 hr.	Proper tapering rates/weaning parameters prevent hypoglycemia. Hypoglycemia is less common with the TNA 3-in-1 solutions.

▼

NURSING DIAGNOSIS: HIGH RISK FOR INJURY

Risk Factors

- Central venous catheter insertion and removal
- Bleeding
- Pneumothorax, hemopneumothorax
- Air emboli, thromboemboli

Patient Outcomes

Patient is not harmed during catheter insertion, catheter usage, or removal, as evidenced by

- unlabored symmetrical respirations
- bilateral breath sounds
- normal chest x-ray
- chest x-ray confirmation of proper catheter placement
- patent catheter
- no evidence of catheter emboli

Nursing Interventions	Rationales
Maintain patient in Trendelenburg position with rolled towel between the scapulae while physician, using a sterile technique, inserts the CVC.	The Trendelenburg position increases venous pressure in the subclavian vein, thus distending it for easier cannulation. This helps to prevent air from entering the venous system during catheter insertion. A sterile technique minimizes the potential for infectious complications.

Nursing Interventions	Rationales
Observe for signs/symptoms of shock and respiratory distress during CVC insertion, including tachycardia, hypotension, tachypnea, dyspnea, use of accessory muscles, and absent or decreased breath sounds on affected side.	Shock and/or respiratory distress can occur with complications. The lung may be punctured during insertion and a pneumothorax may occur. An artery may be cannulated, in error, during line insertion. Bleeding may compress the trachea.
After the CVC is inserted, arrange for an immediate chest x-ray. Auscultate lungs in all fields postinsertion and at least once a shift.	The x-ray confirms catheter tip placement in the superior vena cava and rules out pneumo-, hemo-, or chylothorax. Comprehensive auscultation of lung fields assures full-lung aeration. A pneumothorax may not manifest itself immediately on the initial postinsertion x-ray.
Begin TPN only after CVC tip placement is confirmed by x-ray in the superior vena cava.	The hyperosmolar TPN solution can be irritating to smaller vessels (subclavian, innominate, jugular) and can cause thrombophlebitis.
Securely tape all TPN tubing connections and/or use a standardized male-female leur-lock connector system.	Prevents accidental disconnections. Disconnections could result in air emboli, bleeding, clot formation, loss of catheter patency, contamination, and sepsis.
Assess for signs/symptoms of air emboli: sharp chest pain, sudden in nature, extreme anxiety, cyanosis, and churning precordial murmur.	Large amounts of air in the venous circulation may cause an air lock in the heart with subsequent cardiac arrest related to blocked blood flow and ischemia.
If air emboli are suspected, immediately place patient in Trendelenburg with left side down. Administer oxygen and notify physician immediately.	This position allows air to collect at the apex of the right ventricle. Small amounts of air may pass into the pulmonary circulation and be reabsorbed. Air may need to be aspirated by the physician from the right atrium with a needle to relieve the air lock. This is a *medical emergency*.

Nursing Interventions	Rationales
If the CVC intravenous system must be opened to air (e.g., cap changes, catheter repair), instruct the patient to perform a Valsalva maneuver by taking a deep breath, holding it, and bearing down as if having a bowel movement, before opening the CVC intravenous system. Use any CVC clamps provided by the manufacturer to prevent air from entering the system.	The Valsalva maneuver increases intrathoracic pressure and prevents air from entering the IV system and the bloodstream.
Assess chest wall for presence of visible collateral circulation.	This is a sign of venous thrombosis.
Observe for the presence of a suture at the insertion site of a temporary CVC, or if a more permanent, long-term CVC was placed (Broviac, Hickman, Groshong), the suture will be at the exit site. Observe the catheter for any notable increase in external catheter length.	Sutures stabilize the catheter, and an increased external length indicates catheter movement with potential displacement.
Assess for swelling around the CVC insertion site, shoulder, clavicle, and upper extremity. Note any complaints of chest pain, burning, or fluid leaking at the insertion site. Any inability to withdraw blood from a previously patent CVC warrants further investigation.	May indicate vein thrombosis and/or catheter displacement.
When catheter removal is indicated:	
1. Assist patient to supine position.	Allows optimal visualization for suture removal and application of occlusive dressing.
2. Instruct patient to perform the Valsalva maneuver prior to CVC removal.	
3. Immediately after catheter removal, apply ointment (betadine or antibiotic) to exit hole and a sealed, airtight, occlusive dressing.	If ointment and an airtight sealed dressing is not applied, the CVC sinus tract allows air to enter the venous system during inspiration, potentially causing air emboli.
4. Measure catheter length and observe integrity of catheter.	Ensure entire catheter was completely removed.

▼

NURSING DIAGNOSIS: HIGH RISK FOR INFECTION

Risk Factors

- Indwelling (CVC)
- Administration of contaminated TPN solution

Patient Outcomes

Patient is without infection as evidenced by

- normal white blood cell (WBC) count
- afebrile response
- normal serum blood glucose
- negative blood cultures
- negative catheter tip culture
- CVC site without redness, swelling, drainage, warmth, or tenderness

Nursing Interventions	Rationales
Monitor WBC, blood glucose levels, temperature, and pulse rate. Notify physician of any increases (subtle or more dramatic) that may be above the patient's established baseline.	Increases may indicate impending line infection/sepsis.
Monitor results of blood cultures if obtained.	
Assess CVC site daily and as needed. Observe for redness, swelling, drainage, or tenderness.	
Change CVC dressing following institution protocol or any time dressing is damp or nonocclusive using sterile technique.	
Adhere to institution protocol for TPN tubing changes and antibacterial preparation of all IV tubing connector sites.	
Refrigerate TPN until ready to use. Each TPN solution should not hang longer than 24 hr.	
Never add any additional substances to the TPN solutions specially prepared in the pharmacy.	

Nursing Interventions	Rationales
Do not infuse any cloudy or precipitated TPN solutions. Notify the pharmacy if cloudy or precipitated TPN solutions are found.	
Infuse only TPN solutions through the dedicated TPN line. Do not use a dedicated TPN CVC for drawing blood samples or administering medications.	Minimizes chance of infection.

▼

NURSING DIAGNOSIS: KNOWLEDGE DEFICIT

Related To
- New information
- No previous experience

Defining Characteristics
Verbalizes a lack of knowledge about use of TPN at home
Willing to learn procedure

Patient Outcomes
The patient/family will
- infuse TPN solution aseptically using an infusion pump.
- test blood glucose accurately.
- perform CVC care, dressing change, and cap change and flush correctly.
- state signs, symptoms, and problems to report.

Nursing Interventions	Rationales
Collaborate with physician, dietitian, pharmacist, certified nutrition support nurse, nutrition support team, and/or discharge planning nurse to establish a discharge plan that is reasonable with clear expectations: 1. Assure insurance coverage is verified and/or authorization of benefits is obtained prior to discharge. 2. Determine how home care supplies can be ordered and delivered on a regular basis.	

Nursing Interventions	Rationales
Provide educational materials about: 1. TPN–storage; setup and administration; proper technique for adding additional medications to premade TPN solution as prescribed, if needed, at home (e.g., vitamins). 2. CVC care—dressing change, cap change; site assessment; signs and symptoms of infection; flushing technique to maintain catheter patency, if/when catheter not in use (e.g., heparinized saline or normal saline). 3. infusion pump—operation and programming; trouble shooting alarms. 4. blood glucose monitoring—signs and symptoms of hypo-/hyperglycemia; technique for self-testing of blood sugars; administration of insulin, as needed, if prescribed.	
Incorporate teaching into patient's daily routine by having patient/family member perform infusion skills, gradually adding new pieces of information, but taking care not to overwhelm patient/family with too much information.	
Increase patient/family independence with infusions, testing, and catheter care on a daily basis and document progress.	
Investigate potential for establishing a cyclic TPN schedule with physician, dietitian, pharmacist, or nutrition support team.	Allows patient some time off of TPN. Many patients prefer a nighttime cycle.

Nursing Interventions	Rationales
Investigate potential for placing an external long-term CVC (Hickman, Groshong) when home TPN is necessary and patient has a short-term CVC in place.	Long-term external CVCs are uniquely designed for safer extended usage. Infection rates and thromboembolitic events are reduced.

▼

DISCHARGE PLANNING/CONTINUITY OF CARE

- Assure patient/family understands self-care management plan and demonstrates competency with TPN self-care skills, e.g., CVC dressing changes, equipment setup, and when to call the physician.
- Refer to a home care agency if continued nursing care, teaching, or assistance with self-care management is needed.
- Arrange for follow-up with physician or nurse for continued management postdischarge.
- Assist patient with obtaining TPN supplies, equipment, and prescriptions; establish a plan for replacing, restocking, and refilling.
- Assure patient/family understands the financial arrangements (cost and reimbursement) of home TPN equipment, supplies, and nursing care as outlined by the patient's payment source.

REFERENCES

American Society For Parenteral And Enteral Nutrition. (1988). Standards for home nutrition support. *Nutrition In Clinical Practice, 3*, 202–205.

Keithley, J. K. & Kohn, C. L. (1992). Advances in nutritional care of medical-surgical patients. *Medical Surgical Nursing, 1*, 13–21, 67.

Lewis, S. M. & Collier, I. C. (1992). *Medical surgical nursing: Assessment and management of clinical problems* (3rd ed). St. Louis, MO: Mosby.

Shekleton, M. E. & Litwack, K. (1991). *Critical care nursing of the surgical patient.* Philadelphia, PA: Saunders.

Worthington, P. H. & Wagner, B. A. (1989). Total parenteral nutrition. *Nursing Clinics of North America, 24*, 355–370.

▼

PAIN MANAGEMENT: PATIENT-CONTROLLED ANALGESIA

Deborah R. Johnson, RN, MS, CNSN

Patient-controlled analgesia (PCA), or "demand analgesia," is a useful clinical tool that represents a major advancement in the treatment of acute, chronic, or postoperative pain. Patient-controlled analgesia is designed so that patients self-administer a predetermined therapeutic amount of narcotic (referred to as the incremental dose) through a patent venous access system within preset time intervals (referred to as the delay) at times of discomfort. The most common medications used are morphine sulfate, hydromorphone, and meperidine. Intravenous narcotics administered in smaller dosages and at a greater frequency create a more optimal serum analgesic level when compared to the conventional intermittent intramuscular (IM) injection dosing regimes.

ETIOLOGIES

See individual plans of care.

CLINICAL MANIFESTATIONS

See individual plans of care.

CLINICAL/DIAGNOSTIC FINDINGS

See individual plans of care.

▼

NURSING DIAGNOSIS: KNOWLEDGE DEFICIT—USE OF PCA

Related To

- New experience
- No previous information

Defining Characteristics

Verbalizes a lack of knowledge
Demonstrates inaccurate follow-through of instructions

Patient Outcomes

The patient will

- demonstrate an understanding of PCA principles.
- demonstrate accurate follow-through with plan of care while hospitalized.

Nursing Interventions	Rationales
Distribute PCA teaching materials.	
Explain principles of PCA to patient/family. Also include the following: 1. No IM narcotics or "hypos" given while on PCA. 2. May receive antiemetics or smooth-muscle relaxants to treat any nausea or vomiting that occassionally occurs postoperatively. 3. No pain management modality can relieve all discomfort. An optimal comfort level is that which permits participation in activities to promote recovery. 4. May notice an increased level of alertness.	Titration of comfort and sedation is more difficult when IM and intravenous (IV) administration routes are combined.
Dispel fears of overdosage: 1. Modality is controlled by the patient (and not other family members) in response to an individualized discomfort level. 2. Dose is titrated and monitored by the nurse and physician. 3. Computerlike system with programmed safety delays is used.	
Reinforce that there is no addiction potential with short-term usage.	

Nursing Interventions	Rationales
Teach patient to use PCA button in anticipation of activity (cough, turn, ambulation), special treatments (dressing changes), and procedures.	
Reassess patient understanding of PCA principles and reinforce concepts as necessary.	
Respect and support patient's decision to discontinue PCA if requested.	

▼

NURSING DIAGNOSIS: PAIN

Related To

- Inflammation
- Surgical incision
- Surgical manipulation
- Reflex muscle spasm

Defining Characteristics

Muscle tension, guarded body posture
Inability to participate in activities to facilitate recovery
Facial grimacing, moaning, irritability, restlessness
Diaphoresis, blood pressure and pulse changes
Verbal complaints of pain

Patient Outcomes

- Patient expresses satisfaction with pain relief.
- Patient participates in activities that facilitate recovery.

Nursing Interventions	Rationales
Assess comfort level using verbal and nonverbal cues.	
Assess patency of IV and assure correct setup of PCA equipment.	An infiltrated IV will not allow infusion of medication into the bloodstream.

Nursing Interventions	Rationales
If patient experiences little or no pain relief: 1. Assess/monitor the number of attempts and injections. • If attempts are much more frequent than injections, consider increasing incremental dose or giving a bolus dose. • If attempts and injections are infrequent, encourage patient to press PCA button more often.	Attempts should about equal injections for optimal comfort. This may be necessary to increase analgesic therapeutic blood levels for optimal comfort. Smaller dosages at a greater frequency may create a more optimal serum analgesic level.
Plan or contract with patient for nighttime usage to maintain an optimal analgesic blood level throughout the night and in anticipation of next day's activities. Options include: 1. Nurse pushes PCA button for patient on hourly rounds. 2. Patient continues self-administration throughout the night and nurse encourages increased usage in the early morning hours (5:00–6:30 a.m.) 3. The PCA/basal mode may be prescribed by the physician for nighttime use. This is a continuous analgesic infusion with the patient having the capability to use additional incremental doses for "breakthrough" pain when the button is pushed. If the PCA/basal mode is prescribed, assess the total amount of narcotic administered via basal rate and incremental dose with delay for appropriateness/safety.	
Position patient for optimal comfort.	
Encourage/teach/reinforce relaxation techniques.	
Maintain optimal room temperature according to patient preferences.	

Nursing Interventions	Rationales
Minimize environmental stimuli, for example, a quiet room, dim lights, TV off, monitor visitors, and close the door.	
Investigate other sources of potential discomfort, for example, a distended bladder, antiembolic stockings, nasogastric tubes, Foley catheter, tape, drains, and dressings.	
Assess/reassess efficacy of pharmacological and nonpharmacological interventions.	
Advise patient that PCA can/will be discontinued at any time if the patient is not satisfied with comfort level; more traditional narcotic dosing can be resumed.	
Notify physician if unrelieved pain persists.	

▼

NURSING DIAGNOSIS: HIGH RISK FOR INEFFECTIVE BREATHING PATTERN

Risk Factors

- Excessive narcotic self-administration
- Obesity
- Anesthesia
- Other medications

Patient Outcomes

- Patient is alert or easily aroused.
- Patient will maintain clear open airways as evidenced by easy, spontaneous respirations with an acceptable rate, depth, and pattern.
- Patient maintains an effective cough.
- Patient skin and nailbeds are pink, warm, and dry.

Nursing Interventions	Rationales
Assess level of consciousness, respiratory rate, pattern, pupil size, muscle tone, and skin color with vital signs and as needed.	

Nursing Interventions	Rationales
Do not give IM narcotics while on PCA.	
Examine total medication regime for substances that may foster relaxation or potentiate PCA narcotics, for example, droperidol, Fentanyl, hydroxyzine, Versed, and diphenhydramine HCl.	
Decrease the incremental dose as prescribed if assessment suggests early signs of oversedation.	
If signs of overdosage occur, stop the PCA, administer 0.4 mg naloxone IV in 0.1-mg increments as prescribed. Stay with patient and notify physician.	Naloxone is short acting; reevaluate for reoccurrence of signs/symptoms of overdosage 30–45 min after naloxone is given.

▼

NURSING DIAGNOSIS: HIGH RISK FOR PAIN (ITCHING)

Risk Factors

Systemic histamine release more commonly associated with morphine sulfate administration

Patient Outcomes

Skin redness, swelling, and/or itching is minimal, tolerable, or nonexistent.

Nursing Interventions	Rationales
Administer diphenhydramine HCl as prescribed.	Antihistamine will minimize itching.
Suggest changing PCA narcotic from morphine sulfate to hydromorphone.	Hydromorphone produces a lesser systemic histamine release compared to morphine sulfate.
If symptoms persist may need to discontinue PCA and resume more traditional IM narcotic regime.	

▼

NURSING DIAGNOSIS: KNOWLEDGE DEFICIT—WEANING FROM PCA AND ADVANCING TO ORAL ANALGESICS

Related To
- New experiences
- No previous information

Defining Characteristics
Verbalizes a lack of knowledge
Demonstrates inaccurate follow-through of instructions

Patient Outcomes
The patient will
- state the reasons for advancement to oral medication.
- participate in the process of discontinuing PCA.
- describe the differences in onset/length of action between oral and IV narcotics (PCA) for pain control.

Nursing Interventions	Rationales
Attempt to wean from PCA when the patient has bowel sounds, a soft belly, and no nausea or vomiting, the patient is tolerating clear liquids, and the nasogastric (NG) tube is removed.	These are the same assessments used to transition from IM analgesics to oral (PO) analgesics.
Explain that the above assessments are normal, expected, positive progressions in the clinical course of recovery.	
Explain the differences in onset/length of action between IV (PCA) pain medication and the oral pain medication.	

Nursing Interventions	**Rationales**
The weaning process is: 1. Direct patient to self-administer a PCA incremental dose; then give the oral analgesic as prescribed. 2. Take the PCA button from the patient, but do not remove the PCA machine from the room. 3. Monitor frequently to assess comfort level. 4. Reinforce the differences in oral vs. IV analgesic action. 5. If patient is uncomfortable after oral medication is given (rare), it is acceptable for patient to administer another PCA incremental dose. Take PCA button away from patient after this PCA dose is given and monitor comfort level. 6. Administer second dose of oral analgesic at earliest prescribed frequency to maximize analgesic blood level. 7. Discontinue PCA if patient is comfortable after second dose of oral analgesic is given.	A successful weaning process is built on a trusting relationship between the patient and the nurse.

▼

DISCHARGE PLANNING/CONTINUITY OF CARE

- Refer to individual plans of care.
- Assure that oral analgesics control discomfort so that patient can participate in activities that facilitate recovery.
- Reinforce that patient should not drive or operate machinery when taking prescribed oral analgesics.
- Assist patient with obtaining prescription and establish a plan for refilling prescriptions.

REFERENCES

Jacox, A., Ferrel, B., Heidrich, G., Hester, N., & Miaskowski, C. (1992). A guideline for the nation: Managing acute pain. *American Journal of Nursing*, 92(5), 49–55.

Kaiser, K. (1992). Assessment and management of pain in the critically ill trauma patient. *Critical Care Nursing Quarterly, 15*(2), 14–34.

McCaffery, M. & Beebe, A. (1989). *Pain: Clinical manual for nursing practice.* St. Louis, MO: Mosby.

Sheidler, V. (1987). Patient controlled analgesia. *Current Concepts In Nursing, 1* (1), 13–16.

U.S. Department of Health and Human Services (DHHS), Public Health Service, Agency for Health Care Policy and Research (AHCPR). (1992). *Acute pain management: Operative or medical procedures and trauma, clinical practice guideline*, publication No. 92–0032. Washington, DC: DHHS.

▼

Common Cardiovascular Conditions and Procedures

▼

ANGINA PECTORIS

Linda A. Briggs, RN, MS, CCRN

Angina pectoris is related to acute ischemic syndromes secondary to several pathophysiological processes most often associated with coronary artery disease (CAD). These acute ischemic syndromes result from rapid progression of atherosclerosis. A myriad of events complicate the impact of the atheromatous plaque. Occurring independently or in combination, they include hemorrhage or rupture of the plaque, thrombus formation, platelet aggregation, vasospasm, and impaired vascular endothelium. While other disease processes may cause angina, the common denominator of these processes is a decrease in myocardial oxygen supply and/or an increase in myocardial demands. While there is no death of myocardial muscle cells, angina represents a warning sign of critical oxygen imbalance. Table 5.1 lists the types of angina.

ETIOLOGIES

- Atherosclerosis
- Cardiomyopathy
- Hypertension
- Aortic stenosis
- Marked anemia
- Shock syndromes
- Stress

CLINICAL MANIFESTATIONS

Chest discomfort

- Substermal, may radiate to neck, jaw, arms, teeth, elbows, shoulders
- Usually lasts under 15 min (average 3 min)
- Discribed as pain, pressure, tightness, heaviness, burning
- Poorly localized, nontender
- Associated symptoms often shortness of breath, fatigue, diaphoresis

Table 5.1 • Types of Angina

Stable Angina
Due to significant coronary artery stenosis.

Symptoms
- Predictable
- Controllable
- Usually initiated by exertion
- Relieved by nitroglycerine and/or rest

Unstable Angina
Due to atheromatous plaque that ruptures, causing a partial occlusion and platelet aggregation. Rupture may progress to myocardial infarction.

Symptoms
- Similar to stable angina, but usually more severe
- Sudden onset of symptoms at rest or with exertion
- Change in the pattern of symptoms, i.e., increased frequency, severity, or duration
- Recurrence of symptoms within 4 weeks of an acute MI

Variant Angina
Due to coronary vasospasm

Symptoms
- Severe, prolonged discomfort without precipitating factors
- Frequently noted at rest or on early morning rising
- May have a circadian pattern

Silent Ischemia
Due to transient reduction in coronary blood flow

Symptoms
- Absence of typical chest discomfort symptoms
- Greater than 1 mm horizontal or downsloping ST-segment depression 60–80 ms after J point
- May have vague symptoms of fatigue, weakness, need for greater rest
- May require continuous ST-segment and/or ECG monitoring at home

▼

CLINICAL/DIAGNOSTIC FINDINGS

- Tachycardia
- Dyspnea
- Diaphoresis
- Pulsus alternans
- Transient ST-segment flattening or depression found in leads that correspond to affected coronary artery distribution [one third to one fourth of patients may have a normal electrocardiogram (ECG)]
- Transient T-wave change

- Cardiac enzymes within normal limits
- Vital signs that show little or minor changes in heart rate, blood pressure, and respiratory rate

▼

NURSING DIAGNOSIS: PAIN (CHEST)

Related To myocardial ischemia, decreased myocardial blood flow, or increased oxygen demand

Defining Characteristics

Patient describing and reporting own characteristics of chest discomfort
Transient ST/T-wave changes (if ECG monitored)
Anxiety, restlessness
Diaphoresis, nausea
Blood pressure, heart rate, and respiratory rate changes

Patient Outcomes

- Patient will verbalize relief of pain or discomfort.
- Electrocardiogram changes will return to normal.
- Patient will verbalize description of own unique pain characteristics.
- Patient will appear less anxious.

Nursing Interventions	Rationales
Assess patient's pain characteristics and precipitating factors thoroughly, including location, radiation, intensity, and duration. Assess associated symptoms: nausea, fatigue, shortness of breath, diaphoresis, etc.	Knowledge of precipitation may aid in differentiation of angina.
Utilize pain scale (0–10) for pain intensity as appropriate: 0 is no pain; 10 is the worst pain imaginable.	Pain intensity scale is useful to objectify discomfort, assess effectiveness of pain-relieving measures, and provide patient awareness and education. Patients need to be reminded there is no RIGHT answer. Some patients may not find this question helpful, and other assessment techniques will need to be used.

Nursing Interventions	Rationales
Obtain baseline hemodynamic status, including 1. blood pressure 2. heart rate 3. level of consciousness	Sympathetic nervous system response may cause hypertension, tachycardia, and tachypnea, all of which will increase myocardial oxygen demands.
Assist patient in recognition of own unique symptoms and prompt reporting.	Helping patient verbalize and acknowledge own symptoms aids in early recognition and begins the educational process. Autonomic nervous system stimulation may cause sensations that the patient may not connect with the ischemic process.
For monitored patients: Monitor ECG for rate, rhythm, and ST-wave changes. Monitor in leads that correspond with known patient pathology: II, III, and AFV to monitor the inferior left ventricle, V_1–V_4 the anteroseptal left ventricle, V_5–V_6 the anterolateral left ventricle, and I, and AVL the lateral left ventricle.	The ECG changes may accompany angina or appear without patient complaint of pain. Characteristic changes to monitor include transient horizontal or downsloping ST-segment depression, T-wave inversion, and ST-segment elevation for variant angina. Rhythm disturbances can include atrioventricular (AV) conduction problems, premature ventricular contraction (PVC), ventricular tachycardia (VT), and ventricular fibrillation.
Obtain order for 12-lead ECG.	Documents associated ECG changes in all leads.
Modify environment, as appropriate, to decrease myocardial oxygen demand, e.g., restrict activity, encourage bedrest, decrease stimulation, control traffic, and elevate head of bed.	
Stay with patient. Offer calm, reassuring explanations of interventions and their effectiveness.	Anxiety and fear may cause further oxygen demands by increasing catecholamine release and increasing or prolonging ischemic pain.

Nursing Interventions	Rationales
Administer oxygen and medications as prescribed:	
1. To eliminate chest discomfort: • oxygen • nitroglycerin sublingual • nitroglycerin IV • morphine sulfate IV	Oxygen availability may increase myocardial uptake. Nitrates reduce myocardial demand by venous vasodilatation (decreasing preload) and increase myocardial oxygen supply by coronary vasodilatation. Intravenous nitroglycerin allows quick titration to therapeutic blood levels. Morphine sulfate decreases myocardial workload by promoting venous vasodilatation and decreasing anxiety. As long as a chest discomfort exists, myocardial ischemia exists.
2. Calcium channel antagonists to prevent coronary spasm and reduce the number of ischemic events: • diltiazem • nifedipine • verapamil	
3. Antiplatelet/anticoagulant therapy to prevent thrombus formation • aspirin (ASA) • heparin	Aspirin has been found to reduce the risk of myocardial infarction (MI) and death in unstable angina by 50%. Aspirin decreases platelet aggregation. Heparin may also increase protection against thrombosis and will decrease the incidence of MI post unstable angina.
4. Thrombolytic therapy	Since the incidence of thrombus formation has frequently been identified in unstable angina patients, the use of thrombolytic therapy in this group of patients is under current investigation.
Offer alternative pain-relieving measures: relaxation, deep breathing, imagery, and massage.	Alternative measures may offer patient more control or distraction from pain. Muscular tension increases myocardial oxygen demands.
Assess and document response to pain-relieving measures.	

NURSING DIAGNOSIS: HIGH RISK FOR DECREASED CARDIAC OUTPUT

Risk Factors

- Left ventricular failure
- Alteration in cardiac rate or rhythm
- Increased myocardial demands

Patient Outcomes

- Vital signs will be within normal limits.
- Patient will state absence of chest pain/discomfort.
- Patient will demonstrate normal mentation.
- Patient will demonstrate absence of dyspnea, fatigue, shortness of breath (SOB), and peripheral constriction.

Nursing Interventions	Rationales
Assess vital signs every 10–15 minutes. Observe systolic blood pressure (SBP) and diastolic blood pressure (DBP) as indices of left ventricular (LV) afterload.	Obtain baseline data for comparison and treatment effectiveness. Diastolic blood pressure optimally 60–90 mmHg. DBP > 90 mmHg increases LV afterload. DBP < 60 mmHg may decrease coronary artery perfusion pressure. Afterload significantly increases myocardial oxygen demands.
Document mental status to include level of alertness, response to environment, memory, and restlessness	Baseline mental status is necessary to compare with changes. Subtle changes in organ perfusion often occur first.
Monitor fluid and electrolyte status, that is, intake, output, daily weights, laboratory values, and diuretic treatment.	Efforts to decrease preload will decrease myocardial workload.
Ausculate heart sounds for presence of S_3, S_4, and murmurs.	Due to atrial filling against a noncompliant left ventricle, an S_3 is an early warning sign of LV failure. New murmurs may be due to papillary muscle dysfunction and resultant regurgitant flow.
Ausculate lung sounds, with concentration on dependent posterior lung fields.	Early signs of LV failure include end inspiratory crackles audible in bibasilar posterior lung fields.

Nursing Interventions	Rationales
Monitor effects of drug combinations for example, beta blockers, calcium antagonists, and class IA antiarrhythmics (quinidine, procainamide)	Potent medical regimens are often employed to produce overall effects of decreasing myocardial workload and increasing oxygen supply. Negative inotropic effects of drug combinations can further lower cardiac output to unacceptable levels. Vasodilators may decrease diastolic blood pressure to critical levels, thus decreasing coronary artery perfusion pressure and decreasing myocardial blood flow. Additionally, vasodilators may cause a reflex tachycardia, further decreasing coronary blood flow and increasing myocardial demands.

▼

NURSING DIAGNOSIS: KNOWLEDGE DEFICIT—DIAGNOSIS AND TREATMENT PLAN

Related To

- Lack of previous experience
- Misinformation
- New diagnosis

Defining Characteristics

Asks questions
Requests information
Follows instructions

Patient Outcomes

Patient will

- begin to demonstrate some awareness of diagnosis
- ask for clarification of information
- follow guidelines
- ask for written information
- begin to participate in educational process

Nursing Interventions	Rationales
Assess patient/family level of understanding once per shift. Ask questions like: 1. "What has your physician told you?" 2. "What do you understand about why you're here?"	A patient/family educational program begins with the patient's current level of understanding. With a new diagnosis, the patient needs clarification, repeated information, and correction of misinformation.
Devise a teaching plan based on readiness to learn, physical condition, and realistic outcomes.	A teaching plan should begin with what the patient wants to know and because of shortened hospitalization and should include at least basic survival information.
Develop and institute a teaching program for patient and family to include 1. basic disease process 2. risk factors 3. medications 4. dietary instructions 5. exercise guidelines 6. pulse taking 7. how to recognize symptoms 8. what to report 9. follow-up plans	Any educational program is multidisciplinary. The extent of any program will be affected by available resources, patient condition, length of hospitalization, and patient readiness.
Assess understanding of treatment plan and explain tests and procedures to be performed.	A variety of procedures may be recommended to include repeat 12-lead ECGs, exercise stress thallium tests, cardiac catheterization, percutaneous transluminal coronary angioplasty, and/or coronary artery bypass surgery.
Explore activity limitations, including 1. spacing activities 2. resting when tired 3. avoiding activities causing discomfort 4. delegating activities to others	

NURSING DIAGNOSIS: FEAR/ANXIETY

Related To

- New diagnosis

- Fear of dying
- Fear of unknown
- Fear of hospitalization

Defining Characteristics

Decreased verbalization
Inability to concentrate
Restlessness/insomnia
Muscle rigidity

Patient Outcomes

Patient will
- discuss feelings
- utilize relaxation techniques
- identify coping strategies

Nursing Interventions	Rationales
Maintain consistent nurse-patient relationship.	
Give repeated orientation to environment, procedures, and treatment.	Patients who are informed about hospitalization, routines, interventions, etc., will have more realistic perspectives. Anxiety may also be decreased.
Instruct in relaxation exercises and deep-breathing techniques. Utilize touch or music therapy as appropriate.	Relaxation and deep-breathing exercises will decrease muscular tension and provide distraction and a sense of control over one's environment.
Assess patient's prior experience with illness and hospitalization.	Utilizing past coping skills increases effectiveness.
Assess patient's concerns, expectations, and perspectives: 1. Listen to patient's feelings. 2. Help distinguish realistic concerns from unrealistic fears. 3. Allow patient to deny certain aspects of illness he or she is yet unable to cope with.	Adaptive denial can assist in relieving situational anxiety. Patients come to terms with their illness in individual and unique ways.
Assess need for sedation.	

DISCHARGE PLANNING/CONTINUITY OF CARE

- Assure understanding of actions to take for recurrent angina to include rest and nitroglycerine guidelines. Encourage use of "anginal diary" to outline symptoms, precipitating factors, and symptoms and related effectiveness of treatment. Assure understanding of medications, activity restrictions, dietary guidelines, symptoms to report, and risk factors that need to be modified (e.g., smoking).
- If patient is on a complex medication regime, has several risk factors to be modified, or has had difficulty learning self-management techniques during hospitalization, refer to home health care agency for follow-up.
- Arrange follow-up with physician for continued management postdischarge.
- Assist patient in obtaining prescriptions, establishing a realistic medication schedule, and establishing a plan for refilling medications.
- Provide information on local support or educational groups to assist with specific risk factor modification to include stop smoking programs, exercise programs, education programs on diet and cholesterol, and cardiopulmonary resuscitation classes, if appropriate.
- Refer to a local chapter of the American Heart Association for further information.

REFERENCES

Enger, E. Schwertz, D. (1989). Mechanisms of myocardial ischemia. *Journal of Cardiovascular Nursing, 3*(4), 1–15.

Epstein, C. (1992). Changing interpretations of angina pectoris associated with transient myocardial ischemia. *Journal of Cardiovascular Nursing,* 7(1), 1–13.

Gottlieb., S. & Flaherty, J. (1991). Medical therapy of unstable angina pectoris. *Cardiology Clinics,* 9(1), 89–97.

Guzzetta, C. & Dossey, B. (1992). *Cardiovascular nursing.* St. Louis, MO: Mosby Year Book.

Thadani, U. (1991). Medical therapy of stable angina pectoris. *Cardiology Clinics,* 9(1), 73–85.

▼

ARTERIOGRAPHY (ANGIOGRAM)

Penny M. Bernards, RN, MS, GNP

An arteriogram is an invasive procedure involving insertion of a catheter into an artery and injecting contrast dye. The contrast dye allows x-ray pictures to be taken of the arterial blood flow to demonstrate the passage as well as any occlusions or abnormalities. A digital subtraction angiogram (DSA) is used more often than conventional arteriograms to evaluate the arterial system, since a better image is obtained with subtraction of overlying bone and less contrast dye is used, which results in less trauma to the kidneys. Possible entry sites include the femoral artery at the groin, the axillary artery, the brachial artery, and the abdominal aorta via the translumbar approach. An arteriogram usually takes between 1 and 2 hr.

ETIOLOGIES (INDICATIONS)

- Symptomatic peripheral arterial occlusive disease
- Extracranial vascular disease
- Preoperative assessment of arterial aneurysm disease
- Screening of hypertensive patients for renal artery disease
- Screening of potential donors for renal transplant
- Evaluation for pulmonary emboli
- Access for interventional radiology such as angioplasty and embolization

CLINICAL MANIFESTATIONS

- Intermittent claudication
- Rest pain
- Nonhealing ulcers
- Uncontrolled hypertension
- Acute shortness of breath
- Transient ischemic attacks

CLINICAL/DIAGNOSTIC FINDINGS

- Absent or diminished Doppler pulse signal
- Ankle-brachial index < 0.4 or higher if patient has functional deficits
- Dampening of pulse waveforms
- Increased velocities in an artery or bypass graft per ultrasound
- Presence of a large arterial aneurysm on ultrasound or computerized tomography (CT) scan

▼

NURSING DIAGNOSIS: FEAR

Related To
- Unknown procedure
- Diagnosis
- Anticipated pain

Defining Characteristics
Apprehension
Verbalization of fear
Diaphoresis
Tachycardia
Avoidance behavior
Tenseness

Patient Outcomes
The patient will
- express fears related to the procedure and diagnosis.
- describe some of the sensations experienced during the procedure.
- utilize methods of coping to reduce anxiety.

Nursing Interventions	Rationales
Assess level of anxiety.	
Evaluate understanding of the procedure to clear up any misconceptions.	

Nursing Interventions	Rationales
Describe the sensations often felt during an angiogram such as the hardness of the examining table, coolness of the radiology room and the cleansing soap, burning of the local anesthetic, pressure of the catheter and warmth of the dye. Occasionally straps are used to hold an extremity in place while films are obtained or the head during carotid arteriograms.	Preparing patients for procedures using sensory events that they can expect decreases stress.
Encourage verbalization of feelings to help identify source of anxiety.	
Assess understanding and level of anxiety in family members and significant others and include them in patient teaching.	Patients can have increased anxiety when people around them are anxious or are providing conflicting information.
Explore successful coping strategies in previous experiences and relevance to current situation.	Drawing on past experiences with coping with stresses may help determine which intervention will be most beneficial.
Alert the radiology and medical staff if patient appears excessively anxious.	The physician may choose to use an antianxiety medication prior to the procedure.

▼

NURSING DIAGNOSIS: KNOWLEDGE DEFICIT—PREPARATION AND POSTPROCEDURE CARE

- Lack of exposure to information

Defining Characteristics

Verbalization of inadequate understanding or misconception
Anger
Anxiety

Patient Outcomes

The patient will

- describe the procedure.
- identify the purpose of the procedure.
- verbalize understanding of preprocedure routines.
- verbalize understanding of postprocedure routines.

Nursing Interventions	Rationales
Evaluate understanding of the procedure.	Some patients confuse the procedure arteriogram with the surgery.
Explain that the purpose of the arteriogram is to provide a definitive diagnosis necessary to assess treatment options.	
Describe the different steps of the arteriogram procedure, including positioning on the examining table, preparation of the injection site, (most commonly femoral artery), placement of the catheter, injection of the dye, obtaining pictures, repositioning of the catheter and more pictures, removal of the catheter, and holding pressure at the site.	
Instruct patients on what will be expected of them during the arteriogram, such as holding their breath, deep breathing, and holding still.	
Instruct the patients that they will be on complete bedrest for 4–8 hr postprocedure with punctured extremity straight.	Care is provided to prevent dislodgement of a clot at the arterial injection site which may result in formation of a hematoma or hemorrhage.
Explain that vital signs will be monitored frequently for changes in blood pressure, pulse, and respiration, presence of discomfort, swelling or bleeding at the injection site, and circulation, movement, and sensation of involved extremity.	Frequent assessments are done to evaluate for bleeding or hemorrhage from the injection site that may not be apparent through visualization of the insertion site.

Nursing Interventions	Rationales
Instruct patient that intravenous fluids will be used before and after the arteriogram and that it is important to push oral fluids. A regular meal can be ordered postprocedure if there is no problem with nausea.	Hydration is used to flush dye out of kidneys.
Inform patient that ambulation can be resumed after 4–8 hr although prolonged sitting should be avoided.	
Instruct patient regarding care of the arterial puncture site after discharge. Wash area with soap and water, place a Band-Aid if desired, and monitor for signs of infection, swelling, or bleeding at the site.	
Inform patient of any follow-up care with the physician.	

NURSING DIAGNOSIS: HIGH RISK FOR INJURY

Risk Factors

- Chronic renal failure
- Allergy to contrast dye, iodine, or seafood
- Osmolarity of contrast dye
- Poor hydration
- Cardiovascular disease
- Diabetes

Patient Outcomes

The patient will have

- no allergic reaction to the contrast dye
- creatinine level within 0.2 of preprocedure
- a balanced intake and output
- blood glucose levels ranging from 80 to 200 if diabetic

Nursing Interventions	Rationales
Obtain list of all allergies and sensitivities and report them to the physician.	Patients with an allergy to iodine or seafood may be sensitive to the contrast dye.

Nursing Interventions	Rationales
Administer antihistamines and/or corticosteroids as prescribed prior to an arteriogram for patients with suspected allergy to contrast dye.	
Obtain renal history and baseline blood urea nitrogen (BUN) and creatinine. Repeat BUN and creatinine the following day or at clinic visit.	Patients with chronic renal disease or renal transplants may require alternative interventions such as decreased hydration, corticosteroids, or a dopamine drip. Laboratory values are used to evaluate damage to kidneys from the contrast dye.
Maintain intravenous (IV) hydration as prescribed pre- and postprocedure. Encourage oral fluids postprocedure if patient is not nauseated.	Hydration is used to flush dye from kidneys.
Monitor urine output.	Low urine output may be an indicator of acute renal failure.
Assess cardiopulmonary status ongoing.	Patients with cardiovascular or renal disease are at risk for fluid overload due to IV hydration during and after procedure.

▼

NURSING DIAGNOSIS: HIGH RISK FOR ALTERED PERIPHERAL OR CEREBRAL TISSUE PERFUSION

Risk Factors

- Atherosclerosis
- Embolus
- Hypotension
- Bleeding from injection site

Patient Outcomes

The patient will have

- stable vital signs
- a flat, dry puncture site
- baseline peripheral pulses distal to insertion site
- absence of petechia distal to insertion site
- no neurological deficits
- no changes in functional status

Nursing Interventions	Rationales
If patients are on anticoagulation therapy, consult with physician on when to discontinue medication and when to resume postprocedure. Warfarin should be discontinued for 48–72 hr prior to the angiogram.	Anticoagulation therapy increases risk of hemorrhage postprocedure.
Monitor vital signs frequently postprocedure.	Elevated pulse and respirations with drop in blood pressure may indicate acute blood loss.
Assess insertion site for bleeding or swelling with vital signs. Apply continuous pressure for 10 min if bleeding is noted and contact physician immediately.	
Check pulses distal to insertion site with vital signs.	Diminished pulses may indicate bleeding at the site or acute occlusion.
Maintain proper positioning with extremity straight to prevent dislodgement of newly formed clot.	
Monitor for changes in sensation and movement of extremity with vital signs.	Embolus to extremity or thrombosis at insertion site may alter sensation and movement.
Obtain a hematocrit prior to the arteriogram	A baseline hematocrit is used to help estimate blood loss in suspected hemorrhage or hematoma.
Obtain serial hematocrit levels when translumbar approach is used or when bleeding is suspected.	A large hematoma can be concealed retroperitoneal in the abdomen. The use of sandbags at the puncture site is not always recommended due to risk of internal bleeding.
Administer IV fluids at prescribed rate and encourage oral fluids to replace fluid loss by diuresis.	The osmolarity of the dye may cause diuresis and a fluid deficit.
Check for color or temperature changes in extremities.	An embolus to the extremity may cause acute occlusion or petechia on skin.

Nursing Interventions	Rationales
Perform neurological exam, including extremity strength and function, speech, swallowing, visual acuity, facial symmetry, peripheral sensation, pupil reactivity, and mentation with vital signs after carotid arteriogram.	One risk of the carotid arteriogram is dislodgement of plaque during the procedure.

▼

DISCHARGE PLANNING/CONTINUITY OF CARE

- Assure understanding of puncture site care.
- Instruct patient to call physician if bleeding, swelling, or signs and symptoms of infection are noted at the puncture site
- Review signs and symptoms of transient ischemic attacks for patients with carotid artery disease and impress importance of reporting these symptoms.
- Instruct patient to call physician if there are sudden changes in sensation and movement in extremity.
- Coordinate follow-up care, which may include surgical intervention, other procedures, consultations, or clinic visits.

REFERENCES

Rice, V. H., Sieggreen, M., Mullin, M., & Williams, J. (1988). Development and testing of an arteriography information intervention for stress reduction. *Heart & Lung*, *17*, 23–28.

Vogelzang, R. L. (1988). Vascular imaging techniques and percutaneous vascular intervention. In V. A. Fahey (Ed.), *Vascular nursing*. Philadelphia, PA: Saunders.

Waugh, J. R. & Sacharias, N. (1992). Arteriographic complications in the DSA era. *Radiology*, *182*, 243–246.

▼

CARDIAC CATHETERIZATION

Linda Wonoski, RN, MSN

Cardiac catheterization is a diagnostic procedure used to obtain information about the structure and function of the cardiac chambers, valves, and vessels. Almost every type of cardiac anatomic or pathological condition or defect can be detected, quantified, and documented by the procedure. The technique involves inserting a radiopaque catheter and contrast dye into a vein or artery (femoral or brachial) and passing it through the various chambers and vessels. Pressure readings and oxygen concentrations are measured in the chambers and vessels of the heart.

ETIOLOGIES (INDICATIONS)

- Confirm the presence of valvular heart disease, myocardial disease, and/or coronary artery disease.
- Determine location and severity of disease process.
- Preoperative assessment for cardiac surgery.
- Evaluate ventricular function.
- Evaluate effect of medical treatment on cardiovascular function.
- Access for coronary angioplasty.

CLINICAL MANIFESTATIONS

- Angina, chest pain
- Myocardial infarction (MI)
- Hypertension
- Fatigue, weakness
- Dyspnea

CLINICAL/DIAGNOSTIC FINDINGS

- Presence of occlusions or partial occlusion in coronary arteries
- Presence of insufficient and/or stenotic heart valves

- Decreased cardiac output
- Areas of decreased contractility of myocardium
- Ventricular aneurysm
- Cardiac anomalies

NURSING DIAGNOSIS: KNOWLEDGE DEFICIT—PROCEDURE

Related To lack of previous exposure to information

Defining Characteristics

Expression of anxiety about the procedure
Statement of lack of knowledge and need for information
Asking many questions
Procedure new for the patient

Patient Outcomes

Patient will

- state reason for procedure
- describe pre- and postprocedure routine
- describe what to expect during the procedure
- state ways to cope with anxiety during the procedure

Nursing Interventions	Rationales
Assess patient/family understanding of the procedure and willingness to learn.	
Provide available teaching materials (pamphlets, videos) to supplement teaching.	
Explain preprocedure routine, including 1. consent for procedure 2. identification of allergies or sensitivities, especially to contrast media, iodine, or seafood, to identify risk for allergic reaction	Contrast material used contains a hypertonic solution with iodine. Patients may be at risk for an allergic reaction. Physician may premedicate with prednisone or diphenhydramine.
3. chest x-ray, blood work, and electrocardiogram (ECG) 4. nothing by mouth, or clear liquids only, prior to procedure to reduce risk of vomiting or aspiration	

Nursing Interventions	Rationales
5. intravenous (IV) fluids to be started before the procedure to decrease dehydration caused by contrast medium 6. pedal pulses marked if femoral site used 7. vital signs obtained 8. voiding prior to procedure 9. mild sedative given prior to procedure	
Explain routine and sensations experienced during catheterization: 1. Patient will be awake and may be able to see x-ray monitor.	Understanding that certain sensations are expected during the procedure and are not complications will help to alleviate anxiety.
2. A local anesthetic will be administered at catheter puncture site. Pressure but no sharp or severe pain may be felt when the catheter is inserted.	
3. Notify physician or nurse of any sharp or severe pain experienced during the procedure. Nitroglycerin may be administered.	Contrast medium displaces coronary blood flow and may create transient ischemia.
4. Palpitations may be felt as the catheter is advanced because catheter manipulation can irritate the endocardium and produce ectopic beats.	
5. Contrast medium injection may create a warm, flushing sensation for a few seconds. Nausea and lightheadedness may also be experienced briefly at this time.	
6. May be asked to make a deep, abdominal cough.	Coughing clears contrast material from the coronary arteries and acts as a mechanical stimulus to the heart if ectopic beats occur.
7. Blood samples and pressure readings will be obtained to assess the condition of the cardiac chambers and valves and to determine oxygen saturation values.	

Nursing Interventions	Rationales
Explain postprocedure routine: 1. Catheters are removed at end of procedure. Manual pressure is applied for 20–30 min; then a pressure dressing is applied. A sandbag may be used on the puncture site. 2. Vital signs will be checked frequently to prevent bleeding and hematoma formation. 3. Bedrest will be maintained for 6–8 hr, with affected extremity held straight to prevent postprocedure bleeding. If femoral site is used, the head of the bed will be kept elevated to at most 30°. 4. Patient may eat and drink soon after procedure; fluids are encouraged. 5. Patient is instructed to notify the nurse if warmth or wetness is felt in the groin area because it may indicate bleeding. 6. Mild discomfort/pain may be experienced at puncture site. Patient is told to inform nurse; pain medication may be given. 7. Patient is told when results of procedure will be discussed.	

▼

NURSING DIAGNOSIS: HIGH RISK FOR DECREASED CARDIAC OUTPUT

Risk Factors

- Hypotension
- Tachypnea
- Dyspnea
- Angina
- Dysrhythmia
- Oliguria
- Hematoma at puncture site

Patient Outcomes

Cardiac output is adequate, as evidenced by

- vital signs within normal limits for patient
- absence of angina
- absence of dysrhythmias
- urine output > 30 mL/hr
- skin warm and dry
- no bleeding or hematoma at puncture site

Nursing Interventions	Rationales
Assess vital signs prior to procedure for baseline.	
Assess postprocedure vital signs and puncture site dressing every 15 min for first hour; every 30 min for 2 hr; hourly for 4 hr; and then every shift.	
Record amount of drainage, and/or size of hematoma giving date, time, and drawing lines around drainage on dressing for future comparison.	
Immediately apply pressure to puncture site if bleeding is noted. A sandbag may be used. Notify physician if bleeding is significant.	
Place patient in Trendelenburg position if a sudden drop in blood pressure and heart rate (vasovagal response) is noted. Notify physician. Be prepared to administer IV fluid.	A vasovagal response is caused by parasympathetic stimulation which reduces the heart rate and blood pressure, adversely affecting cardiac output and peripheral perfusion.
Maintain bedrest for 6–8 hr with affected extremity held straight. Prevent flexion of hip by keeping head of bed elevated at most 30°, if femoral site used.	
Encourage fluids. Monitor intake and output.	Contrast medium has a diuretic effect and may cause hypovolemia and hypotension.

NURSING DIAGNOSIS: HIGH RISK FOR DECREASED PERIPHERAL TISSUE PERFUSION TO AFFECTED EXTREMITY

Risk Factors

- Edema
- Vessel occlusion
- Bleeding/hematoma

Patient Outcomes

Peripheral perfusion is adequate, as evidenced by

- palpable peripheral pulses
- circulation, movement, sensation, temperature (CMST) within normal limits with capillary refill < 3 s
- absence of pain, numbness, tingling
- absence of peripheral edema

Nursing Interventions	Rationales
Assess and mark pedal pulses prior to procedure if femoral site is used.	
Assess CMST of affected extremity and pulses every 15 min for first hour, every 30 min for 2 hr, hourly for 4 hr, and then every shift. Use Doppler if pulses are difficult to feel.	
Encourage frequent deep breathing and passive and active exercises of the unaffected extremities.	Reduces the possibility of atelectasis in the lungs and thrombus formation in the deep veins of the legs.

NURSING DIAGNOSIS: KNOWLEDGE DEFICIT—SELF-CARE AFTER CATHETERIZATION

Related To lack of previous exposure to information

Defining Characteristics

Verbalizes lack of knowledge of self-care after catheterization

Asks questions regarding heart disease and long-term management (if results are positive for heart disease)

Patient Outcomes

Patient will

- describe normal appearance and healing process of the puncture site.

- define activity restrictions.
- state what to do if bleeding occurs.
- state what to do if chest pain occurs.
- state when to notify physician.

Nursing Interventions	Rationales
Review activity restrictions of strenuous activity for 24 hr. Encourage patient to discuss return to work with physician.	
Review puncture site healing process: 1. Skin will be discolored for several weeks. 2. Tenderness and a small grape size lump in the area are normal. 3. No ointment or special care of the site is necessary.	
Instruct on what to do if bleeding occurs: 1. Lie down. 2. Apply pressure to site. 3. Call ambulance for transfer to hospital.	
Instruct patient on what to do if chest pain occurs: 1. Rest. 2. Take nitroglycerin (up to 3 tablets over 15 min) if prescribed. 3. If pain continues, call ambulance for transfer to hospital.	
Instruct patient to notify physician if the following occur: 1. bleeding 2. signs of infection, inflammation, or drainage at puncture site or body temperature > 100. 3. changes in color, temperature, or sensation of extremities 4. chest pain or pressure.	

▼

DISCHARGE PLANNING/CONTINUITY OF CARE

- Assure understanding of catheterization results and self-management plan.
- If the patient was found to have heart disease, discuss a referral to a cardiac rehabilitation program with physician and patient.
- Provide information about risk factor management and review plan to minimize risk factors.
- Assist in obtaining prescriptions and establishing a medication schedule and a plan for refilling prescriptions.
- Provide information on local educational programs on heart disease or risk factor management.
- Provide information on local support groups and the local chapter of the American Heart Association.

REFERENCES

Damlt, L. H., Groene, J., & Herick, R. (1992). Helping your patient through cardiac catheterization. *Nursing 92*, 22(2), 52–55.

Guzzetta, C. & Dossey, B. (1992). *Cardiovascular nursing—Body mind tapestry*. St. Louis, MO: Mosby Year Book.

Kinney, M., Packa, D., & Andreoli, K., Zipes, D. (1992). *Comprehensive cardiac care* (7th ed). St. Louis, MO: Mosby Year Book.

Perdue, B. (1990). Cardiac catheterization before and after. *Advancing Clinical Care, 5*(2), 16–19.

▼

CARDIOMYOPATHY

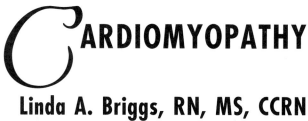

Linda A. Briggs, RN, MS, CCRN

Cardiomyopathy refers to diseases that affect the heart muscle rendering it dysfunctional and resulting in myocardial enlargement and failure. When classifying cardiomyopathies according to etiology, the terms *primary* or *idiopathic* and *secondary* are identified. Primary cardiomyopathy refers to disease of unknown cause, although viral diseases, autoimmunity, and lymphocytic myocarditis have all been implicated. Secondary cardiomyopathies occur secondary to a systemic disease process such as coronary artery disease, valvular disease, or hypertension. When classifying cardiomyopathies according to function, the terms hypertrophic, dilated, or restrictive are used (Table 8.1).

ETIOLOGIES

- Primary or idiopathic
  - autoimmunity
  - lymphocytic myocarditis
- Secondary
  - artery disease
  - valvular disease
  - hypertension

CLINICAL MANIFESTATIONS

- Manifestations of left ventricular failure (LVF)
  - dyspnea
  - orthopnea
  - coughing
  - fatigue
  - bibasilar crackles
  - tachycardia
  - murmurs, S_3, S_4
  - hypertension, hypotension
  - wheezes
  - worsening peripheral perfusion

- Manifestations of right ventricular failure (RVF)
  - jugular vein distention (JVD)
  - tachycardia
  - hypotension
  - peripheral edema
  - ascites
  - S_3
  - hepatomegaly
  - splenomegaly
  - nausea
  - anorexia
  - abdominal distension

Table 8.1 • Types of Cardiomyopathy

Hypertrophic cardiomyopathy	A genetically transmitted disease, hypertrophic cardiomyopathy is characterized by widespread cellular hypertrophy, especially involving the interventricular septum. This septal hypertrophy often renders the mitral valve incompetent, causing mitral regurgitations. The resulting myocardial muscle becomes stiff and noncompliant, resisting diastolic filling and causing decreased cardiac output.
Dilated cardiomyopathy	This cardiomyopathy is characterized by gross ventricular dilatation without hypertrophy. This dilatation caused myocardial fibril dysfunction resulting in decrease contractility, elevated ventricular filling pressures, congestive symptoms, and poor cardiac output. Dilatation occurs in all four chambers creating atrial and ventricular dysrhythmias and embolus formation.
Restrictive cardiomyopathy	A less common cause of cardiomypathy, this category is marked by ventricular infiltration of fibroelastic tissue, causing extensive muscular rigidity. Diastolic filling is impaired, and thus this form of cardiomyopathy is similar to constrictive pericarditis. Resistence to ventricular filling not only causes poor cardiac output, but also causes backward congestive symptoms.

CLINICAL/DIAGNOSTIC FINDINGS

- Chest x-ray
  - pulmonary congestion
  - enlarged cardiac silhouette

- Electrocardiogram (ECG)
  - left ventricular hypertrophy (exception: restrictive cardiomyopathy)
  - dysrhythmias: tachycardias, atrial and ventricular dysrhythmias, conduction disturbances
  - ST-T wave abnormalities
- Echocardiogram
  - left ventricular (LV) dilatation (hypertrophic and dilated cardiomyopathy)
  - increased LV wall thickness (restrictive cardiomyopathy)
  - mitral valve dysfunction
- Hemodynamics
  - elevated filling pressures
  - decreased cardiac output
  - decreased ejection fraction

▼

NURSING DIAGNOSIS: DECREASED CARDIAC OUTPUT

Related To

- Decreased contractility
- Increased preload
- Increased afterload
- Alterations in cardiac rate or rhythm

Defining Characteristics

See signs of LVF or RVF.

Patient Outcomes

Patient will

- demonstrate vital signs within acceptable parameters.
- demonstrate improved mentation.
- increase urine output.
- report decreased level of symptoms.
- report increased activity tolerance.

Nursing Interventions	Rationales
Assess patient's baseline symptomatology to include	Compensatory sympathetic stimulation causes tachycardia, vasoconstruction, and fluid retention.

Nursing Interventions	Rationales
1. pulse: rate, rhythm	Atrial dysrhythmias [premature atrial contractions, atrial fibrillation (PACs, A. Fib.)] occur as fluid overload from failing ventricle caused atrial irritability. Ventricular dysrhythmias occur due to ischemia, hypoxia, electrolyte imbalance, and acid-base disturbances.
2. blood pressure	In early cardiac failure, blood pressure is elevated from compensatory vasoconstriction. Later, as compensatory mechanisms fail, hypotension ensues.
3. peripheral circulation	
4. mentation	Changes in mentation occur with decreased cerebral perfusion, hypoxia, hypercarbia, acidosis, and fluid and electrolyte imbalances.
5. heart sounds	An S_3, indicative of an exacerbation of failure, occurs as a result of atrial contraction against a noncompliant left or right ventricle. Murmurs may be audible as valvular dysfunction accompanies ventricular failure.
6. urine output	Kidney response to decrease perfusion from vasoconstriction is to release renin, which in turn activates an enzyme, angiotensin I, which activates angiotensin II, which is a potent vasoconstrictor and also produces aldosterone. Aldosterone causes kidney reabsorption of sodium and water, thus creating a concentrated urine.

Nursing Interventions	Rationales
Institute measures to decrease myocardial oxygen demand to include	An important therapeutic goal is to decrease preload, thus optimizing myocardial stretch.
1. keeping head of bed elevated	Head elevation decreases venous return, or preload, thus decreasing myocardial oxygen demand. Ventilation will also be facilitated.
2. monitoring fluid status	Fluids must be monitored to prevent overload.
3. providing environmental control (visitors, rest, diagnostic scheduling, etc.)	
4. providing emotional rest	A variety of physical as well as psychosocial variables may increase the work of the heart. Fear, anxiety, stress, lack of sleep, etc., must be minimized. Reducing anxiety and other stress responses will limit catecholamine release.
5. assisting with physical cares as necessary	
6. instructing patient to avoid Valsalva maneuvers	Valsalva maneuvers increase myocardial oxygen demand.
Administer prescribed medications as indicated:	
1. preload reducing agents • diuretics • nitrates • morphine sulfate	Reducing preload assists in relieving the congestive symptoms of heart failure. Nitrates are effective venous vasodilators which assist in pooling venous blood. Morphine not only will cause venous vasodilation therapy, decreasing preload, but also will decrease myocardial oxygen demand by relieving anxiety.

Nursing Interventions	Rationales
2. afterload reducing agents • vasodilators • angiotensin converting enzyme (ACE) inhibitors	Afterload is a major contributor to myocardial workload. By reducing systemic vascular resistance, afterload is reduced and contractility enhanced. The ACE inhibitors block the action of angiotensin II, which will promote vasodilation and decrease afterload.
3. inotropic agents • digoxin	
Monitor electrolytes and supplement as necessary. Include sodium, potassium, calcium, and magnesium.	Inadequate nutrition, fluid shifts, vomiting, diarrhea, and use of diuretics may alter electrolytes that affect cardiac contractility and electrical conduction.
Monitor organ function through laboratory studies and clinical assessment: 1. blood urea nitrogen (BUN), creatinine (renal function) 2. serum glutamic oxaloacetic transaminase (SGOT), lactic dehydrogenase (LDH) (liver function)	Compensatory vasoconstriction eventually takes its toll on organ perfusion. As kidneys deal with hypoperfusion, prerenal causes of acute renal failure ensue. Systemic elevation in pressure overloads the liver, spleen, and mesenteric systems. Medical therapy must often be adjusted as organ failure becomes evident.
Prepare patient for intravenous drug therapy and probable transfer to intensive care unit if condition rapidly deteriorates.	When usual measures of improving cardiac output are not effective, the patient may require more aggressive therapy to improve ventricular function to include intravenous inotropes and vasodilators as well as intra-aortic balloon counter pulsation.

▼

NURSING DIAGNOSIS: FLUID VOLUME EXCESS

Related To sympathetic response to decreased cardiac output

Defining Characteristics

Pulmonary congestion: decreased breath sounds, crackles, wheezes
Systemic congestion: JVD, peripheral edema

Orthopnea
Weight gain
Hypertension
Tachycardia
Intake greater than output

Patient Outcomes

Patient will

- demonstrate improved fluid balance
- experience decreased pulmonary and systemic congestion
- lose weight or experience no further weight gain
- have blood pressure and heart rate that decreases toward normal

Nursing Interventions	Rationales
Auscultate anterior and posterior breath sounds for adventitious sounds.	As pulmonary interstitial fluid accumulates, alveoli are unable to fully expand and eventually collapse. This fluid accumulation is first evidenced by decreased breath sounds, which leads to crackles audible at end inspiration, especially evident in posterior bases (dependent edema). Audible wheezes present as fluid accumulation causes airway spasms.
Monitor weight daily.	Daily weights effectively assess fluid accumulation and distribution among fluid compartments. Approximately 1 kg weight gain is equivalent to 1 L of fluid accumulation.
Monitor intake and output.	
Restrict sodium and fluid intake. Establish patient preferences.	
Monitor serum electrolytes.	

Nursing Interventions	Rationales
Monitor mentation.	Mental changes may occur as fluid shifts, causing hyponatremia. Fluid moves by osmosis from areas of low concentration to those of high concentration. With hyponatremia, therefore, fluid will move into cells. Brain cells are especially sensitive to fluid changes. Intracellular fluid accumulation may be assessed by observing for signs of increased restlessness or altered sensorium, irritability, and lethargy.
Assess for presence and/or exacerbation of peripheral edema: 1. Change position frequently. 2. Elevate feet.	As right-sided heart failure occurs, elevated systemic pressure causes transudation of fluid and venous circulation, causing JVD and dependent pitting edema (ankles, sacrum, feet). Positional efforts to mobilize fluid will promote patient comfort and prevent skin breakdown.
Monitor central venous pressure (CVP) as indicated.	Normal CVP is 2–10 mmHg. As CVP rises, it is indicative of inability of the right side of the heart to handle incoming fluid.
Assess gastrointestinal system for evidence of anorexia, nausea, distension, and hepaxomegaly: 1. Provide nutritional supplementation. 2. Enlist patient preferences. 3. Provide small, pallatable meals at more frequent intervals. 4. Consult with dietitian as indicated. 5. Monitor drug levels as necessary. 6. Provide emotional support for altered physical appearance.	In progressive right-sided heart failure, venous engorgement eventually creates altered gastrointestinal function, liver failure, and nutritional compromise.

Nursing Interventions	Rationales
Administer medications as prescribed: 1. diuretics: furosemide, bumetanide 2. potassium-sparing agents: Aldactone 3. potassium supplements	Diuretics enhance urine output by inhibiting sodium and chloride reabsorption in the renal tubules.
Monitor effects of diuretic therapy.	Long-term diuretic therapy can cause hypokalemia and hyponatremia

▼

NURSING DIAGNOSIS: IMPAIRED GAS EXCHANGE

Related To ventilation perfusion inequality secondary to pulmonary interstitial fluid accumulation

Defining Characteristics

Restlessness
Confusion
Hypoxia
Hypercapnia
Pulmonary congestion

Patient Outcomes

Patient will experience

- improved mentation
- decreased hypoxia, hypercarbia
- decreased pulmonary congestion

Nursing Interventions	Rationales
Assess mentation changes.	Hypoxia and/or hypercarbia causes mental deterioration such as restlessness, confusion, irritability, and lethargy.
Monitor arterial blood gases (ABGs) as appropriate.	Arterial blood gas analysis periodically reveals level of hypoxia and hypercarbia and depth of compensatory responses.
Monitor pulse oximetry if hypoxemia is present.	
Position patient in semi-Fowler's.	

Nursing Interventions	Rationales
Intervene to assist in preventing hyperventilation: 1. Provide calm, reassuring approach. 2. Explain all interventions. 3. Teach techniques to slow breathing. 4. Administer morphine sulfate as appropriate. 5. Elevate head of bed.	Fear and anxiety contribute to the work of breathing, which in turn contributes to increasing myocardial workload. Breathing techniques that promote alveolar opening and promote effective cough efforts will aid maximum lung inflation. Breathing techniques also allow patient control.

▼

NURSING DIAGNOSIS: ACTIVITY INTOLERANCE

Related To decreased cardiac output

Defining Characteristics

Weakness
Fatigue
Dyspnea
Ischemic pain
ECG changes (if monitored)
Vital sign changes: heart rate 30 bpm > baseline, heart rate 15 bpm > baseline for patients on beta blockers or calcium channel blockers

Patient Outcomes

Patient will

- participate in activities of daily living
- increase level of activity without symptoms
- have vital signs within acceptable limits during activity: heart rate elevations < 20 bpm above baseline
- experience heart rate that returns to normal 5 min after activity

Nursing Interventions	Rationales
Assess response to activity: 1. dyspnea 2. tachycardia 3. fatigue 4. chest pain	Activity may increase oxygen demand at a time when the myocardium is unable to deliver. Heart rate increases to compensate, thus creating fatigue, dyspnea, and vital sign changes. Appearance of symptoms will limit patient's activity level.

Nursing Interventions	Rationales
Assess vital signs before and after activity.	
Assess medication regime.	Medications such as diuretics, vasodilators, beta blockers, and calcium antagonists may cause vital sign changes especially evident during exercise.
Assess changes in activity level.	Decrease activity, fatigue, and chest discomfort all contribute to muscular atrophy and weakness. Muscle strengthening can increase endurance and quality of activity.
Devise an activity schedule that clusters activities, allows for frequent rest periods, and incorporates patient choices.	
Consult occupational therapy and/or physical therapy as necessary for muscle-strengthening exercises, strategies for energy conservation, and exercise guidelines.	
Instruct in passive range-of-motion exercises while in bed.	Joints can remain more flexible and muscles stretched.

▼

NURSING DIAGNOSIS: ALTERED NUTRITION—LESS THAN BODY REQUIREMENTS

Related To
- Weakness
- Anorexia

Defining Characteristics
Weight loss of > 10% of body weight
Serum albumin < 3.5 g/100 mL
Negative nitrogen balance
Total lymphocyte count < 1500
Fatigue
Caloric intake less than requirements

Patient Outcomes

Patient will demonstrate

- stable weight
- serum albumin > 3.5 g/mL
- total lymphocyte count > 1500
- positive nitrogen balance
- increased energy and endurance
- caloric intake equal to requirements

Nursing Interventions	Rationales
Assess for signs of nutritional deficit.	Poor nutrition will exacerbate any infectious process and retard the healing process. Early attention will promote recovery.
Monitor laboratory data: 1. serum protein or transferrin 2. urinary urea nitrogen 3. total lymphocytes 4. nitrogen balance (estimated by subtracting excertion from intake)	Among the components of nutritional assessment is the evaluation of protein status. The breakdown of protein can be estimated by the renal excretion of urea nitrogen. Nitrogen balance determines nutritional adequacy. When intake exceeds output, a positive nitrogen balance exists. When output exceeds intake, a negative nitrogen balance exists, which will require nutritional adjustment. Serum albumin or transferrin reflects changes in amino acid availability. Malnourishment affects our immune system. Monitoring lymphocytes is one measurement of nutritional state.
Compare weight daily.	Loss of lean body mass may be assessed by monitoring daily weights. Effective nutritional therapy can also be monitored by daily weight comparisons.
Monitor nutritional intake: 1. Provide high-calorie, high-protein foods. 2. Monitor calorie counts daily.	To provide adequate nutrients for anabolism.
Monitor environment to ensure adequate rest.	To decrease metabolic demands and nutritional needs.

▼

NURSING DIAGNOSIS: HOPELESSNESS/POWERLESSNESS

Related To failing or deteriorating physical condition

Defining Characteristics

Passive, apathetic
Lack of participation in decision making, conversations, etc.
Irritable, angry
Verbalization of frustration and lack of improvement
Increased sleep

Patient Outcomes

Patient will

- participate in decisions, care, and conversations
- appear more relaxed
- verbalize progress
- sleep during more normal intervals

Nursing Interventions	Rationales
Provide consistent nurse-patient relationship. Assess patient perception of stage of illness and treatment plan.	
Encourage expression of feelings, concerns, frustrations, etc.	Giving permission to express dissatisfaction builds trust and communication outlets.
Help develop realistic short-term goals.	Reinforces sense of accomplishment and lessens frustrations.
Involve patient in care planning as much as possible, for example, activity schedule, visitors, or personal cares. Encourage as much independence as possible.	Allowing some control over environment and life.
Involve family and close friends as patient desires. Encourage them to allow patient to do as much as he or she can independently. Provide support and realistic outcomes.	
Answer patient and family questions honestly.	

▼

NURSING DIAGNOSIS: KNOWLEDGE DEFICIT—DIAGNOSIS AND TREATMENT PLAN

Related To

- Lack of previous experience
- New diagnosis
- Misinformation

Defining Characteristics

Asks questions
Verbalizes inadequate knowledge
Demonstrates behaviors inconsistent with treatment plan

Patient Outcomes

Patient will

- verbalize knowledge of disease process, limitations, and self-management guidelines
- demonstrate skills that are necessary for treatment compliance

Nursing Interventions	Rationales
Assess patient understanding of disease process and treatment plan. Begin educational process with assessment of patient readiness to learn and stage of acceptance of disease and disease progression.	
Provide information on basic disease process and realistic outcomes.	
Assist in understanding activity restrictions.	
Instruct in signs and symptoms to report: 1. weight gain of more than 2 lb in 1 day 2. increased shortness of breath 3. chest discomfort 4. decreased activity tolerance	
Reinforce dietary restrictions to include low-sodium and low-cholesterol guidelines.	Dietary restrictions may change as disease progresses.

Nursing Interventions	Rationales
Instruct on daily weights and pulse taking.	
Explore treatment options and role in decision making with patient and family 1. Provide information and support on advanced directives. 2. Assist family in obtaining cardiopulmonary resuscitation (CPR) training if desired. 3. Assist in devising appropriate questions to discuss with physician.	With the progression of the disease process and limitation of treatment options, discussions may center on long-term mortality and decisions regarding the dying process. With information and support introduced slowly, patients and families can together explore these difficult issues while the patient is still competent.

DISCHARGE PLANNING/CONTINUITY OF CARE

- Assure understanding of self-management plan, including activity restrictions, signs and symptoms to report, and medications.
- Refer to a home health agency or hospice, if needed, for monitoring, education, or assistance with care or the dying process.
- Arrange for follow-up with physician for continued management.
- Assist in filling prescriptions, devising medication schedule, and establishing a system for refilling prescriptions.
- Refer family to local agencies for CPR education if desired.
- Refer to a local chapter of the American Heart Association for further information.

REFERENCES

Canobbio, M. (1990). *Cardiovascular disorders.* St. Louis, MO: Mosby.

Guzzetta, C. & Dossey, B. (1992). *Cardiovascular nursing.* St. Louis, MO: Mosby Year Book.

Purcell, J. (1990). Advances in the treatment of dilated cardiomyopathy. *AACN Clinical Issues*, 1(1), 31–45.

CONGESTIVE HEART FAILURE

Linda A. Briggs, RN, MS, CCRN

Congestive heart failure is a complex clinical syndrome initiated by poor myocardial contractility. The resultant cardiac output is inadequate to meet the body's metabolic needs, thus causing a host of systemic responses to occur in an effort to compensate. It is these very compensatory mechanisms that proceed to increase heart rate, myocardial preload, afterload, and contractility, creating an increase in myocardial oxygen demand that further burdens an already stressed heart. It is ironic that while these compensatory responses initially succeed in masking the disease process, they terminate in worsening peripheral perfusion. Acute failure of the heart creates little time for compensatory responses, and circulatory compromise occurs immediately. At the other extreme, chronic heart failure allows years of compensatory responses to occur and a long and often smoldering clinical course.

ETIOLOGIES

- Decreased myocardial contractility
  - coronary artery disease
  - cardiomyopathies
  - myocarditis
  - collagen vascular disorders (systemic lupus erythematosus)
  - tumors
  - medications (beta blockers, calcium antagonists)
- Increased myocardial workload
  - hypertension (systemic, pulmonary)
  - valvular heart disorders
  - intracardiac shunting
  - anemia
  - hyperthyroidism
  - pulmonary embolism
  - systemic infection

- Decreased preload (decreased myocardial fibril stretch)
  - cardiac tamponade
  - constrictive precarditis
  - tachydysrhythmias
  - loss of atrial contraction

CLINICAL MANIFESTATIONS

Left ventricular failure (LVF)

- dyspnea
- orthopnea
- daytime coughing
- fatigue
- wheezes
- worsening peripheral perfusion: weak pulses, cool diaphoretic skin, altered mentation, and decreased urine output
- tachycardia
- S_3, S_4
- hypertension
- moist bibasilar crackles

Right ventricular failure (RVF)

- jugular vein distention (JVD)
- hypotension
- ascites
- hepatomegaly
- nausea
- abdominal distention
- tachycardia
- peripheral edema
- S_3
- splenomegaly
- anorexia

Clinical Clip

Mechanisms of Heart Failure

Left Ventricular Failure (LVF) As the left ventricle fails, left ventricular end-diastolic pressure (LVEDP) rises. This pressure elevation is transmitted backward to the pulmonary vasculature, eventually causing transudation of fluid into the pulmonary interstitium, interfering with oxygen exchange.

Right Ventricular Failure (RVF) As the right ventricle fails, right ventricular end diastolic pressure (RVEDP) rises. This pressure elevation is transmitted to the systemic circulation, causing transudation of fluid into the peripherial tissues as well as organ congestion. Right ventricular failure results from primary lung disorders (COPD), from disorders of right ventricular dynamics (RV myocardial infarction), or as the eventual sequelae of LVF.

CLINICAL/DIAGNOSTIC FINDINGS

- Chest x-ray
  - pulmonary congestion

- Laboratory values
  - hyponatremia
  - hypo- or hyperkalemia
  - hypochloremia
  - elevated blood urea nitrogen (BUN), creatinine
  - arterial blood gases (ABGs): decreased PaO_2, increased $PaCO_2$
- Electrocardiogram (ECG)
  - left ventricular hypertrophy
  - right ventricular hypertrophy
  - atrial hypertrophy
- Hemodynamics
  - decreased cardiac output
  - decreased ejection fraction (normal > 60%)
  - elevated pulmonary artery systolic, diastolic, and wedge pressures

NURSING DIAGNOSIS: HIGH RISK FOR DECREASED CARDIAC OUTPUT

Risk Factors

- Decreased contractility
- Increased preload
- Increased afterload
- Alterations in cardiac rate or rhythm

Patient Outcomes

- Vital signs are within acceptable parameters.
- Mentation is improved.
- Urine output is greater than 30 mL/hr.
- Patient reports decreased level of symptoms.
- Activity tolerance is increased.

Nursing Interventions	Rationales
Assess patient's baseline symptomatology to include	Compensatory sympathetic stimulation causes tachycardia, vasoconstriction and fluid retention.
1. pulse: rate, rhythm	Atrial dysrhythmias [premature atrial contractions, atrial fibrillation (PACs, A.Fib.)] occur as fluid overload from failing ventricle caused atrial irritability. Ventricular dysrhythmias occur due to ischemia, hypoxia, electrolyte imbalance, and acidbase disturbances.

Nursing Interventions	Rationales
2. blood pressure	In early congestive heart failure (CHF), blood pressure is elevated from compensatory vasoconstriction. Later, as compensatory mechanisms fail, hypotension ensues.
3. peripheral circulation	
4. heart sounds	An S_3, indicative of an exacerbation of failure, occurs as a result of atrial contraction against a noncompliant left or right ventricle. Murmurs may be audible as valvular dysfunction accompanies ventricular failure.
5. urine output	Kidney response to decreased perfusion from vasoconstriction is to release renin, which in turn activates an enzyme, angiotensin I, which activates angiotensin II, which is a potent vasoconstrictor and also produces aldosterone. Aldosterone causes kidney reabsorption of sodium and water, thus creating a concentrated urine.
6. mentation	Mentation changes occur with changes in cerebral perfusion, hypoxia, hypercarbia, acidosis, and fluid and electrolyte imbalances.
Institute measures to decrease myocardial oxygen demand, including:	An important therapeutic goal is to decrease preload, thus optimizing myocardial stretch.
1. Keep head of bed elevated.	Head elevation decreases venous return, or preload, thus decreasing myocardial oxygen demand. Ventilation will also be facilitated.
2. Monitor fluid status.	Fluids must be monitored to prevent overload.
3. Provide environmental control (visitors, rest, diagnostic scheduling, etc.).	

Nursing Interventions	Rationales
4. Provide emotional rest.	
5. Assist with physical care as necessary.	A variety of physical as well as psychosocial variables may increase the work of the heart. Fear, anxiety, stress, lack of sleep, etc. must be minimized. Reducing anxiety and other stress responses will limit catecholamine release.
Administer prescribed medications:	
1. preload reducing agents • diuretics • nitrates • morphine sulfate	Reducing preload assists in relieving the congestive symptoms of heart failure. Nitrates are effective venous vasodilators which assist in pooling venous blood. Morphine will not only cause venous vasodilation therapy, decreasing preload, but will also decrease myocardial oxygen demand by relieving anxiety.
2. afterload reducing agents • vasodilators • angiotension converting enzyme ACE inhibitors	Afterload is a major contributor to myocardial workload. By reducing systemic vascular resistance, afterload is reduced and contractility enhanced. The ACE inhibitors block the action of angiotensin II, which will promote vasodilation and decrease afterload.
3. inotropic agents • digoxin	Positive inotropic agents increase myocardial contractility.
Monitor electrolytes, including sodium, potassium, calcium, and magnesium. Supplement as necessary.	Inadequate nutrition, fluid shifts, vomiting, diarrhea, and use of diuretics may alter electrolytes that affect cardiac contractility and electrical conduction.

Nursing Interventions	Rationales
Monitor renal and liver function through laboratory studies and clinical assessment: 1. BUN, creatinine (renal function) 2. serum glutamic oxaloacetic transaminase (SGOT), lactic dehydrogenase (LDH) (liver function)	Compensatory vasoconstriction eventually takes its toll on organ perfusion. As kidneys deal with hypoperfusion, prerenal causes of acute renal failure ensue. Systemic elevation in pressure overloads the liver, spleen, and mesenteric systems. Medical therapy must often be adjusted as organ failure becomes evident.

▼

NURSING DIAGNOSIS: FLUID VOLUME EXCESS

Related To sympathetic response to decreased cardiac output

Defining Characteristics

Pulmonary congestion: decreased breath sounds, crackles, wheezes
Systemic congestion: JVD, peripheral edema
Orthopnea
Weight gain
Hypertension
Tachycardia
Intake greater than output

Patient Outcomes

Patient will

- have improved fluid balance.
- have decreased pulmonary and systemic congestion.
- lose weight or experience no further weight gain.
- have normal blood pressure and heart rate.

Nursing Interventions	Rationales
Auscultate anterior and posterior breath sounds for adventitious sounds.	As pulmonary interstitial fluid accumulates, alveoli are unable to fully expand and eventually collapse. This fluid accumulation is first evidenced by decreased breath sounds, which leads to crackles audible at end inspiration, especially evident in posterior bases (dependent edema). Audible wheezes present as fluid accumulation cause airway spasms.

Nursing Interventions	Rationales
Monitor daily weight.	Daily weights effectively assess fluid accumulation and distribution among fluid compartments. Approximately 1 kg weight gain is equivalent to 1 L of fluid accumulation.
Monitor intake and output.	
Restrict sodium and fluid intake. Establish patient's preferences in food selections.	
Monitor mentation.	Mental changes may occur as fluid shifts, causing hyponatremia. Fluid moves by osmosis from areas of low concentration to those of high concentration. With hyponatremia, therefore, fluid will move into cells. Brain cells are especially sensitive to fluid changes. Intracellular fluid accumulation may be assessed by observing for signs of increased restlessness or altered sensorium, irritability, and lethargy.
Assess for presence and/or exacerbation of peripheral edema. To reduce edema, change position frequently and elevate feet.	As right-sided heart failure occurs, elevated systemic pressure causes transudation of fluid and venous circulation, causing JVD and dependent pitting edema (ankles, sacrum, feet). Positional efforts to mobilize fluid will promote patient comfort and prevent skin breakdown.
Monitor central venous pressure (CVP), if available.	Normal CVP is 2–10 mmHg. As CVP rises, it is indicative of inability of the right side of the heart to handle incoming fluid.

Nursing Interventions	Rationales
Assess gastrointestinal system for evidence of anorexia, nausea, distention, and hepatomegaly. If present: 1. Provide nutritional supplementation. 2. Enlist patient preferences. 3. Provide small, palatable meals at more frequent intervals 4. Consult with dietitian as indicated. 5. Monitor drug levels as necessary. 6. Provide emotional support for altered physical appearance.	In progressive right-sided heart failure, venous engorgement eventually creates altered gastrointestinal function, liver failure, and nutritional compromise.
Administer medications as prescribed/indicated: 1. diuretics: furosemide, bumetanide 2. potassium-sparing agents: aldactone 3. potassium supplements	Diuretics enhance urine output by inhibiting sodium and chloride reabsorption in the renal tubules.
Monitor effects of diuretic therapy.	Long-term diuretic therapy can cause hypokalemia, hyponatremia, and hypomagnesemia.

▼

NURSING DIAGNOSIS: IMPAIRED GAS EXCHANGE

Related To ventilation perfusion inequality secondary to pulmonary interstitial fluid accumulation

Defining Characteristics

Restlessness
Confusion
Hypoxia
Hypercapnia
Pulmonary congestion

Patient Outcomes

Patient will

- experience improved mentation.
- experience decreasing hypoxia and hypercarbia.
- experience decreased pulmonary congestion.

Nursing Interventions	Rationales
Auscultate breath sounds for adventitious sounds.	As pulmonary interstitial fluid accumulates, decreased breath sounds, crackles, and wheezes may become audible. Monitoring lung sounds will also give some index of effectiveness of therapy.
Monitor ABGs as appropriate.	Arterial blood gas analysis periodically reveals level of hypoxia, level of hypercarbia, and depth of compensatory responses.
Monitor pulse oximetry when borderline hypoxia is present.	
Administer oxygen as indicated.	
Position patient in semi-Fowler's.	
Intervene to assist in preventing hyperventilation by	Fear and anxiety contribute to the work of breathing, which in turn contributes to increasing myocardial workload.
1. providing calm, reassuring approach.	
2. explaining all interventions.	
3. teaching breathing techniques.	Breathing techniques that promote alveolar opening and promote effective cough efforts will aid maximum lung inflation. Breathing techniques also allow patient control.
4. administering morphine sulfate as appropriate.	
5. elevating head of bed.	

NURSING DIAGNOSIS: ACTIVITY INTOLERANCE

Related To decreased cardiac output

Defining Characteristics

Weakness
Fatigue
Dyspnea

Ischemic pain
ECG changes (if monitored)
Vital sign changes: heart rate 30 bpm > baseline
Vital sign changes: heart rate 15 bpm > baseline for patients on beta blockers or calcium channel blockers

Patient Outcomes

Patient will

- participate in activities of daily living.
- increase level of activity without symptoms.
- have vital signs within acceptable limits during activity: heart rate elevations < 20 bpm above baseline.
- experience a heart rate return to normal 5 min after activity.

Nursing Interventions	Rationales
Assess patient response to activity, including dyspnea, tachycardia, fatigue, and chest pain.	Activity may increase oxygen demand at a time when the myocardium is unable to deliver. Heart rate increases to compensate, thus creating fatigue, dyspnea, and vital sign changes. Appearance of symptoms will limit patient activity level.
Assess vital signs before and after activity.	
Assist to maintain regular activity as able, but to recognize activity limitations, incorporate rest periods and methods of conserving energy.	
Assess medication regime.	Medications such as diuretics, vasodilators, beta blockers, and calcium antagonists may cause vital sign changes especially evident during exercise.
Assess changes in activity level.	Decreased activity, fatigue, and chest discomfort all contribute to muscular atrophy and weakness. Muscle strengthening can increase endurance and quality of activity.
Consult occupational therapy and/or physical therapy as necessary for muscle-strengthening exercises, strategies for energy conservation, and exercise guidelines.	

Nursing Interventions	Rationales
Instruct in passive range-of-motion exercises while in bed.	Joints can remain more flexible and muscles stretched.

▼

NURSING DIAGNOSIS: KNOWLEDGE DEFICIT—DIAGNOSIS AND TREATMENT PLAN

Related To
- Lack of previous experience
- New diagnosis
- Misinformation

Defining Characteristics
- Asks questions
- Verbalizes inadequate knowledge
- Demonstrates behaviors inconsistent with treatment plan

Patient Outcomes
Patient will
- describe treatment plan and signs and symptoms to report.
- demonstrate skills that are necessary for treatment compliance.

Nursing Interventions	Rationales
Assess patient understanding of stage of disease process and prior education.	Patient education in this area is an ongoing endeavor. Each new hospitalization affords an opportunity to provide new information, clarify old information, assess compliance, and offer new strategies for coping and living with chronic illness.

Nursing Interventions	Rationales
Prioritize information to be taught. Concentrate on the most important information the patient should know (i.e., "survival information"). Topics include 1. basic disease process 2. signs/symptoms to report • weight gain > 2 lb in 24 hr • decreased activity tolerance • dyspnea on exertion • chest discomfort uncontrolled by usual methods 3. activity guidelines 4. dietary instructions: low sodium 5. daily weights and pulse taking 6. basic medication information	A variety of issues may limit the accomplishment of a thorough teaching plan. Short hospitalizations, patient's mentation, and motivation are among these variables. Consider what is most important to be taught for patient safety.
Inform of potential sleep disturbance related to nocturia, dyspnea, and orthopnea: 1. Teach to alter diuretic dose schedule. 2. Teach to elevate head of bed or sleep in recliner.	Sleep disturbances are common in CHF patients. Nocturia may be caused by drug therapy taken too close to bedtime. Orthopnea and dyspnea occur as recumbent position allows increased venous return and decreased myocardial contractility, causing pulmonary congestion
Provide written information whenever possible.	
Explore, with patient and family, treatment options and role in decision making: 1. Provide information and support on advanced directives. 2. Assist family in obtaining cardiopulmonary resuscitation (CPR) training if desired. 3. Assist patient in devising appropriate questions to discuss with physician.	With chronic CHF, repeated exacerbations and hospitalizations may leave many questions related to long-term mortality and desire for continued treatment. With information and support introduced slowly, patients and families can together explore these difficult issues while the patient is still competent.
Include family/significant others in teaching plan.	

Nursing Interventions	Rationales
Assess factors that may impact on patient's ability to learn.	Psychological state of adaptation to chronic illness, activity intolerance, learning ability, patient priorities, and motivation are all variables impacting on ability to learn.

▼

DISCHARGE PLANNING/CONTINUITY OF CARE

- Assure understanding of self-management plan, including activity restrictions, dietary guidelines, pulse taking, daily weights, medications, and symptoms to report.
- Arrange for home oxygen equipment or other medical equipment if appropriate.
- Refer to home health agency if patient has had difficulty understanding treatment plan.
- Arrange follow-up with physician for continued management.
- Assist in obtaining prescriptions, devising medication schedule, and establishing a plan for refilling prescriptions.
- Provide patient/family with information on stop-smoking programs, educational programs, and CPR classes.
- Refer to local chapter of the American Heart Association for further information.

REFERENCES

Guzzetta, C. & Dossey, B. (1992). *Cardiovascular nursing*: St. Louis, MO: Mosby Year Book.

Letterer, R., Carew, B., Reid, M., & Woods, P. (1992). Learning to live with congestive heart failure. *Nursing* 92, *(5)*, 34–41.

Thelan, L., Davie, J., & Urden, L. (1990). *Textbook of critical care nursing*. St. Louis, MO: Mosby.

▼

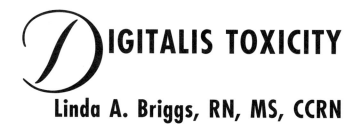

DIGITALIS TOXICITY

Linda A. Briggs, RN, MS, CCRN

As one of the most common cardiac medications, digitalis is prescribed to increase myocardial contractility and decrease heart rate. It is indicated for a wide variety of cardiac disorders, given for extended periods of time, and commonly administered to the elderly. The therapeutic-to-toxic dose is very narrow, thus creating a frequent clinical phenomenon of overdose or toxicity.

ETIOLOGIES

- Advanced or long-standing cardiac disease
- Electrolyte imbalance, specifically potassium and magnesium
- Decreased renal function
- Coadministration of other drugs (calcium antagonists, quinidine, beta blockers, diuretics, laxatives, antacids)
- Acid-base imbalances
- Hypoxia
- Hypothyroidism
- Altered drug absorbency

CLINICAL MANIFESTATIONS

- Gastrointestinal
  - anorexia
  - nausea
  - vomiting
  - diarrhea
- Central nervous system
  - visual disturbances (difficulty with red and green color perception, halos around objects)
  - fatigue
  - confusion

  - depression
  - psychosis
- Cardiac
  - any dysrhythmia
  - atrial tachycardia with block
  - accelerated junctional rhythms
  - sinus tachycardia and bradycardia
  - atrioventricular (AV) blocks, progressive
  - atrial fibrillation
  - ventricular dysrhythmias

CLINICAL/DIAGNOSTIC FINDINGS

- Serum digoxin level
  - usually elevated above therapeutic range (0.5–2.0 ng/mL)
  - patients with risk factors may show signs of toxicity at low or normal serum levels
- Electrolytes
  - hypokalemia, hypomagnesemia, hypocalcemia
  - may aggravate digitalis toxicity
- Electrocardiogram
  - variety of rhythm disturbances which may not be specific

OTHER PLANS OF CARE TO REFERENCE

Congestive heart failure (CHF)

▼

NURSING DIAGNOSIS: HIGH RISK FOR DECREASED CARDIAC OUTPUT

Risk Factors

- Preexisting, advanced cardiac disease
- Electrolyte imbalance
- Decreased renal function
- Increased sensitivity with other drugs

Patient Outcomes

Patient will

- have heart rate and rhythm within acceptable range.
- have rhythm status within normal limits or controlled.
- have normal renal status [blood urea nitrogen (BUN), creatinine].
- have normal electrolytes.

Nursing Interventions	Rationales
Assess patient hemodynamic status to include 1. blood pressure 2. heart rate, including apical assessment 3. heart rhythm: • Monitor and document rhythm status (if monitored). • Investigate new rhythm disturbances; monitor on telemetry or obtain 12-lead ECG.	Rhythm disturbances frequently accompany digitalis toxicity. However, rhythm disturbances are not uncommon in the patient population requiring digitalis treatment. New dysrhythmias should be investigated. Many digitalis-related dysrhythmias may decrease cardiac output and result in decreased peripheral organ perfusion. Other dysrhythmias may lead to more lethal, life-threatening situations.
Assess for other signs of heart failure (see CHF).	Digitalis toxicity may aggravate preexisting cardiac conditions.
Monitor electrolyte status and treat imbalances.	Hypokalemia will increase the potential for digitalis toxicity. Potassium and digitalis compete for similar cellular binding sites. Less potassium allows digitalis to bind with greater sites. Hypomagnesium causes refractory hypokalemia, and hypercalcemia potentials cause digitalis toxicity.
Monitor serum digoxin levels.	
Monitor renal function to include urine output, BUN, and creatinine values.	Digitalis is excreted through the kidneys, and altered renal function will potentiate digitalis toxicity.
Assess other prescribed or over-the-counter medications for potential drug interactions to include 1. antacids, neomycin 2. drugs containing calcium (quinidine, verapamil) 3. drugs that cause potassium wasting (steroids, diuretics) 4. beta blockers	Drugs such as antacids, laxatives, and neomycin may alter bowel absorption and decrease digitalis effectiveness. Calcium preparations and hypokalemia enhance digitalis toxicity. Beta blockers may decrease heart rate and potentiate digitalis-induced bradycardias

Nursing Interventions	Rationales
Prepare patient for treatment of dysrhythmias that may include temporary pacing and antiarrhythmic drug therapy and transfer to critical care unit.	
Administer digoxin-immune Fab (antigen-binding fragments) as prescribed. During administration, monitor potassium levels.	The digoxin-immune Fab binds antibodies with digoxin binding sites, thus minimizing the effects of existing digitalis. A 13-year multicenter trial has proved the drug's effectiveness. Serum digoxin levels will rise and will not be a reliable indicator. Potassium levels will elevate during administration and may need to be treated with other measures temporarily.

▼

NURSING DIAGNOSIS: HIGH RISK FOR FLUID VOLUME DEFICIT

Risk Factors

- Gastrointestinal side effects of digitalis toxicity
- Diuretic therapy
- Malnutrition

Patient Outcomes

Patient will

- verbalize relief from nausea, vomiting, and diarrhea.
- have balanced intake and output.

Nursing Interventions	Rationales
Monitor closely for gastrointestinal symptoms of nausea, vomiting, anorexia, and diarrhea.	Gastrointestinal side effects occur in approximately 80% of patients with digitalis toxicity. These symptoms may often be overlooked and related to other factors such as the underlying disease process or medications. The appearance of one new symptom should be investigated.

Nursing Interventions	Rationales
Monitor fluid status to include intake, output, and daily weights.	
Provide adequate fluids and foods as tolerated.	
Administer antiemetics as prescribed.	

▼

NURSING DIAGNOSIS: HIGH RISK FOR ALTERED THOUGHT PROCESSES

Risk Factors

- Age
- Underlying cardiac disease
- Underlying mental status

Patient Outcomes

Patient will demonstrate

- return to baseline mental status
- usual visual acuity

Nursing Interventions	Rationales
Obtain baseline mental status, incorporating information from family as appropriate.	Understanding patient baseline mentation is important in evaluating any observed changes. Many underlying conditions, including advancing age, may render the normal exam.
Assess patient closely for mentation changes to include fatigue, confusion, and depression.	
Protect the patient from harm by frequent orientation, monitoring closely, or assisting with ambulation.	
Provide emotional support to patient and family.	Many digitalis-induced changes in mentation completely resolve once the body is cleared of high digitalis levels.

▼

NURSING DIAGNOSIS: KNOWLEDGE DEFICIT—DIGITALIS USE

Related To
- Lack of information
- Misinformation

Defining Characteristics

Lack of knowledge regarding digitalis and risk factors for toxicity
Does not follow prescribed treatment
Unable to identify side effects of toxicity

Patient Outcomes

Patient will
- verbalize risk factors for toxicity.
- follow recommendations for drug administration.
- verbalize side effects of toxicity.

Nursing Interventions	Rationales
Provide information on purpose of digitalis and administration guidelines.	Knowledge may increase compliance with treatment and avoid the potential for side effects.
Instruct patient to adhere to medication schedule and the importance of not omitting doses or taking extra doses.	
Instruct in pulse taking and to notify physician if pulse is less than the physician's predetermined rate.	Digitalis and associated drug combinations may cause bradycardias. Although a heart rate below 60 bpm may indicate toxicity, the physician may prescribe other heart rate guidelines.
Encourage patient to check with physician or pharmacist before taking any over-the-counter medications.	To avoid drug interactions with digitalis.

Nursing Interventions	Rationales
Inform of the following side effects to report to the physician: 1. nausea 2. vomiting 3. diarrhea 4. change in heart rate 5. visual disturbances 6. change in mentation	

▼

DISCHARGE PLANNING/CONTINUITY OF CARE

- Assure understanding of self-management plan, including medication schedule, pulse taking, and symptoms to report.
- Refer to a home health agency for medication monitoring, compliance with treatment plan, and further education.
- Arrange follow-up with physician for continued management.
- Assist in obtaining prescriptions, devising medication schedule, and establishing a plan for refilling prescriptions.

REFERENCES

Bayer, M., (1992). When drugs turn against the heart. *Emergency Medicine*, August 15, 1992, pp. 119–136.

Guzzetta, C. & Dossey, B. (1992). *Cardiovascular nursing*. St. Louis, MO: Mosby Year Book.

McDonnell-Cooke, D. (1992). Shielding your patient from digitalis toxicity. *Nursing 92*, 7, 44–47.

▼

ENDOCARDITIS

Linda A. Briggs, RN, MS, CCRN

The endothelial layer of the heart may become infected by microorganisms, creating a condition called endocarditis. This inflammation extends to the cardiac valves as well. While the incidence is low, the treatment requires a long course of antibiotic therapy and close monitoring for complications. Acute endocarditis develops rapidly on usually normal valvular structures and causes widespread destruction. Subacute endocarditis is more insidious, develops on previously damaged structures, and is more responsive to treatment. After the onset of bacteremia from a multitude of causes, colonization occurs on valve leaflets. The bacteria is well protected in a fibrin shell, increasing its resilience. Thrombi form on the damaged structures, leading to scarring of the leaflets and valvular dysfunction as well as abscess formation. These patients are additionally at risk for septic embolization, especially to the aorta, cerebral vessels, and systemic arterioles of the lung, kidney, or spleen.

ETIOLOGIES

- Streptococcal bacteria
- Staphylococcal bacteria
- Predisposing factors to bacteriemia
  - cardiac surgery (including prosthetic valve replacement and aortic grafts)
  - rheumatic heart disease
  - congenital heart disease
  - degenerative heart disease
  - mitral valve prolapse
  - immunosuppression
  - dental manipulations (extractions, teeth cleaning, periodontal disease)
  - intubation, bronchoscopy
  - gastrointestinal (GI) procedures (colonoscopy, barium enema)
  - intravenous (IV) drug use

- cannulation of systemic vessels (arterial lines, transvenous, pacemakers, etc.)

CLINICAL MANIFESTATIONS

- Fever (low grade with subacute)
- Malaise, weakness, fatigue
- Heart murmurs, change in preexisting murmurs
- Signs of heart failure
- Signs of peripheral embolization
  - Osler nodes: small raised and tender lesions on fingers and toes
  - petechial: conjunctivae, extremities
  - hematuria
  - Roth's spots: fibrin accumulations leading to retinal hemorrhages
  - sensorium changes: behavior changes, parasthesias, etc.
  - Janeway lesions: hemorrhagic lesions on palms, soles
- Splenomegaly (more common in subacute)

CLINICAL/DIAGNOSTIC FINDINGS

- Laboratory
  - elevated white blood cell (WBC) count
  - elevated sedimentation rate
  - anemia
  - positive blood cultures
  - proteinuria
  - elevated blood urea nitrogen (BUN) and creatinine (in renal compromise)
- Echocardiogram
  - visualization of valvular vegetations
  - valvular incompetence
  - impaired ventricular performance

OTHER PLANS OF CARE TO REFERENCE

Long-term venous access devices

▼

NURSING DIAGNOSIS: ALTERED BODY TEMPERATURE

Related To inflammation

Defining Characteristics

Fever: high grade if acute (39–40 °C), low grade if subacute (<39.4 °C)
Malaise

Weakness
Fatigue
White blood cell count elevated
Positive blood culture
Signs of dehydration

Patient Outcomes

Patient will

- have normal body temperature.
- report less fatigue, weakness, or malaise.
- have normal WBC count and cultures.
- be free of signs of inflammation in wounds and IV sites.
- have adequate hydration.

Nursing Interventions	Rationales
Monitor vital signs every 4 hr.	Early signs of infection include tachycardia, narrowed pulse pressure, tachypnea, and elevated temperature.
Monitor patient energy level.	Malaise, weakness, and fatigue may indicate early inflammation.
Monitor lab data: WBCs and blood cultures	Elevated WBC count with a shift to the left may indicate early infection. Blood cultures will eventually isolate the organism. Chronically abnormal laboratory values may indicate persistent infection and require reevaluation of antibiotic therapy.
Monitor intake and output every 8 hr. Encourage fluids.	
Maintain aseptic technique during access device insertion and/or maintenance: 1. Assess sites daily for signs of infection. 2. Protect sites from contamination from other body dramage. 3. Report early signs of infection.	Antibiotic therapy may place any IV access site at risk for inflammation and infection. During the course of treatment the patient should be protected from any additional organisms that may cause a recurrence of the infection.
Administer antibiotic and antipyretic therapy as prescribed.	

▼

NURSING DIAGNOSIS: HIGH RISK FOR ALTERED TISSUE INTEGRITY

Risk Factors

- Valvular heart disease
- Systemic embolization to brain, kidney, and GI system
- Pulmonary embolization (with right-sided endocarditis)

Patient Outcomes

Patient will

- demonstrate normal neurological function.
- not have petechiae of conjunctive, mucosa, or extremities.
- have normal renal, lung, and GI function.
- not have other signs of peripheral embolization: Osler's nodes, Roth's spots.

Nursing Interventions	Rationales
Assess neurological system once per shift and as needed. Obtain baseline information on patient's mentation, behavior, response to environment, and motor and sensory function.	Deviations may suggest cerebral embolization. The incidence of cerebral emboli is 6–31%
Assess pulmonary status for signs of sudden chest pain, dyspnea, and tachypnea.	The potential for valvular embolization to peripheral arteries as well as venous status from immobilization may predispose patient to deep-vein thrombosis and, consequently, pulmonary embolization. Additionally, right-side endocarditis may cause embolization directly to the lungs.
Assess extremities for signs of embolization to include Osler's nodes and Roth's spots.	
Assess renal status for signs of hematuria, oliguria, and flank pain. Monitor laboratory data.	Embolization to kidneys may compromise normal renal function.
Assess GI status for complaints of abdominal pain, tenderness, or rigidity.	May indicate embolization to abdominal organs such as the spleen.

Nursing Interventions	Rationales
Report any changes to physician.	
Promote rest with active/passive range-of-motion exercises and antiembolism stockings as indicated.	Patient activity level must be limited to conserve energy and promote recovery. However, bedrest may contribute to venous stasis and circulatory compromise. Range-of-motion exercises will promote venous return. Antiembolism stockings may assist with venous return and are most effective when combined with activity.
Administer anticoagulants as prescribed.	May be used prophylactically.

▼

NURSING DIAGNOSIS: ALTERED NUTRITION—LESS THAN BODY REQUIREMENTS

Related To infection and increased metabolic rate

Defining Characteristics

Weight loss of 10% of body weight
Serum albumin <3.5 g/100 mL
Negative nitrogen balance
Total lymphocyte count <1500
Fatigue: lack of energy
Caloric intake less than requirements

Patient Outcomes

- Patient weight loss will stabilize, with gradual weight gain.
- Patient serum albumin will be greater than 3.5 g/dL.
- Patient total lymphocyte count will be greater than 1500.
- Patient will demonstrate positive nitrogen balance.
- Patient will have increased energy and endurance.
- Patient will demonstrate intake equal to caloric requirements.

Nursing Interventions	Rationales
Assess for signs of nutritional deficit.	Poor nutrition will exacerbate any infectious process and retard the healing process. Early attention will promote recovery.

Nursing Interventions	Rationales
Monitor laboratory data: 1. serum protein or transferrin 2. urinary urea nitrogen 3. total lymphocytes	Among the components of nutritional assessment is the evaluation of protein status. The breakdown of protein can be estimated by the renal excretion of urea nitrogen. Nitrogen balance is estimated by substracting excretion from intake. When intake exceeds output, a positive nitrogen balance exists. When output exceeds intake, a negative nitrogen balance exists. Serum albumin or transferrin reflect changes in amino acid availability. Malnourishment affects our immune system. Monitoring lymphocytes is one measurement of nutritional state.
Weigh daily.	Loss of lean body mass may be assessed by monitoring daily weights. Effective nutritional therapy can also be monitored by daily weight comparisons.
Monitor nutritional intake. 1. Provide high-calorie, high-protein foods. 2. Monitor calorie counts daily.	To provide adequate nutrients for anabolism.
Monitor environment to ensure adequate rest.	To decrease metabolic demands and nutritional needs.

▼

NURSING DIAGNOSIS: HIGH RISK FOR DECREASED CARDIAC OUTPUT

Risk Factors

- Impaired valvular function
- Left ventricular failure

Patient Outcomes

- Patient will demonstrate no new murmurs.
- Patient's lungs will be clear.
- Patient will demonstrate vital signs within normal limits.
- Patient will not have peripheral edema.

Nursing Interventions	Rationales
Assess patient baseline symptomatology to include	Compensatory sympathetic stimulation causes tachycardia, vasoconstriction, and fluid retention.
1. pulse: rate, rhythm	Atrial dysrhythmias [premature atrial contractions, atrial fibrillation (PACs, A. Fib.)] occur as fluid overload from failing ventricle causes atrial irritability. Ventricular dysrhythmias occur due to ischemia, hypoxia, electrolyte imbalance, and acid-base disturbances.
2. blood pressure	
3. peripheral circulation	
4. mentation	Mentation changes occur with changes in cerebral perfusion, hypoxia, hypercarbia, acidosis, and fluid and electrolyte imbalances.
5. heart sounds	An S_3, indicative of an exacerbation of failure, occurs as a result of atrial contradiction against a noncompliant left or right ventricle. Murmurs may be audible as valvular dysfunction accompanies ventricular failure.
6. urine output	Kidney response to decreased perfusion from vasoconstriction is to release renin, which in turn activates an enzyme, angiotensin I, which activates angiotensin II, which is a potent vasoconstrictor and also produces aldosterone. Aldosterone causes kidney reabsorption of sodium, thus creating a concentrated urine.
Institute measures to decrease myocardial oxygen demand:	An important therapeutic goal is to decrease preload, thus optimizing myocardial stretch.

Nursing Interventions	Rationales
1. Keep head of bed elevated.	Head elevation decreases venous return, or preload, thus decreasing myocardial oxygen demand. Ventilation will also be facilitated.
2. Monitor fluid status.	Fluids must be monitored to prevent overload.
3. Provide environmental control (visitors, rest, diagnostic scheduling, etc.). 4. Provide emotional rest. 5. Assist with physical care as necessary.	A variety of physical as well as psychosocial variables may increase the work of the heart.Fear, anxiety, stress, lack of sleep, etc., must be minimized. Reducing anxiety and other stress responses will limit catecholamine release.
Assess response to activity, noting complaints of fatigue and dyspnea.	Blood pressure, heart rate, rhythm, and respiratory changes may occur as untoward effects of activity in patients with compromised contractility.
Plan activity that allows for optimal rest and gradual resumption of activities of daily living (ADLs).	Bedrest is imperative to promote healing and conserve energy, but guided activity is necessary to avoid the complications of bedrest and slowly return patient to normal health.
Administer oxygen as needed. Administer medications as prescribed:	
1. preload reducing agents • diuretics • nitrates • morphine sulfate	Reducing preload assists in relieving the congestive symptoms of heart failure. Nitrates are effective venous vasodilators which assist in pooling venous blood. Morphine will not only cause venous vasodilation therapy, decreasing preload, but will also decrease myocardial oxygen demand by relieving anxiety.

Nursing Interventions	Rationales
2. afterload reducing agents • vasodilators • angiotension converting enzyme (ACE) inhibitors	Afterload is a major contributor to myocardial workload. By reducing systemic vascular resistance, afterload is reduced and contractility enhanced. The ACE inhibitors block the action of angiotensin II, which will promote vasodilation and decrease afterload.
3. inotropc agents • digoxin	
Monitor electrolytes and supplement as necessary. Include sodium, potassium, calcium, and magnesium.	Inadequate nutrition, fluid shifts, vomiting, diarrhea, and use of diuretics may alter electrolytes that affect cardiac contractility and electrical conduction.
Monitor organ function through laboratory studies and clinical assessment: 1. BUN, creatinine (renal function) 2. serum glutamic oxaloacetic transaminase (SGOT), lactic dehydrogenase (LDH) (liver function)	Compensatory vasoconstriction eventually takes its toll on organ perfusion. As kidneys deal with hypoperfusion, prerenal causes of acute renal failure ensue. Systemic elevation in pressure overloads the liver, spleen, and mesenteric systems. Medical therapy must often be adjusted as organ failure becomes evident.

▼

NURSING DIAGNOSIS: KNOWLEDGE DEFICIT—ENDOCARDITIS AND TREATMENT PLAN

Related To

- New diagnosis
- Lack of information
- Misinformation

Defining Characteristics

Asks questions related to diagnosis
Unaware of symptoms to report or prophylactic measures
Lack of participation in measures that would improve outcomes
Unaware of purpose or importance of medications

Patient Outcomes

Patient will

- verbalize knowledge and treatment of disease process.
- verbalize importance of avoidance of precipitating factors and prophylactic measures.
- state signs/symptoms to report.
- verbalize understanding of medications.
- obtain Medic-Alert bracelet.

Nursing Interventions	Rationales
Explain the basic disease process and treatment objectives.	Understanding the relationship between endocarditis and normal heart function is important for understanding the treatment plan and prophylactic measures.
Explain factors that may precipitate recurrent infection to include: 1. infectious situations (colds, flu, etc.) 2. poor oral care 3. dental work (cleaning, extractions) 4. surgical procedures 5. invasive diagnostic procedures	Once damaged, the endocardium remains susceptible to recurrent injury. Awareness of precipitating factors is necessary to alert the health care professional to the need for prophylactic antibiotics. Oral penicillin is indicated for most patients. Intravenous therapy may be warranted for high-risk groups (valve replacements). Vancomycin or erythromycin may be used for those allergic to penicillin.
Explain importance of alerting physicians and dentists of history of endocarditis prior to any procedures.	
Teach patient signs/symptoms of recurrent inflammation and when to notify the physician.	To allow for prompt antibiotic therapy.
Explain the purpose of a Medic-Alert bracelet and assist in completing application form.	The Medic-Alert bracelet will allow any health care professional to recognize patients' history of endocarditis and take appropriate actions.
Explain the basic purpose, action, and precautions of all discharge medications. Provide written information as available.	Patient must understand the need for completion of all antibiotic therapy, regardless of absence of symptoms.

DISCHARGE PLANNING/CONTINUITY OF CARE

- Assure understanding of self-management plan, including avoidance of risk factors for infections, symptoms to report, attainment of Medic-Alert bracelet, and completion of all antibiotics
- Refer to a home health agency if needed for monitoring treatment effectiveness and further education
- Arrange for follow-up with physician for continued management
- Assist in filling prescriptions, devising medication schedule, and establishing a system for refilling prescriptions.

REFERENCES

Canabbio, M. (1990). *Cardiovascular disorders.* St. Louis, MO: Mosby Co.

Guzzetta, C. & Dossey, B. (1992). *Cardiovascular nursing.*, St. Louis, MO: Mosby Year Book.

Thelan, L., Davie, J., & Urden, L. (1990) *Textbook of critical care nursing.* St. Louis, MO: Mosby.

Hypertension

Linda A. Briggs, RN, MS, CCRN

Hypertension, defined as a blood pressure greater than 160/95 mmHg, is a major cause of cerebrovascular accidents, cardiac disease, and renal failure. Those with blood pressures between 140/90 and 160/95 are considered borderline hypertensive. Hypertension is classified as primary(essential) (90% of all cases), secondary (occurring as a consequence of another identifiable pathological condition), or malignant (a diastolic blood pressure greater than 120 mmHg). The maintenance of normal blood pressure is accomplished through complex interactions that involve factors affecting peripheral vascular resistance (cardiac output, heart rate, blood volume, vasomotor tone) baroreceptor response and sympathetic reflex, and renal production of renin, an enzyme that leads to the activation of angiotensin II, a potent vasoconstrictor and aldosterone stimulant.

ETIOLOGIES

Primary hypertension

Cause is unknown; cardiac risk factors may stimulate the disease process:

- family history
- age
- race
- obesity
- cigarette smoking
- stress
- high-sodium and high-saturated-fat diet

Secondary hypertension

- Renal impairment (infections, tumors, transplant, atherosclerosis, diabetes, embolism)
- Metabolic disorders (pheochromocytoma, aldosteronism, myedema, hypercalcemia, oral contraceptives)
- Central nervous system disorders (tumors, increased intracranial pressure, neurogenic, psychogenic)

CLINICAL MANIFESTATIONS

- Borderline hypertensive: 140/90–160/95; may be asymptomatic
- Moderate hypertensive
- Cardiac
  - blood pressure ≥ 160/95 lying, sitting, and standing and bilateral assessments made over at least two visits may have postural hypotension related to medical regime
  - tachycardia: bounding central pulses, diminished distal pulses
  - angina
  - dysrhythmias
  - heart sounds: accentuated S_2, S_4 (due to ventricular hypertrophy), systolic or diastolic murmurs, S_3 [early congestive heart failure (CHF)]
  - peripheral vascular vasoconstriction: skin cool, pale, discolored; delayed capillary refill; cyanosis
- Central nervous system
  - dizziness, syncope
  - headaches
  - visual disturbances
  - numbness/weakness episodes
  - epistaxis
  - mental status changes
  - optic fundi: retinal changes range from minimal arterial narrowing to spasms, tortuosity, hemorrhages, and edema
- Respiratory
  - dyspnea
  - signs/symptoms of respiratory distress

CLINICAL/DIAGNOSTIC FINDINGS

- Electrocardiogram (ECG): evidence of left ventricular hypertrophy and ischemia
- Chest x-ray (CXR): enlarged heart, aortic atherosclerosis
- Laboratory
  - urine: proteinura, hematuria
  - blood: elevated blood urea nitrogen (BUN), and creatinine, elevated potassium if renal failure, decreased potassium on diuretic therapy, elevated cholesterol and lipid levels if hyperlipidemic

▼

NURSING DIAGNOSIS: HIGH RISK FOR DECREASED CARDIAC OUTPUT

Risk Factors

- Increased afterload
- Ventricular hypertrophy
- Myocardial ischemia

Patient Outcomes

Patient will

- have blood pressure within acceptable limits.
- have heart rate within acceptable limits.
- have no dysrhythmias.
- follow medical regimen to reduce blood pressure.
- have adequate peripheral perfusion.
- have no pulmonary congestion.

Nursing Interventions	Rationales
Monitor blood pressure. Observe systolic and diastolic values.	Blood pressure should initially be assessed bilaterally for comparison. Thereafter, assess blood pressure in same arm. Systolic elevations increase risk of cerebrovascular compromise. Diastolic elevation increases cardiac workload and ischemic complications.
Monitor for signs and symptoms of increased peripheral vascular resistance to include 1. diminished peripheral pulses 2. pale, cool, moist skin 3. delayed capillary refill 4. tachycardia 5. decreased urine output	Elevated peripheral vascular resistance causes vasoconstrictive complications, resulting in decreased perfusion to the skin and kidney.

Nursing Interventions	Rationales
Auscultate heart and lungs for abnormal sounds: S_3, S_4, murmurs, crackles, and wheezes.	Hypertension creates an increase in afterload for the left side of the heart. To compensate, atrial and ventricular hypertropy occur. An S_4 is indicative of atrial filling against a noncompliant left ventricle. An S_3 may become audible as the left ventricle continues to fail and atrial contraction occurs into a noncompliant left ventricle. Increased afterload further causes valvular dysfunction and impaired capillary muscle function. Eventually, the left ventricle becomes dysfunctional, creating a backward pressure elevation, causing pulmonary interstitial fluid accumulation.
Assist patient in adhering to activity restrictions: bed/chair rest, assistance with activities of daily living (ADLs), rest periods, and so on.	To conserve energy and decrease oxygen demand.
Assist patient in modifying his or her environment as appropriate: limitation of visitors, calm surroundings, and relaxation techniques.	Stress and anxiety increase catecholamine release and may exacerbate hypertension.
Monitor intake and output. Report output less than 30 mL/hr.	Fluids need to be carefully monitored to avoid further overload. Restrict as ordered. Output monitoring is important to assess renal function.
Monitor electrolytes, BUN, and creatinine.	To continue to assess renal function.
Assist patient in adhering to all components of medical plan of care. (See Knowledge Deficit.)	
Administer antihypertensive agents as prescribed and monitor effects.	

Nursing Interventions	Rationales
1. diuretics • thiazides: chlorothiazide, hydrochlorothiazide, bendroflumethiazide	These commonly used diuretics decrease vascular volume and decrease peripheral vascular resistance.
• loop diuretics: furosemide, ethacrynic acid, bumetanide	Producing marked diuresis, these potent diuretics reduce fluid retention by promoting sodium excretion via renal tubules.
• potassium-sparing diuretics: spironolactone, triamterene, amiloride	Given to minimize potassium loss.
2. beta blockers: • nonselective: propranolol, nadolol, pindolol • selective: metoprolol, acebutolol, atenolol	While individual beta blockers have specific actions, overall they reduce blood pressure by inhibiting sympathetic outflow and suppressing renin release from the kidney. Selective blockers primarily block $beta_1$ receptors on the heart to decrease heart rate and contractility. Nonselective blockers additionally block $beta_2$ receptors on bronchi and peripheral blood vessels.
3. vasodilators • minoxidil • hydralazine	Vasodilatation decreases peripheral vascular resistance, thus decreasing afterload.
4. alpha-adrenergic blockers: • prazosin • terazosin	Decrease peripheral vascular resistance.
5. centrally acting alpha inhibitors • clonidine • guanabenz • methyldopa	Block sympathetic outflow from the brain.
6. peripheral adrenergic inhibitors • reserpine	
7. angiotensin converting enzyme inhibitors • captopril • enalapril • lisinopril	Block the conversion of angiotensin I to angiotensin II, thus minimizing the effects of this potent vasoconstrictor.

Nursing Interventions	Rationales
8. calcium antagonists • nicardipine • nifedipine • diltiazem • verapamil	Coronary and peripheral vasodilatation negative inotrope.

▼

NURSING DIAGNOSIS: PAIN (HEADACHE)

Related To increased intracranial pressure

Defining Characteristics

Suboccipital throbbing headache, more apparent upon awakening
Dizziness, blurred vision, nausea, vomiting

Patient Outcomes

Patient will

- report discomfort is relieved/controlled.
- deny dizziness, blurred vision, nausea, and vomiting.

Nursing Interventions	Rationales
Assess characteristics of pain to include associated symptoms	
Initiate immediate measures to relieve headache. Limit all activities that may further increase intracranial pressure: 1. Maintain quiet, darkened environment. 2. Maintain bedrest; change positions. 3. Monitor environment: limit visitors; decrease noise. 4. Utilize relaxation and imagery techniques; neck and back massage. 5. Eliminate other activities that promote vasoconstriction: coughing, Valsalva maneuvers, and bending over.	Decreasing stress and anxiety limits catecholamine release and thus sympathetic vasoconstriction.

Nursing Interventions	Rationales
Ensure patient's safety: 1. Assist with ambulation as necessary. 2. Monitor for postural hypotension.	Dizziness, blurred vision, and postural blood pressure changes that may accompany headache may cause patient to be unsteady with ambulation.
Administer pain-relieving medications as indicated: 1. analgesics 2. tranquilizers	

▼

NURSING DIAGNOSIS: ACTIVITY INTOLERANCE

Related To

- Decreased cardiac output
- Weakness.

Defining Characteristics

Heart rate response to activity of greater than 30 bpm over baseline
Heart rate response to activity of greater than 15 bpm over baseline for patient on beta blockers or calcium channel blockers
Weakness
Fatigue
Dyspnea
Ischemic pain
ECG changes (if monitored): ST-, T-wave changes

Patient Outcomes

Patient will

- be able to participate in ADLs.
- increase level of activity without symptoms.
- demonstrate vital signs within acceptable limits during activity: heart rate elevations greater than 30 bpm above baseline.
- demonstrate heart rate return to normal 5 min after activity

Nursing Interventions	Rationales
Assess patient's response to activity: 1. dyspnea 2. fatigue 3. tachycardia 4. chest pain	Activity may increase oxygen demand for an already stressed myocardium. Heart rate increases to compensate, thus creating fatigue, dyspnea, and vital sign changes. Symptoms will limit patient's activity level.

Nursing Interventions	Rationales
Assess vital signs before and after activity.	
Assess and evaluate medication regimen with physician.	Medications such as diuretics, vasodilators, beta blockers, and calcium antagonists may cause vital sign changes especially evident during exercise.
Assess changes in patient activity level.	Decreased activity and fatigue contribute to muscular atrophy and weakness. Muscle strengthening can increase endurance and quality of life.
Consult occupational/physical therapy as necessary for muscle-strengthening exercises, strategies for energy conservation, and exercise guidelines.	

▼

NURSING DIAGNOSIS: KNOWLEDGE DEFICIT—TREATMENT PLAN, SELF-MONITORING AND LIFESTYLE CHANGES

Related To

- New diagnosis
- Lack of exposure to information

Defining Characteristics

Unwilling to express feelings
Angry, irritable
Unwilling to discuss lifestyle modifications
Unwilling to participate in self-monitoring techniques
Lack of knowledge regarding medications

Patient Outcomes

Patient will

- express feelings related to chronic illness.
- discuss participation in lifestyle changes.
- discuss appropriate exercise routine.
- demonstrate self-monitoring techniques.
- state basic medication information and related side effects.

Nursing Interventions	Rationales
Assess patient current coping strategies and willingness to adhere to prescribed treatments and lifestyle changes. Encourage expression of feeling regarding diagnosis.	Dealing with chronic illness is individual and unique. Allowing the patient time to adapt to the impact of the disease will promote trust and eventual readiness to learn. Investigate potential coping mechanisms that may contribute to hypertension, for example, anger, inability to problem solve, and irritability.
Investigate other factors that may influence patient ability to learn and comply with treatment recommendations, for example, finances, age, culture, occupation, and misconceptions. Make referrals as indicated.	Concern over the impact of the disease may take precedence over the need to learn. Assist patient as appropriate in working through other issues.
Devise a teaching plan that includes definition of hypertension and potential complications.	
Identify risk factors:	
1. obesity	Obesity increases myocardial workload.
2. diet high in sodium and saturated fats	Sodium intake is one of the most significant modifiable risk factors. Consistent sodium restriction may result in decreased need for medications. Saturated fats contribute to atherosclerotic process.
3. smoking	
4. lack of activity	Nicotine increases catecholamine release, promoting vasoconstriction and hypoxia.
5. stress	
Assist patient in selecting risk factors that he or she is willing to begin to modify.	

Nursing Interventions	Rationales
Explain dietary restrictions to include sodium, unsaturated fats, cholesterol, calories, caffeine, and alcohol. Initiate dietary referral as needed.	Research shows that even modest reductions in both table salt and salt in preservatives can lower blood pressure. Excess saturated fats, cholesterol, alcohol, and calories are nutritional risks for hypertension.
Explain relationship between exercise and blood pressure control. Refer for exercise counseling.	Studies show that weight loss results in lowered blood pressure. Aerobic exercise programs improve cardiovascular efficiency and can lower systolic and diastolic blood pressure by 10 mmHg. Avoid isometric exercises which can increase catecholamine levels.
Explain role of stress in hypertension. Explore areas of life stress with patient. Suggest relaxation therapy.	Relaxation therapy has been found to be successful in blood pressure reduction. Techniques include imagery, breathing exercises, muscle relaxation, and biofeedback.
Instruct in self-monitoring techniques to include blood pressure measurements, pulse taking, daily weights, and symptoms to report: 1. sudden increase in blood pressure 2. chest pain 3. visual disturbance 4. sudden weight gain 5. frequent nose bleeds	Teaching self-monitoring techniques increases patient reinforcement and compliance and aids in evaluating therapy. Complications of the disease or medication side effects must be detected and reported early to prevent progression.
Obtain previous medication history.	
Explain antihypertensive therapy: 1. name 2. dose 3. purpose	Adequate knowledge of medication aids in compliance and early reporting of disturbing and harmful side effects.

Nursing Interventions	Rationales
Encourage exploration of undesirable medication side effects and influence on quality of life.	Any antihypertensive agent may produce unwanted side effects. As multiple-drug therapy is initiated, the risk for side effects increases. Medications can be changed or dose regulated to avoid side effects. Drugs that cause a disturbance in patient's sex life, activity or work should be avoided.
Encourage patient to consult pharmacist regarding interactions and over the counter drugs to avoid, including 1. cold and allergy drugs 2. nonsteroidal anti-inflammatory agents 3. appetite suppressants 4. laxatives and antacids 5. cimetidine	Various cold and allergy products may inhibit response to antihypertensives. Nonsteroidal anti-inflammatory drugs and appetite suppressants inhibit hypotensive actions. Various laxatives and antacids are high in sodium. Cimetidine potentiates the actions of some beta blockers and calcium antagonists.
Explain the need for close follow-up with physician or clinic.	

▼

DISCHARGE PLANNING/CONTINUITY OF CARE

- Assure understanding of self-management plan, including blood pressure measurements, pulse taking, risk factor modification, dietary restrictions, exercise program, symptoms to report, and medications.
- Refer to a home health agency for education or monitoring of blood pressure if needed.
- Arrange follow-up with physician for continued management.
- Assist in obtaining prescriptions, devising a medication schedule, and establishing a plan for refilling prescriptions.
- Provide patient/family with information on stop-smoking programs, exercise programs, hypertension clinics, and other available education.
- Refer to a local chapter of the American Heart Association for further information.

REFERENCES

Blake, G. H. & Beebe, D. (1991). Management of hypertension: Useful nonpharmacologic measures. *Postgraduate Medicine, 90*(1), 151–154.

Deglin, J. & Deglin, S. (1992). Hypertension: Current trends and choices in pharmacotherapeutics. *AACN Clinical Issues, 3*(2), 507–525.

Guzzetta, C. & Dossey, B. (1992). *Cardiovascular nursing*. St. Louis, MO: Mosby Year Book.

Hockenberry, B. (1991) Multiple drug therapy in the treatment of essential hypertension. *Nursing Clinics of North America, 26*(2), 417–435.

▼

MYOCARDIAL INFARCTION

Linda A. Briggs, RN, MS, CCRN

Myocardial ischemia results when myocardial oxygen demand exceeds related coronary artery blood flow. When this ischemia is severe enough to cause irreversible cellular death, a myocardial infarction (MI) results. The wavefront of cellular death begins in the subendocardium and moves slowly to the epicardium, a process taking approximately 3–6 hr. This wavefront process creates the window of opportunity for optimal intervention. Although much progress has been made in the treatment of this disorder, there are currently over a half million deaths per year with approximately 30% of those prior to hospitalization. And despite significant advances in the treatment and prevention of MI, there remains a great deal to be learned. While most infarctions occur in the left ventricle, it is important to appreciate that approximately 25–46% of all inferior wall MIs have concomitant right ventricular involvement. Myocardial infarctions are classified according to the presence or absence of Q waves on the electrocardiogram (ECG) (Table 13.1) as well as the location on the ventricular myocardium (Table 13.2).

ETIOLOGIES

- Atherosclerosis: coronary artery narrowing and reduced blood flow to myocardium
- Thrombosis (80–90% of all cases)
- Plaque hemorrhage
- Coronary artery spasm

CLINICAL MANIFESTATIONS

- Chest pain/discomfort: prolonged, severe
- Anxiety, restlessness, agitation
- Tachycardia
- Tachypnea

- Nausea, vomiting, diaphoresis
- Normal or hypotensive
- Heart sounds: S_3 or S_4
- With left ventricular dysfunction: signs of decreased cardiac output

Table 13.1 • Classification of Myocardial Infarctions

	Q-Wave Infarct	Non-Q-Wave Infarct
Thrombus	Occlusive	Nonocclusive
Size of infarct	Large, usually transmural	Smaller, often nontransmural
Reinfarction	5–10%	10–30%
Postinfarct angina	10–20%	50%
CK-MB peak activity	Frequently high	Usually lower

Table 13.2 • Anatomic Location of Myocardial Infarctions

Type of MI	Coronary Artery Affected	Leads Showing ECG Changes of MI
Anterior left ventricle	Left anterior descending (LAD)	V_1–V_6
Anteroseptal left ventricle	Usually LAD	V_1–V_3
Inferior left ventricle	Right coronary artery	II, III, AVF
Lateral left ventricle	Circumflex	I, AVL
Posterior left ventricle	Usually RCA (circumflex in 10%)	Reciprocal changes: V_1, V_2
Right ventricular	Right coronary artery (RCA)	V_4R, V_5R, V_6R

CLINICAL/DIAGNOSTIC FINDINGS

ECG

- Acute process: (occur in leads that face the area of damage)
  - ST-segment elevation with peaked T waves
  - Q waves (>0.03 s in duration) if transmural damage exists
- Evolutionary
  - ST segments return to baseline (usually within 2–3 days)
  - T-wave inversion
  - Q waves persist

- Reciprocal changes
  - Seen in leads that are opposite the area of damage, to include ST-segment depression, tall T wave, and tall R wave. Presence usually indicates increased severity of infarction process.

Laboratory
- Enzymes: With cell damage, enzymes are released into the circulation:

	Onset	Peak	Return
CPK/CKMB isoenzyme	4–12 hr	24 hr	3–4 days
LDH/LDH isoenzyme	24–48 hr	3–6 days	7–14 days

Note: CPK = creatinine phosphokinase, CKMB = creatine kinase myocardial band, LDH = lactic dehydrogenase.

- Complete blood count (CBC): elevated white blood cell (WBC) count and sedimentation rate
- Thallium scintigraphy: shows decreased blood flow, areas of decreased uptake, or "cold spots" are visualized (may be used to confirm diagnosis)
- Technetium-99m imaging: permits localization and estimation of size of MI if performed within 2–6 days of the event

OTHER PLANS OF CARE TO REFERENCE

Pericarditis

▼

NURSING DIAGNOSIS: PAIN

Related To myocardial ischemia

Defining Characteristics

Severe substernal chest pain or discomfort
Radiation to arms, back, and jaw
Anxiety, diaphoresis, and nausea

Patient Outcomes

Patient will
- report pain or discomfort appropriately.
- will verbalize relief of pain or discomfort.
- will verbalize own unique pain characteristics.
- Patient ECG will remain normal or return to normal.
- Patient will exhibit less anxiety.

Nursing Interventions	Rationales
Assess patient pain characteristics and precipitating factors thoroughly, including location, radiation, intensity, duration, and aggravating or alleviating factors. Associated symptoms: nausea, fatigue, shortness of breath, diaphoresis, and so on.	Pain related to MI is prolonged (>30 min) and severe. Often described as a discomfort rather than pain, it is located substernally, and may radiate to back, jaw, and arms. Sensations the patient may describe include heaviness, squeezing, or crushing. It is unrelieved by rest, position changes, or sublingual nitroglycerin. It may be precipitated by activity or stress, or occur without obvious cause. The reoccurrence of chest discomfort indicates myocardial ischemia and requires immediate intervention. The MI may extend anytime throughout the hospital course. A thorough investigation of the recurrent chest discomfort may assist in the identification of other causes to include postmyocardial pericarditis.
Utilize pain scale (0–10) for pain intensity as appropriate. If 0 is no pain at all, and 10 is the worst pain imaginable.	Pain intensity scale is useful to objectify discomfort, assess effectiveness of pain-relieving measures, and provide patient awareness and education. Patients need to be reminded there is no RIGHT answer.
Assist in recognition of own unique symptoms of chest discomfort and importance of prompt reporting.	Helping the patient verbalize and acknowledge own symptoms aids in early recognition and begins the educational process.
Obtain baseline hemodynamic status, including 1. blood pressure 2. heart rate 3. level of consciousness	
Obtain order for 12-lead ECG	To document associated changes in all leads.

Nursing Interventions	Rationales
For monitored patients: Monitor ECG for rate, rhythm, and ST changes. Monitor in leads that correspond with known patient pathology: leads II, III, and AFV to monitor the inferior left ventricle, V_1–V_4 the anteroseptal left ventricle, V_5–V_6 the anterolateral left ventricle, and I and AVL the lateral left ventricle.	The ECG changes may accompany angina to include ST-segment elevation or depression, T-wave changes, or pathological Q waves. These changes will only be evident in leads that face the area of damage or coronary artery involved.
Modify environment, as appropriate, to decrease myocardial oxygen demand, for example, restrict activity, encourage bedrest, decrease stimulation, control traffic, elevate head of bed.	
Stay with patient. Offer calm, reassuring explanations of interventions and their effectiveness.	Anxiety and fear may cause further oxygen demands by increasing catecholamine release and increasing or prolonging ischemic pain.
Administer the following as prescribed to include	
1. oxygen	Oxygen availability may increase myocardial uptake, especially in patients who are hypoxemic.
2. nitrates	Nitrates reduce myocardial oxygen demand by decreasing preload and increase myocardial oxygen supply by coronary vasodilatation and relief of coronary spasm. Intravenous nitroglycerin has been shown to decrease mortality by 35% in patients with evolving MI.
3. morphine	Morphine sulfate intravenously decreases pain, provides sedation, and decreases myocardial oxygen demand for decreasing preload and afterload.

Nursing Interventions	Rationales
4. calcium antagonists 5. diltiazem	Although the efficacy of calcium antagonists for all MI patients is controversial, diltiazem is indicated for non–Q wave infarctions, due to its ability to reduce postinfarction angina and reinfarction in these patients.
6. beta blockers: timolol, propranolol, metoprolol	Intravenous beta blockers may be given within the first 4 hr of acute infarction to limit myocardial damage and mortality. Oral beta blockers are indicated for long-term therapy to decrease long-term mortality.
7. anticoagulants: heparin, warfarin	Mortality and recurrent MI are reduced if patients are given intravenous or high-dose subcutaneous heparin. Other goals of therapy include prevention of venous thrombosis and ventricular thrombi. Warfarin for months post-MI is indicated for patients with evidence of mural thrombi.
8. antiplatelets: aspirin	Daily aspirin has been shown to decrease mortality and recurrent infarction.
9. thrombolytics	Thrombolytic agents are indicated for patients with confirmed MI to assist with clot dissolution. Therapy is most effective when given within 3–6 hr of symptom onset. Patient will need to be transferred to the intensive care unit.
Offer alternative pain-relieving measures: relaxation, deep breathing, imagery, and massage	Alternative measures may offer patient more control or distraction from pain. Muscular tension increases myocardial oxygen demands.
Assess and documents patient response to pain-relieving measures.	

NURSING DIAGNOSIS: HIGH RISK FOR DECREASED CARDIAC OUTPUT

Risk Factors

- Left ventricular failure
- Aneurysm formation
- Cardiac rupture
- Dysrhythmias
- Pericarditis

Patient Outcomes

Patient will

- have optimal ventricular function.
- not have dysrhythmias.
- show absence of signs of aneurysm formation, cardiac rupture, or pericarditis.

Nursing Interventions	Rationales
Assess and report signs of decreased cardiac output: 1. hypotension 2. tachycardia 3. fatigue 4. decreased urinary output 5. decreased mentation 6. abnormal heart sounds (S_3, S_4, murmurs) 7. posterior, bibasilar dependent crackles	A decrease in cardiac output may occur for a variety of reasons post-MI to include aneurysm formation, cardiac rupture, valvular dysfunction, dysrhythmias, and left ventricular failure.
Assess and report signs of pericarditis to include 1. chest pain that increases with inspiration 2. pericardial friction rub 3. fever	Inflammation of the pericardium may occur 3 days to 6 months post-MI, especially related to transmural infarctions. (See Pericarditis.)
Investigate assessment of irregular pulse: 1. Obtain order for 12-lead ECG. 2. Implement telemetry monitoring if available. 3. Investigate potential causes of dysrhythmias (e.g., hypoxia, electrolyte imbalance, ischemia).	Irregular pulse may indicate a variety of post-MI dysrhythmias to include supraventricular tachycardias, bradyarrhythmias, atrioventricular (AV) conduction disturbances, and ventricular dysrhythmias.

Nursing Interventions	Rationales
Monitor fluid and electrolyte status: 1. daily intake and output 2. daily weights 3. laboratory values 4. diuretic therapy	Fluid overload increases preload, thus increasing myocardial oxygen demand and compromising left ventricular function.
Restrict activity and progress ambulation as appropriate (see High Risk for Activity Intolerance).	
Monitor effects of drug combinations, for example, beta blockers, calcium antagonists, and class I antiarrhythmias.	The negative inotropic effects of drug combinations can lower cardiac output. Vasodilators may decrease coronary artery perfusion pressure and decrease myocardial blood flow.

▼

NURSING DIAGNOSIS: HIGH RISK FOR ACTIVITY INTOLERANCE

Risk Factors

- Myocardial dysfunction
- Pulmonary congestion

Patient Outcomes

- Patient will not experience weakness, fatigue, or dyspnea during activity.
- Patient will gradually increase activity without symptoms.
- Patient will engage in graded excercise program.
- Vital signs will be within acceptable limits during activity (heart rate elevations < 20 bpm above baseline).
- The ECG will be normal (if monitored).

Nursing Interventions	Rationales
Assess baseline response to activity to include 1. dyspnea 2. fatigue 3. tachycardia 4. chest pain 5. vital signs	Activity may increase oxygen demand at a time when the myocardium is unable to deliver. Heart rate increases to compensate, thus creating fatigue, dyspnea, and vital sign changes. Appearance of symptoms will limit patient's activity level.

Nursing Interventions	Rationales
Enlist in graded exercise program: 1. Consult occupational/physical therapy and cardiac rehabilitation program as appropriate. 2. Muscle-strengthening exercises may be needed to increase endurance and quality of activity.	Patient will need to increase activity gradually, learning to monitor signs of intolerance.
Instruct in passive range-of-motion exercises while in bed.	Joints can remain more flexible and muscles stretched.
Assess medication regime.	Medications such as diuretics, vasodilators, beta blockers, and calcium antagonists may cause vital sign changes especially evident during exercise.

▼

NURSING DIAGNOSIS: KNOWLEDGE DEFICIT—DIAGNOSIS AND TREATMENT

Related To
- Lack of previous experience
- Misinformation
- New diagnosis

Defining Characteristics
Asks questions
Requests information
Lack of compliance with treatment guidelines

Patient Outcomes
Patient will
- begin to demonstrate awareness of diagnosis.
- ask for clarification of information.
- follow treatment guidelines.
- begin to participate in educational plan.

Nursing Interventions	Rationales
Assess level of understanding of diagnosis and treatment plan once per shift: 1. "What has your physician told you?" 2. "What do you understand about why you're here?"	A patient/family educational program begins with the patient current level of understanding. With a new diagnosis, the patient needs clarification, repeated information, and correction of misinformation.
Devise a teaching plan based on patient readiness to learn, physical condition, and realistic outcomes.	A teaching plan should begin with what the patient wants to know and, because of shortened hospitalizations, should include at least basic survival information.
Develop and institute teaching program for patient and family to include: 1. basic disease process 2. risk factors 3. medications 4. dietary instructions 5. exercise guidelines 6. pulse taking 7. symptoms to report Consult cardiac rehabilitation program as appropriate.	Any educational program is multidisciplinary. The extent of any program will be affected by available resources, patient condition, length of hospitalization, and patient readiness.
Assess understanding of treatment plan and explain tests and procedures to be performed to include 1. daily ECGs 2. nuclear scans 3. cardiac catheterization 4. percutaneous transluminal coronary angioplasty 5. coronary artery bypass surgery	

▼

NURSING DIAGNOSIS: ANXIETY/DENIAL

Related To threat to biological, psychological, or social integrity

Defining Characteristics

Frequent expressions of concerns, fears
Difficulty sleeping
Verbalizes sense of impeding doom

Feels apprehensive
Muscular tension
Restless
Does not participate in treatment plan
Does not verbalize understanding of diagnosis

Patient Outcomes

Patient will

- appear relaxed, less tense.
- express positive plans for future.
- sleep regularly.
- verbalize reduction in apprehension.
- state some understanding of diagnosis.
- participate in treatment plan.
- practice relaxation techniques.

Nursing Interventions	Rationales
Provide a consistent nurse-patient relationship.	
Assess current level of perception regarding diagnosis and individual response.	A variety of psychological reactions to the diagnosis of MI is normal and expected. However, exaggerated or prolonged responses can influence cardiovascular stability and quality of life. Anxiety is a universal response to this life-threatening diagnosis, peaking on admission, on transfer from the critical care unit, on discharge from hospital, and during the first few weeks at home. Excessive anxiety and fear trigger the autonomic nervous system, increasing myocardial oxygen demand. Denial, another coping mechanism, may be adaptive, that is, helpful in assisting the patient with gradually accepting the diagnosis or maladaptive, creating lack of participation in treatment objectives.
Encourage expressions of feelings, concerns, and fears regarding diagnosis and future.	Creating an open environment for expression will promote trust and validation that feelings are important and normal.

Nursing Interventions	Rationales
Inform patient and family that a variety of reactions arc normal and may continue through the posthospitalization period.	
Provide clear explanations of routines and normal events.	
Provide reassurrance on patient's progress.	
Allow patient to deny certain aspects of disease he or she is yet unable to deal with.	
Instruct in relaxation strategies to include relaxation exercises, deep-breathing exercises, imagery, and music therapy.	
Allow input into daily schedule as appropriate.	To allow for control and increasing self-esteem.
Administer anxiolytic medications as prescribed. Assess and document patient response and need for medication.	Since anxiety is a frequent patient response, these medications are often prescribed. However, some patients feel more anxious or out of control on these medications.
Consult other professionals if appropriate.	

▼

DISCHARGE PLANNING/CONTINUITY OF CARE

- Assure understanding of self-management plan to include activity restrictions, excercise program, dietary limitations, risk factor modification, medications, and symptoms to report.
- Refer to a home health agency if patient is having any difficulty with treatment plan objectives.
- Arrange follow-up with physician for continued management postdischarge.
- Assist in obtaining prescriptions, devising a medication schedule, and establishing a plan for refilling prescriptions.
- Provide with information on local cardiac rehabilitation programs, support groups, stop-smoking programs, and other educational programs.

- Refer to a local chapter of the American Heart Association for further information.

REFERENCES

Guzzetta, C. & Dossey, B. (1992). *Cardiovascular nursing*. St. Louis, MO: Mosby Year Book.

Malan, S. (1992) Psychosocial adjustment following MI: Current views and nursing implications. *Journal of Cardiovascular Nursing, 6*(4), 57–70.

Rossi, L. & Leary, E. (1992). Evaluating the patient with coronary artery disease. *Nursing Clinics of North America, 27*(1), 171–186.

Stewart, S. L. (1992). Acute MI: A review of pathophysiology, treatment and complications. *Journal of Cardiovascular Nursing, 6*(4), 1–24.

Wingate, S. (1990). Post-MI patient's perceptions of their learning needs. *Dimensions of Critical Care Nursing, 9*(2), 112–118.

PERICARDITIS

Linda A. Briggs, RN, MS, CCRN

Pericarditis is an inflammation of the pericardium, the double-walled sac that surrounds the heart. The inner membrane, the visceral pericardium, surrounds the heart, whereas the outer membrane, the parietal pericardium, is adherent to the lung pleura. Normally, the pericardial sac contains 20–40 mL of serous fluid. With inflammation, friction between the two layers causes further irritation. Depending on the cause, this inflammation may cause exudation of fluid into the pericardial sac, causing pericardial effusion. Effusions that accumulate slowly allow for pericardial distention and accommodation of up to 1 L of fluid. Rapid accumulations, however, lead to cardiac tamponade with as little as 75 mL of effusion. There is a wide variety of clinical presentations, benign to life threatening. Acute pericarditis, with its concomitant pericardial effusions, may cause serious hemodynamic instability due to impaired diastolic ventricular filling and development of cardiac tamponade. Chronic pericarditis leads to not only chronic effusions but also development of scarring, adhesions, and constructive pathology. Acute pericarditis can occur within 2 weeks of exposure and lasts up to 6 weeks. Chronic pericarditis can follow acute exposures to infection and last up to 6 months or continue as a chronic situation secondary to other conditions.

ETIOLOGIES

- Viral
  - Mycoplasma pneumoniae
  - chickenpox
  - acquired immunodeficiency syndrome (AIDS)
- Infections
  - tuberculosis
  - bacterial
  - fungal (histoplasmosis, aspergillosis)

- Neoplasms
  - primary
  - secondary
- Connective tissue diseases
  - scleroderma
  - systemic lupus erythematosus
  - rheumatoid arthritis
- Uremia (chronic renal failure)
- Chemotherapy
- Postmyocardial infarction (Dressler's syndrome)
- Trauma
  - perforation of right ventricle via catheters, pacers, chest injuries
- Anticoagulants
  - heparin
  - warfarin
- Drugs
  - procainamide
  - dantrolene

CLINICAL MANIFESTATIONS

Acute pericarditis
- Substernal chest pain that increases with inspiration and movement and may be relieved by leaning forward
- Pericardial friction rub
- Tachycardia
- Dyspnea
- Hypotension and cardiovascular dysfunction (if significant pericardial effusion)
- Anxious, restless, frightened
- Low-grade fever, diaphoresis
- Pericardial friction rub (intermittent, loudest during inspiration and with patient leaning forward, varying intensity, may be triphasic)

Constrictive pericarditis
- Dyspnea on exertion
- Orthopnea
- Fatigue
- Jugular vein distention (JVD)
- Kussmaul's sign
- Pulsus paradoxus
- Afebrile
- Signs of elevated venous pressure: JVD, Kussmaul's sign, peripheral edema, hepatomegaly, ascites

CLINICAL/DIAGNOSTIC FINDINGS

- Laboratory
  - elevated white blood cell (WBC) count with shift to left (acute process only)

  - elevated sedimentation rate
  - elevated blood and urine cultures (depending on cause)
- Electrocardiogram (ECG)
  - widespread, diffuse ST-segment elevation
  - T-wave inversions
  - low voltage (with effusion)
  - atrial dysrhythmias
- Chest x-ray
  - enlarged cardiac borders (with significant effusions > 250 mL)
- Echocardiogram
  - verifies presence of pericardial fluid
  - evaluates ventricular performance

OTHER PLANS OF CARE TO REFERENCE

Corticosteroid therapy

▼

NURSING DIAGNOSIS: PAIN

Related To pericardial inflammation

Defining Characteristics

Chest pain that increases with inspiration and movement
Chest pain that may subside with position changes
Chest pain that may not be relieved with narcotics
Chest pain that may radiate

Patient Outcomes

Patient will

- verbalize relief from pain.
- move to positions of comfort.

Nursing Interventions	Rationales
Assess characteristics of chest pain: 1. quality 2. intensity 3. site, radiation 4. precipitating factors (inspiration, movement) 5. alleviating factors (leaning forward)	Clear descriptions of chest pain are helpful to assist in differentiation of other causes of chest discomfort, such as acute myocardial infarction, pulmonary embolism, pleurisy, dissecting aortic aneurysm, and pneumothorax. Pericardial pain may be described in a variety of ways: dull, aching, sharp, or burning. It may be intermittent or constant. Pericardial pain may radiate to left precordium, interscapula, and trapezius areas. This referred pain is produced by stimulation of the phrenic and the intercostal nerves, which both innervate the parietal pericardium. Certain activities that stimulate the pleura will cause increased discomfort, for example, coughing, deep inspiration, and swallowing.
Assist patient to assume positions of comfort such as sitting up and/or leaning forward.	Positional changes may move pericardium and relieve pain sensation temporarily.
Administer prescribed pain medication as indicated:	Typical narcotic medications are ineffective in relieving the pain of pericardial inflammation. Narcotics may dull the sensorium, but when awake, the pain level will be unaffected.
1. anti-inflammatory agents: indomethacin, ibuprofen	Nonsteroidal anti-inflammatory agents are effective in relieving the source of the discomfort. Administer with food or milk to minimize side effects. Indomethacin and ibuprofen may impair healing post–myocardial infarction and may be contraindicated in these situations.
2. analgesics: aspirin (high dose)	
3. corticosteroids	For more rapid relief of pain not relieved by usual methods.

Nursing Interventions	Rationales
4. specific agents to treat cause: chemotherapeutic agents, antituberculosis agents	If the cause of the pericarditis is identified, specific treatment to combat the disease is indicated.
Assess for pericardial friction rub.	As the pericardial layers become irritated, they rub together, causing a squeaking, grating sound audible with each cardiac cycle. This rub may be intermittent, varies with intensity, and often becomes audible after the appearance of pain. Friction rubs are usually loudest during inspiration, may disappear with accumulating effusions, and are best auscultated at the cardiac apex with the patient leaning forward.

▼

NURSING DIAGNOSIS: DECREASED CARDIAC OUTPUT

Related To

- Pericardial effusion
- Cardiac tamponade

Defining Characteristics

Hypotension
Pulse pressure < 20 mmHg
Dyspnea
Tachycardia
Pulsus paradoxus > 12 mmHg
Decreased heart sounds
Elevated central venous pressure (CVP)
Pericardial friction rub

Patient Outcomes

Patient will

- be normotensive.
- show absence of dyspnea, tachycardia, pericardial friction rub.
- have pulsus paradoxus < 10 mmHg.
- have normal CVP.

Nursing Interventions	Rationales
Assess for signs of cardiac tamponade:	If pericardial effusion develops slowly, the pericardial sac can accommodate large volumes of fluid (1–2 L) without cardiac compromise. If effusions develop rapidly, however, there is no compensation and even small amounts of fluid can increase pericardial pressure which interferes with cardiac filling. This leads to hypotension and decreased oxygen delivery.
1. dyspnea 2. decreased heart sounds 3. hypotension 4. tachycardia	Dyspnea may be related to lung compression by expanding pericardium, tachycardia, fever, or anxiety.
5. pulsus paradoxus > 12 mmHg	Pulsus paradoxus is an exaggerated decline in systolic blood pressure during inspiration (>12 mmHg).
6. increased CVP 7. distended neck veins 8. pericardial friction rub	Impedance to diastolic filling from elevated pericardial pressure causes elevated right atrial pressure and systemic venous congestion.
Intervene to reduce fear and anxiety in patient/family: 1. Explain all procedures and environment. 2. Keep patient informed of progress. 3. Inform patient of potential procedures. 4. Provide assurance of close monitoring. 5. Teach relaxation techniques.	Fear and anxiety are common reactions to this threat. Fear of the unknown, constant monitoring, and prolonged waiting contribute to patient and family concerns.

Nursing Interventions	Rationales
Prepare patient for pericardiocentesis if appropriate:	As fluid accumulates in the pericardial sac (pericardial effusion) and acute signs of cardiac tamponade occur, emergency treatment may be needed to remove the offending fluid as a life-saving maneuver. Pericardiocentesis may also be done to evaluate the fluid to determine etiology.
1. Prepare equipment.	
2. Administer fluids as prescribed.	In an emergency situation, fluids may be needed to increase venous return until the procedure can be accomplished.
3. Place patient in high-Fowler's position.	
4. Provide emotional support.	
Prepare patient for pericardiectomy, in case of constrictive pericarditis.	One of the treatments for constrictive pericarditis is the removal of the visceral and parietal pericardium, a procedure that has excellent long-term results. This is a thoracic surgical procedure with the associated surgical preparation required.
Prepare the patient for pericardial window procedure.	Another surgical procedure for recurrent, chronic pericardial effusions. By incising the pericardium, drainage of the pericardial fluid is allowed. Pericardial tissue can also be obtained for culture and clots or fibrin deposits can be removed.

▼

NURSING DIAGNOSIS: KNOWLEDGE DEFICIT—DIAGNOSIS

Related To

- Lack of information
- Misinformation

Defining Characteristics

Asks questions related to diagnosis
Unaware of symptoms to report or prophylactic measures
Unaware of purpose of medications

Patient Outcomes

Patient will

- verbalize knowledge of pericarditis and prophylactic care.
- verbalize signs/symptoms to report.
- verbalize understanding of medications.
- obtain Medic-Alert bracelet, if appropriate.

Nursing Interventions	Rationales
Explain briefly the pathophysiology of pericarditis and associated etiology.	Understanding the anatomic and physiological relationship of the pericardium to normal heart function may increase understanding of limitations, medications, and precautions. Once known, the cause of pericarditis will influence long-term restrictions.
Teach signs/symptoms of recurrent inflammation, prophylactic measures, and when to notify the physician.	Patients should understand their symptoms of pericarditis. They should avoid infectious situations, when possible, that may activate pericarditis. Physician notification of cold symptoms (sore throat, cough) should be emphasized to allow for early treatment with antibiotics. A Medic-Alert bracelet may be indicated for the patient with chronic pericarditis or corticosteroid treatment.
Explain the basic purpose, action, and precautions of all discharge medications. Provide written information as available.	

▼

DISCHARGE PLANNING/CONTINUITY OF CARE

- Assure understanding of self-management plan, including signs of recurrent infection, situations to avoid, and medications. Inform patient of importance of completing all medications.
- Refer to a home health agency, if needed, for further monitoring of recovery.
- Arrange for follow-up with physician for continued management.
- Assist in filling prescriptions, devising a medication schedule, and establishing a system for refilling medications.

REFERENCES

Bresler, M. (1992). Acute pericarditis and myocarditis. *Emergency Medicine*, June 15, 1992, pp. 35–51.

Guzzetta, C. & Dossey, B. (1992). *Cardiovascular nursing*. St. Louis, MO: Mosby Year Book.

Pierce, C. (1992). Acute post-MI pericarditis. *Journal of Cardiovascular Nursing*, 6(4), 46–56.

▼

PERIPHERAL ARTERIAL OCCLUSIVE DISEASE

Penny M. Bernards, RN, MS, GNP

Peripheral arterial occlusive disease is a condition where arterial blood flow is diminished or occluded in the extremities and abdomen. The impedance may be an acute or chronic process. The majority of patients have a chronic process which may require only conservative treatments such as risk factor modifications. The risk factors for peripheral arterial disease are similar to cardiovascular disease risks, and patients often have both conditions. Thus the management of cardiovascular disease is also important in peripheral vascular patients. In addition, diabetic patients may first present with ulcerations. Noninvasive vascular studies such as pulse volume recordings (PVRs) and blood pressure indexes are used for diagnosis and documentation of progression of disease. Surgical and radiological interventions are aimed at limb salvage.

ETIOLOGIES

- Atherosclerosis most common
- Arteritis
- Vasospastic phenomenon
- Embolus
- Trauma
- Radiation arteritis
- Heparin-induced thrombocytopenia
- Arterial aneurysm

CLINICAL MANIFESTATIONS

- Intermittent claudication
- Rest pain
- Numbness and tingling of extremities
- Impotence
- Trophic changes

- Ischemic ulcers usually located on toes, heel, and dorsum of foot
- Dependent rubor and pallor with elevation
- Coolness
- Absent or diminished palpable pulse
- Paralysis

CLINICAL/DIAGNOSTIC FINDINGS

- Absent or diminished pulse by Doppler signal
- Ankle-brachial index (ABI): >1.0 (normal), <0.6–0.7 (claudication), <0.2–0.3 (rest pain), <0.1 (impending gangrene)
- Dampening of pulse waveforms
- Filling defect or abrupt termination of blood flow on angiogram

OTHER PLANS OF CARE TO REFERENCE

- Arteriogram
- Prevention and Care of Pressure Ulcers

NURSING DIAGNOSIS: ALTERED PERIPHERAL TISSUE PERFUSION

Related To interruption in blood flow secondary to atherosclerosis

Defining Characteristics

Claudication
Slow healing ulcers
Lack of lanugo
Dependent blue or purple color of extremity (dependent rubor)
Pallor with elevation of extremity capillary refill > 3 s
Diminished or absent arterial pulsations
Dry brittle nails

Patient Outcomes

The patient will have adequate perfusion to the extremity, as evidenced by

- absence of rest pain
- normal movement of extremity for patient's functional state
- intact skin on extremity
- presence of arterial pulsations

Nursing Interventions	**Rationales**
Palpate and or Doppler peripheral pulses bilaterally and document. Peripheral pulses should include femoral, popliteal, dorsalis pedis, posterior tibial, radial, and carotid. Place a mark over pulsation when difficult to find.	It is important to document pulses to determine changes in status. Sudden loss of pulses may indicate an acute thrombosis or embolic episode.
Assess the presence and location of pain.	Classic pain for peripheral occlusive arterial disease is intermittent claudication which is cramping pain in calf, thigh, hip, or buttock while walking a predictable distance and is relieved with rest. As the disease progresses, pain is present in foot at rest (rest pain). Sudden onset of pain may indicate acute occlusion.
Check for color of extremity.	Lower extremity may be dark red or purple when dependent (dependent rubor) and white when elevated above the heart. Petechia or purple tips of digits may indicate embolic phenomenon.
Check for trophic changes on the extremities which include hair loss, thickened toe nails, thin shiny skin, and ulcerations, especially over bony prominences.	Indication of decreased nutrients and oxygenation saturation of peripheral tissues.
Assess for risk factors for peripheral occlusive arterial disease, which include smoking, hypertension, diabetes, hyperlipidemia, obesity, lack of regular exercise, and family and/or personal history of coronary artery disease.	Modification of risk factors is basis for conservative therapy.
Strongly encourage smoking cessation.	Cigarette smoking contributes to the development of atherosclerosis and increases platelet aggregation.

Nursing Interventions	Rationales
Instruct patient on dietary modifications necessary for desired weight and control of hyperlipidemia and diabetes. Consult dietitian as needed.	Diet is not a strong risk in itself but helps modify the major risk factors such as hyperetension, diabetes, and hyperlipidemia.
Encourage a walking program of 30–60 min a day. Instruct patients to walk until they have to stop due to pain; rest until pain subsides and walk again.	Physical training improves walking distances by training ischemic muscles to function more efficiently.
Monitor ABI: Measure both brachial blood pressures and note the higher pressure. Then place blood pressure cuffs around both ankles and using a Doppler over the dorsalis pedis and posterior tibial artery measure the systolic pressure. Divide ankle by brachial systolic pressure to obtain index.	The ABI is a more objective measure of arterial blood flow than palpation or Doppler signal.

▼

NURSING DIAGNOSIS: HIGH RISK FOR IMPAIRED SKIN INTEGRITY

Risk Factors

- Altered circulation
- Immobilization
- Altered sensation

Patient Outcomes

The patient will maintain intact skin.

Nursing Interventions	Rationales
Follow ischemic foot precautions, including a bed cradle or foot board, sheepskin under legs and feet, and lambswool between toes and boots, which helps prevent heel ulcers. Check shoes and socks for foreign objects. Provide slippers for patient when out of bed.	Bed cradles and foot boards are used to prevent pressure from bed linen over ischemic feet. Sheepskin and lambswool are used to prevent sheering injuries.

Nursing Interventions	Rationales
Demonstrate proper foot care: Inspect feet daily for pressure points, cracks, or blisters; check well between toes and on heel; keep feet clean and dry; apply lotion with lanolin to extremity once or twice a day; and place lambswool between overlapping toes.	Proper foot care is needed to prevent ulcerations by prompt recognition of problem areas and decrease dryness and friction and to assess progression of disease.
Instruct on proper nail care: Trim nails after a bath or shower so nails are soft, cut nails straight across, no shorter than length of toes, and file edges; if the patient's eyesight is poor or the nails are too thick, consult a podiatrist.	There is a potential for injury if nails are cut too short and potential for infection if nails are not kept cleaned.
Avoid use of heating pads or hot water bottles on ischemic feet and instruct patient to test bath water with wrist or elbow before inserting foot.	Patient may have decreased sensation in their feet and are at risk to thermal injuries.
Avoid soaking feet for more than 10 min and use a mild soap such as Dove or Camay.	Soaking feet for longer periods can dry out skin. Harsh deoderant soaps and betadine can also dry skin.
Provide a well-balanced diet and adequate hydration.	Good nutrition and hydration are necessary for maintenance of tissues.
Maintain normal blood glucose levels in patients with diabetes.	Elevated glucose levels increase risk for infection and skin breakdown.
Instruct patient to contact physician when any skin breakdown is noted.	It may be an indication of progression of disease.

▼

NURSING DIAGNOSIS: CHRONIC PAIN

Related To peripheral occlusive arterial disease

Defining Characteristics

Disruption of daily activities
Insomnia

Fatigue
Anger or frustration
Evidence of pain for more than 6 months

Patient Outcomes

The patient will

- identify cause of pain.
- describe various methods to control pain.
- verbalize ability to control pain.
- seek additional intervention for intractable pain.

Nursing Interventions	Rationales
Assess location, intensity, and activity level when pain occurs.	Determine if pain is intermittent claudication or has progressed to rest pain.
Assess what interventions the patient has tried to alleviate pain.	Often patients will discover on their own the positions that are most comfortable. Also they may have some misconceptions regarding what intervention has alleviated pain. For example, patients with rest pain may state that they get out of bed and walk to the bathroom for a pain pill. The act of dangling feet may have provided more relief than the pill.
Explain the cause of their pain.	Understanding the cause of pain may help them understand what interventions are more beneficial.
Teach the importance of daily walking programs for patients with claudication. Stress that the goal is to eventually increase their walking distance before onset of pain.	Patients have difficulty understanding that walking is good when the activity causes pain and progression may be slow.
Explain to patients with rest pain that one method of pain relief is dangling feet. Patients often sleep better when up in a chair with legs dependent.	The blood flow is so diminished that there is ischemia at rest. Dangling feet helps increase blood flow by gravity.
Explore other methods of pain relief such as relaxation, guided imagery, and distraction for patients with rest pain.	Methods used to take their mind off their pain.

Nursing Interventions	Rationales
Explain pharmacological measures such as pentoxifylline and aspirin which may be described to treat their disease and may also decrease their discomfort.	Trental (pentoxifylline) is used to alter the shape of red blood cells, making them more flexible and able to get through narrowed blood vessels. It takes up to 120 days before the effect is seen. It is used for patients with intermittent claudication to help increase their walking distance and with patients with rest pain who are unable to have surgery. Aspirin is used for its antiplatelet effect to help decrease extension of a thrombus.
Explore surgical treatment options for patients with intermittent claudication and rest pain.	Debilitating claudication and rest pain are two indications for peripheral bypass surgery.
Include family members and significant others in patient education.	Peripheral occlusive arterial disease is a chronic disease and may result in life-style changes such as parking closer to desired location or sleeping in a chair. Significant others are usually affected by these changes.

▼

NURSING DIAGNOSIS: KNOWLEDGE DEFICIT—PREVENTION AND TREATMENT OF PAD

Related To lack of exposure to information

Defining Characteristics

Verbalization of the problem

Inaccurate performance of proper foot care and continued high-risk activities

Patient Outcomes

The patient will

- identify own significant risk factors for atherosclerosis.
- state the signs and symptoms of progression of arterial occlusive disease.
- describe ways to protect feet and extremity from injury.
- demonstrate proper foot care and verbalize rationale.

Nursing Interventions	Rationales
Instruct patient about the risk factors for atherosclerosis.	Risk factor modification is the basis for conservative therapy.
Provide information for risk factor modification such as smoking cessation strategies, dietary changes, diabetes management, and medication regimen.	
Describe the signs and symptoms of peripheral occlusive artery disease and when they should seek care. Patients with claudication should be reevaluated when claudication interferes with daily life or when rest pain is present. Patients with ulcerations need regular follow-up visits.	
Instruct patients on ischemic foot precautions and daily foot care.	
Ask patient to demonstrate foot care.	

DISCHARGE PLANNING/CONTINUITY OF CARE

- Assure understanding of ischemic foot precautions and proper foot care at home to prevent injuries and infection.
- Instruct patients on necessary equipment and provide written guidelines.
- Emphasize that they should call their doctor if they develop any skin breakdown which does not heal, worsening of pain, or sudden onset of pain in foot.
- Encourage patients to continue smoking cessation at home.
- Refer patients to a smoking cessation clinic if desired.
- Consult a diabetes educator if needed for counseling on diabetes self-management and education.
- Refer patients to their primary care physician for hypertension monitoring and diabetes management.
- Provide material on necessary dietary changes.
- Coordinate outpatient follow-up to assess progression of disease. Patients with rest pain will need to be monitored for skin breakdown

and scheduled for surgery if recommended. Ischemic ulcers need frequent monitoring for healing and/or development of infection.

- Provide information on new medications and regimen and devise plan for refilling medications and supplies.
- Assess functional status and necessary support systems such as Meals on Wheels and visiting nurse service.

REFERENCES

Bright, L. Georgi, S. Peripheral vascular disease: Is it arterial or venous? *American Journal of Nursing, 92*(9), 34–43.

Graham, L. M. & O'Keefe, M. F. (1988). Arterial disease. In V. A. Fahey (Ed.), *Vascular nursing*, Philadelphia, PA: Saunders.

Robinson, L. C. (1992). Atherosclerotic occlusive disease of the aorta. *Journal of Vascular Nursing, 10*, 17–23.

Williams, L. R., Ekers, M. A., Collins, P. S., & Lee, J. F. (1991). Vascular rehabilitation: Benefits of a structured exercise/risk modification program. *Journal of Vascular Surgery, 14*, 320–326.

THROMBOPHLEBITIS/DEEP-VEIN THROMBOSIS

Penny M. Bernards, RN, MS, GNP

Thrombophlebitis is an inflammation of a vein involving formation of a clot. It may occur in superficial veins or deep veins. Superficial thrombophlebitis is rarely life threatening but may lead to a deep-vein thrombosis (DVT). Patients with a DVT are at risk for a pulmonary embolus which is life threatening. Deep-vein thrombosis may also cause damage to valves resulting in postphlebitic syndrome. Postphlebitic syndrome consists of chronic leg edema, tenderness, hyperpigmentation, stasis dermatitis, scaling, and possibly ulcerations. Thus the most important nursing intervention for DVT is prevention. If a DVT occurs, the key nursing interventions include prevention of progression of the clot, maintaining viability of involved extremity, and monitoring anticoagulation therapy.

ETIOLOGIES

- Venous stasis
- Venous trauma
- Increased blood coagulability
- Hypofibrinolysis

CLINICAL MANIFESTATIONS

Superficial
- Erythema
- Warmth
- Tenderness
- Swelling
- Ecchymosis
- Palpable hard cord

Deep
- Asymptomatic
- Swelling starting distally and progressing proximally

- Dilatation of superficial veins
- Hemosiderin pigment deposition
- Pain in calf on dorsiflexion of foot (Homan's sign)
- Malaise
- Fever
- Phlegmasia cerulea dolens (acute DVT) of the iliofemoral segment resulting in edema, severe pain, cyanosis, blisters, and diminished arterial flow which may lead to ischemia.

CLINICAL/DIAGNOSTIC FINDINGS

- Filling defects or abrupt termination of flow on venogram
- Absence of phasic changes of venous Doppler signal with respirations
- Decreased or absent augmentation of venous Doppler signal with manual compression
- Positive 125I-fibrinogen uptake test
- Congenital or acquired clotting deficits such as antithrombin III, protein C, or protein S deficiencies

▼

NURSING DIAGNOSIS: HIGH RISK FOR ALTERED PERIPHERAL TISSUE PERFUSION

Risk Factors

Venous stasis

- Immobilization
- Obesity
- Age >40
- Congestive heart failure
- Varicose veins
- Estrogen therapy
- Spinal cord injury
- Stroke
- Pregnancy
- Myocardial infarction

Venous trauma

- Intravenous therapy
- Prior incidence of DVT
- Surgical procedures involving the abdomen, pelvis, or extremities
- Lower limb fractures
- Trauma

Hypercoagulability

- Polycythemia
- Leukemia
- Malignancies
- Sickle cell anemia

- Antithrombin III deficiency
- Protein C or S deficiency
- Puerperium
- Nephrotic syndrome
- Polycythemia vera

Patient Outcomes

The patient will

- have no sudden onset of edema or pain in an extremity.
- verbalize and demonstrate preventative measures for DVT.
- have appropriate anticoagulant therapy.

Nursing Interventions	Rationales
Assess for conditions which increase risk for DVT.	Identification of patients at risk is important to increase awareness among nursing staff.
Apply antiembolism stockings and/or intermittent pneumatic compression stockings, as prescribed, for patients who are unable to ambulate.	Stockings are used to reduce venous stasis in lower extremities.
Encourage patients to do dorsiflexion, plantar flexion, and ankle-rolling exercises while in bed or in chair. Perform passive range-of-motion exercises for patients unable to do active exercises.	Exercises help reduce venous statis in lower extremities.
Elevate foot of bed if tolerated. Use caution if pillows are used so veins are not compressed, causing further venous stasis.	Ten degree elevation increases venous blood flow 30%.
Instruct patients to do deep-breathing exercises with or without an incentive spirometer and monitor frequency.	The mechanics of breathing act as a pump which helps with venous return.
Ambulate patients as soon as medically possible.	No mechanical pump works as efficiently as the calf muscles to promote venous return.
Observe intravenous (IV) sites and change at least every 72 hr. (Each practice setting may have its own protocol.)	Rotating IV sites helps reduce venous trauma from direct injury or overuse.

Nursing Interventions	Rationales
Monitor intake and output to maintain proper fluid balance.	Overhydration and underhydration can decrease venous return and cause venous stasis.
Monitor anticoagulant therapy as prescribed by physician:	
1. Heparin is used subcutaneously for prophylactic treatment in the perioperative period and for other high-risk patients.	Heparin neutralizes factor X of the coagulation system which prevents formation of thrombin, which is necessary for formation of a clot.
2. Warfarin is also used for prophylactic treatment although it is usually used postoperatively due to risk of bleeding. An exception is made for orthopaedic patients with hip/knee fractures who are often given warfarin preoperatively as well.	Warfarin inhibits vitamin K, which is necessary to make the clotting factors VII, IX, and X and prothrombin II, which are involved with formation of thrombin.

▼

NURSING DIAGNOSIS: ALTERED PERIPHERAL TISSUE PERFUSION

Related To reduced or disrupted venous flow due to DVT

Defining Characteristics

Edema
Pain
Dilatation of superficial veins
Malaise
Fever

Patient Outcomes

The patient will have

- decreased edema in involved extremity
- decreased pain
- intact skin

Nursing Interventions	Rationales
Maintain bedrest for several days to prevent plaque from breaking off and forming an embolus.	

Nursing Interventions	Rationales
Measure arm or leg circumference at several specific locations to document changes in edema.	
Monitor heparin IV infusions as prescribed. A heparin bolus may be used to establish a therapeutic dose more quickly.	
Monitor the activated partial thromboplastin time (PTT) and platelet count during administration of heparin. The therapeutic range is 1.5–2.0 times the control value.	The laboratory value PTT measures alterations in clotting factors which are used to regulate heparin dose. Patients on heparin are at risk for heparin-induced thrombocytopenia; thus platelet levels are monitored daily.
Monitor PTT every 4–6 hr after changes in heparin drip dose until therapeutic range and then at least twice daily.	It may take several days for the therapeutic range, requiring frequent adjustments. Patients have different tolerances to anticoagulants and require individual dosing.
Apply elastic ace bandages to affected extremity to decrease edema and prevent venous dilatation. Rewrap bandage when loose or at least twice a day to assess skin integrity.	
Elevate affected extremity above the level of the heart if tolerated.	
Apply prescription-strength compression stockings when patients are ambulatory. Stockings are worn during the day and are taken off at night.	Compression stockings are used to prevent venous dilatation. Venous dilatation may cause incompetent valves because they are unable to close completely. This results in backflow of venous blood, which increases venous pressure and may lead to leakage of fluid into interstitial spaces with subsequent venous stasis ulcerations.

Nursing Interventions	Rationales
Warfarin is initiated either with heparin or when heparin is therapeutic depending on physician preference. Instruct patient that warfarin may be continued for at least 3–6 months.	To prevent extension or recurrence of clot.
Monitor prothrombin time (PT) daily while patients are on warfarin. Changes in PT are usually not seen until 48 hr after initiating warfarin. Therapeutic range is 1.5–2.0 times the control.	The PT evaluates defects in prothrombin and factors V, VII, and X.
Monitor any changes in medications or medical condition while on warfarin.	There are numerous medications and medical conditions which can either enhance or inhibit the anticoagulation effect of warfarin.
Observe for signs of bleeding while on anticoagulation therapy. Signs may include hematuria, guaiac positive stools, nosebleeds, coffee ground emesis, coughing up frank blood, unexplained pain, drop in hematocrit and hemoglobin, bleeding gums, and excessive bleeding from incisions.	Bleeding may occur even when patients are subtherapeutic on anticoagulants.

▼

NURSING DIAGNOSIS: HIGH RISK FOR IMPAIRED GAS EXCHANGE

Risk Factors

- Deep-vein thrombosis
- Venous stasis
- Cardiovascular disease
- Previous history of DVT or pulmonary embolus (PE)

Patient Outcomes

The patient will have adequate perfusion to the lung, as evidenced by

- regular unlabored respirations
- absence of chest discomfort
- absence of restlessness

Nursing Interventions	Rationales
Monitor vital signs and report any sudden drop in blood pressure, tachycardia, and tachypnea.	Changes in vital signs are potential signs for PE.
Monitor for signs and symptoms of PE such as shortness of breath, chest pain, fever, cough, hemoptysis, hypotension, syncope, restlessness, and hypoxemia and report them immediately to physician.	
Implement preventative measures for DVT.	The best treatment of pulmonary embolism is prevention.
Instruct patient regarding diagnostic studies used to detect pulmonary emboli, which include ventilation-perfusion scan, chest x-ray, electrocardiogram (ECG), arterial blood gas measurements, and possibly pulmonary arteriogram.	
If a pulmonary embolus is suspected, IV heparin therapy is usually initiated until diagnosis is ruled out or confirmed.	

▼

NURSING DIAGNOSIS: KNOWLEDGE DEFICIT—DIAGNOSIS AND TREATMENT OF DVT

Related To lack of exposure to information

Defining Characteristics

Verbalization of inadequate understanding or misconceptions
Anxiety
Inaccurate demonstration of desired behaviors

Patient Outcomes

The patient will

- describe thrombophlebitis and the DVT healing process, diagnostic tests, and possible complications.
- describe anticoagulation medications regimen and plan for monitoring.
- list precautions to take while on anticoagulation therapy.
- apply and wear compression stockings.
- describe planned walking program.

Nursing Interventions	Rationales
Assess current knowledge of disease process.	Assessment of knowledge base is used to develop teaching plan.
Explain the etiology of DVT and how the identified risk factors contribute to the formation of clot.	Understanding of etiology and risk factors may facilitate changes in behavior that help prevent venous stasis and trauma.
Inform about noninvasive diagnostic tests used to detect DVT, which include	
1. Doppler ultrasound	Doppler ultrasound involves an ultrasonic beam which records an audible signal as moving blood cells pass beneath. The flow characteristics are assessed for patency. No sound is heard over occluded veins and an abnormal signal may be heard over partially occluded veins.
2. impedance plethysmography	Impedance plethysmography is used to detect more proximal DVT. A pneumatic thigh cuff is placed over the thigh, and four electrodes are placed around the calf. The thigh cuff is inflated and then rapidly deflated while the electrodes measure the venous capacitance and outflow. The outflow is decreased when a venous thrombosis is present.
3. duplex imaging	A duplex scan involves use of an ultrasound probe over the skin which provides colored imaging of venous flow and abnormalities such as thrombus.
4. venogram (considered an invasive procedure)	A venogram involves injection of contrast material through a vein in the dorsum of the foot and subsequent filming of venous flow. A filling defect in the vein indicates a thrombus.

Nursing Interventions	Rationales
Instruct regarding potential complications of DVT, especially if left untreated, including extension of clot which increases risk of pulmonary embolus and an ischemic limb if iliofemoral segment is involved and postphlebitic syndrome.	Patients need to be aware of how serious their condition is so that an informed decision can be made regarding treatment.
Assess understanding of anticoagulation therapy, including indications, dosage, target protime levels and frequency of blood draws, regulation of warfarin from protime levels, risks of therapy, and lack of therapy.	
Instruct to take warfarin at the same time daily and to not take an additional dosage, if one is missed, without consultation with their physician.	
Caution about avoiding over-the-counter products which contain aspirin while on warfarin unless directed by physician.	Aspirin enhances the anticoagulation effect of warfarin.
Instruct to wear compression stockings daily even when feeling better to prevent venous dilatation. Stockings are applied in the morning and removed before going to bed. Stockings should be replaced after they lose their elasticity at approximately 3–6 months.	Patients who have had a DVT are at increased risk for development of additional thrombosis.
Emphasize importance of a regular exercise program using leg muscles to promote venous return.	

▼

DISCHARGE PLANNING/CONTINUITY OF CARE

- Coordinate plan for obtaining regular protime levels for regulation of warfarin dose.
- Emphasize importance of monitoring protime levels.

- Review signs and symptoms of bleeding.
- Instruct patient to contact physician if signs and symptoms of recurrent DVT develops.
- Inform patient to seek immediate medical attention if sudden shortness of breath or chest pain occurs.
- Coordinate outpatient follow-up clinic visits and testing to evaluate for reconstitution of vein.
- Assist in obtaining prescriptions and establishing medication time schedule and plan for refilling prescriptions.

REFERENCES

Coffman, J. D. (1989). Deep venous thrombosis and pulmonary emboli: Etiology, medical treatment and prophylaxis. *Journal of Thoracic Imaging*, *4*, 4–7.

Fahey, V. A. (1988). Venous thromboembolism. In V. A. Fahey (Ed.), *Vascular nursing*. Philadelphia, PA: Saunders.

Herzog, J. A. (1992). Deep vein thrombosis in the rehabilitation client. *Rehabilitation Nursing*, *17*, 196–198.

Nunnelee, J. D. (1988). Medications used in vascular patients. In V. A. Fahey (Ed.), *Vascular nursing*. Philadelphia, PA: Saunders.

Ogston, D. (1987). *Venous thrombosis causation and prediction*. Chichester: Wiley Medical.

Common Respiratory Conditions and Procedures

▼

ASTHMA

Ellen M. Jovle, RN, MS

Asthma is a clinical syndrome characterized by airway obstruction, airway inflammation, and airway hyperresponsiveness to a variety of stimuli. Asthma is reversible either spontaneously or with treatment. There are two types of asthma: extrinsic or intrinsic. Extrinsic or allergic asthma is precipitated by external stimuli. Intrinsic or nonallergic asthma is a type of asthma in which specific precipitating factors cannot be identified. Extrinsic asthma often begins in childhood while intrinsic asthma usually begins in person over the age of 35. Since 1980, the rate of asthma-related deaths and hospitalizations has been steadily increasing. The typical hospitalization of the asthmatic patient is related to a severe attack or a less severe attack which is not relieved by self-management or outpatient intervention.

ETIOLOGIES

Extrinsic stimuli that can precipitate an attack of asthma:

- drug and food additives such as aspirin, nonsteroidal anti-inflammatory agents, tartrazine (yellow dye), sulfites (food and beverage preservative), beta-blocking agents including eye drops
- exercise
- emotional stress
- environmental allergens such as dust, pollen, mold, animal dander, house dust mites, tobacco smoke, or occupational triggers
- endocrine factors: menses, pregnancy, or thyroid disease
- respiratory infections
- gastroesophageal reflux
- rhinitis, sinusitis, or nasal polyps
- weather changes (cold air, humidity)

CLINICAL MANIFESTATIONS

- Dyspnea
- Chest tightness, wheezing
- Cough, sputum production

- Increased pulse and blood pressure and respiratory rate
- Pulsus paradoxus
- Anxiety
- Diaphoresis
- Gasping speech
- Use of accessory muscle of or intercostal or supraclavicular retraction

CLINICAL/DIAGNOSTIC FINDINGS

- Alterations in pulmonary function studies
  - decreased forced expiratory volume in one second (FEV_1)
  - decreased peak expiratory flow rate (PEFR)
  - decreased vital capacity (VC)
  - increased total lung capacity (TLC)
  - increased residual volume
- Arterial blood gas (ABG) alterations
  - decreased arterial oxygen partial pressure (PaO_2)
  - arterial carbon dioxide partial pressure ($PaCO_2$), decreased early in attack, progressive increase during prolonged attack
  - pH, increased early in attack, progressive decrease during prolonged attack
- Alterations in chest x-ray showing
  - hyperinflation
  - air trapping
  - flattened diaphragm
  - infiltrates if infection present
- Sinus tachycardia

OTHER PLANS OF CARE TO REFERENCE

- Corticosteroid Therapy
- Chronic Obstructive Pulmonary Disease (COPD)

▼

NURSING DIAGNOSIS: INEFFECTIVE BREATHING PATTERN/ INEFFECTIVE AIRWAY CLEARANCE

Related To
- Bronchospasm
- Tenacious secretions
- Anxiety
- Fatigue

Defining Characteristics

Dyspnea
Dyspneic speech pattern
Pursed lip breathing
Abnormal arterial blood gases
Abnormal breath sounds
Tachypnea
Use of accessory muscles
Altered chest wall excursion
Cough

Patient Outcomes

The patient will exhibit

- decrease in dyspnea level
- respiratory rate, rhythm, and depth comparable to patient's baseline
- normal breath sounds
- normal arterial blood gases
- decreased use of accessory muscles
- decreased chest wall retraction
- ability to mobilize secretions

Nursing Interventions	Rationales
Monitor patient status frequently until stable. Assessment includes respiratory rate, rhythm and depth, use of accessory muscles, presence of chest wall retraction, level of consciousness, presence of cough, character and quantity of sputum, blood pressure and heart rate, degree of pulsus paradoxus, breath sounds, skin color, and skin moisture.	These assessments are indicators of severity of the attack, response to treatment, presence of hypoxemia, and further deterioration of patient status.
Monitor fluid balance by assessing intake and output, weight, skin turgor, and condition of mucous membrane.	Diaphoresis, tachypnea, and decreased oral intake may cause dehydration. Dehydration contributes to thick tenacious secretions which are difficult to expectorate.
Administer oxygen as prescribed. Monitor pulse oximetry for maintenance of arterial oxygen saturation (SaO_2) of 90 mmHg or greater.	Arterial oxygen saturation may intermittently decline during an attack; therefore the goal of 92–93% should be used for patients at risk for adverse consequences of hypoxemia such as the elderly or patients with coronary artery disease.

Nursing Interventions	Rationales
Administer medications as prescribed. Pharmacological management of an acute exacerbation may include	
1. inhaled $beta_2$ agonist (such as albuterol, metaproterenol, or isoetharine) as frequently as every 1–2 hr	Repetitive administration of $beta_2$ agonist is most effective in reversing airflow obstruction and providing incremental bronchodilatation.
2. subcutaneous $beta_2$ agonist such as epinephrine or terbutaline	Subcutaneous $beta_2$ agonist may be used as an alternative bronchodilator and is most often used in the emergency room setting.
3. intravenous or oral methylxanthines such as aminophylline or theophylline (monitoring theophylline levels)	Methylxanthines are mild to moderate bronchodilators at serum levels of 10–20 μg/mL. Levels above 20 μg/mL are considered toxic.
4. systemic corticosteroids such as intravenous methylprednisolone or hydrocortisone or oral prednisone	Systemic corticosteroids speed recovery from an acute attack by reducing airway inflammation.
Avoid medications which are respiratory depressants or beta blockers which can lead to bronchospasm.	
Assist patient into semi- or high Fowler's position leaning forward to maximize the use of respiratory muscles. Support the arms to relieve nonventilatory work of respiratory muscles.	Lying flat causes the abdominal organs to move toward the chest, crowding the lungs and making it more difficult to breathe.
Initiate measures to mobilize secretions such as controlled coughing, chest physiotherapy or suctioning. Monitor arterial oxygen saturation (SaO_2) during chest PT and suctioning to identify the need for supplemental oxygen.	

Nursing Interventions	Rationales
Assist patient to slow respiratory rate by 1. placing one hand on patient's shoulder and one hand on abdomen. 2. initially following patient's respiratory movements while verbally encouraging patient to breathe slower ("breathe in, now breathe in slowly"). 3. speaking in a low, slow voice that is in rhythm with the patient's breathing pattern. 4. once the patient's pattern is established, applying gentle but firm pressure to the abdomen with an up-and-in motion while simultaneously flexing the patient forward. 5. releasing the pressure as patient begins to inhale while keeping hand on patient's abdomen. 6. gradually increasing length of time pressure is exerted, prolonging the expiratory phase. Do not attempt to slow respiratory rate too fast. 7. stopping this intervention if it causes increased anxiety, which is not therapeutic.	This intervention may decrease patient's anxiety and the amount of air trapping.

▼

NURSING DIAGNOSIS: FEAR/ANXIETY

Related To
- Breathlessness
- Lack of control
- Threat of death

Defining Characteristics
Apprehension, tenseness, helplessness
Distress, uncertainty
Feelings of inadequacy
Overexcitedness, jitters
Increased heart rate, palpitations, elevated blood pressure

Increased respiratory rate, increased dyspnea
Trembling
Diaphoresis
Facial tension

Patient Outcomes

The patient will
- use pursed-lip breathing and diaphragmatic breathing during episodes of breathlessness.
- verbalize emotional response to episodes of breathlessness.
- report a decrease in frequency and severity of acute episodes of dyspnea.
- report an increased level of control.
- report decrease in fear and anxiety levels.

Nursing Interventions	Rationales
Assess for level of anxiety and reasons for fear.	Anxiety may range from mild to severe. The level of anxiety guides nursing interventions.
Assess for nonverbal cues of anxiety and fear.	During acute breathlessness patient may be unable to verbalize anxiety and fear but may reveal nonverbal responses.
During severe panic levels of anxiety: 1. Stay with the patient. 2. Acknowledge patient's fear, anxiety, and helplessness. 3. Demonstrate respect for the seriousness of the episode. 4. Reinforce your ability to help and attend. 5. Accept level of dyspnea for what patient says it is. 6. Do not attempt to distract patient from breathing. 7. Be aware of your own anxiety and avoid transferring to patient. 8. Avoid use of empty phrases such as "try to relax" or "try to get in control." 9. Demonstrate breathing techniques that patient can imitate rather than attempting to talk patients through technique.	

Nursing Interventions	Rationales
10. Respect need for increase in personal space. 11. Take charge of the environment, control traffic level of activity and noise.	
When anxiety levels have decreased: 1. Encourage discussion of acute episode, what helped and what did not. 2. Teach patient use of anxiety/fear reducing techniques: pursed-lip breathing, diaphragmatic breathing (see Chronic Obstructive Pulmonary Disease, Tables 19.3 and 19.4). relaxation techniques, and calming self-talk. 3. Assist patient in identifying common antecedents to episodes of dyspnea, strategies to prevent episodes, and effect of anxiety on breathing. 4. Encourage patient to discuss with family behaviors that would be helpful during breathlessness episode.	Learning and problem solving can take place only when anxiety level is reduced to a mild or moderate level. These techniques have shown to reduce anxiety and dyspnea in patients with COPD. Family members often feel helpless and anxious. Learning how to be helpful and supportive in future episodes will assist in reducing patient's and family's anxiety.

▼

NURSING DIAGNOSIS: INABILITY TO SUSTAIN SPONTANEOUS VENTILATION

Related To

- Severe airway obstruction
- Lack of response to treatment
- Fatigue

Defining Characteristics

Dyspnea
Apprehension
Increased use of accessory muscles
Increased heart rate
Decreased cooperation

Decreased PaO_2, increased $PaCO_2$, decreased SaO_2
Decreased PEFR or FEV_1

Patient Outcomes

Patient will maintain adequate gas exchange either spontaneously or with ventilatory support.
NOTE: The medical surgical nurse's role in this diagnosis is assessment and reporting so that early intervention can occur. Intervention with mechanical ventilation will require transferring the patient to a critical care unit.

Nursing Interventions	Rationales
Review patient's history. Note number of hospitalizations and emergency room visits in past year, previous admission to intensive care unit (ICU), prior intubation for asthma, use of systemic corticosteroids, history of sycope or hypoxic seizure, psychiatric disease, or psychosocial problems.	Patients with history of these events are at high risk for asthma-related death and require close monitoring and prompt intervention.
Monitor ABGs and/or SaO_2 with pulse oximetry. Promptly report carbon dioxide ($PaCO_2$) levels less than 45 mmHg and oxygen (PaO_2) greater than 60 mmHg.	Early in the attack $PaCO_2$ is decreased and pH is increased because patient is hyperventilating. The $PaCO_2$ starts to rise and pH decreases as patient fatigues and begins to hypoventilate. This change in ABGs is a sign of deterioration and the need for further intervention to prevent respiratory arrest.
Monitor patient's respiratory status frequently.	Rapid shallow respirations, increased use of accessory muscles, chest wall retraction, asynchronous chest wall movement, and paradoxus abdominal movement indicate respiratory muscle fatigue and impending respiratory failure. Wheezing is an unreliable indicator of obstruction. Severe obstruction may be accompanied by a "silent chest."

Nursing Interventions	Rationales
Assess and report cardiovascular indices of hypoxemia and respiratory effort: tachycardia, abnormal pulse rhythm, elevated blood pressure, and pulsus paradoxus.	Pulsus paradoxus is an exaggeration of the usual fall in systolic pressure during inspiration. A greater than 10 mmHg drop in systolic blood pressure between inspiration and expiration is a sign of increased respiratory effort.
Assess and report neurological indications of hypoxemia (confusion, delirium, loss of judgment and problem-solving ability, combative behavior) or hypercapnea (headache, drowsiness, disorientation, coma).	
Monitor PEFR or FEV_1. Report values 30–50% below baseline values.	Failure of PEFR or FEV_1 to improve by at least 10% after initial treatment indicates patients at risk for life-threatening deterioration.
Provide emotional support to patient and family.	
Anticipate need for ventilatory support to prevent respiratory arrest. Notify respiratory therapy. Prepare for intubation and manual ventilatory assistance with Ambu bag. Sedation is required for intubation. Alert co-workers to situation and potential need for assistance.	
Transfer patient to ICU. Monitor SaO_2, respiratory status, and cardiovascular status during transport.	

NURSING DIAGNOSIS: KNOWLEDGE DEFICIT—ASTHMA SELF-MANAGEMENT

Related To lack of prior exposure to information.

Defining Characteristics

Verbalized lack of knowledge of disease and its treatment
Inappropriate delay in recognizing exacerbation and seeking treatment

Inability to accurately describe use, dosages, schedule, side effects, and complication of medication
Inaccurate technique when using metered-dose inhaler
Inaccurate performance or lack of prior knowledge of PEFR monitoring
Verbalized lack of knowledge of environmental measures to control allergens

Patient Outcomes

Patient will

- state use, side effects, dosage, schedule, and adverse effects to monitor and report.
- demonstrate proper technique when using metered-dose inhaler.
- state measures to avoid infection.
- describe signs and symptoms of exacerbation.
- describe home management of exacerbation and state when to call physician or go to emergency room.
- demonstrate accurate use of peak expiratory flow meter.
- state techniques to reduce anxiety and stress.
- identify environmental allergens and irritants and measures to control them.

Nursing Interventions	Rationales
Assess current knowledge level, readiness to learn, and preferred learning style. Involve patient in establishing learning needs and a plan to meet those needs. Provide written materials.	
Consult available resources such as pharmacist, respiratory therapist, social worker, exercise physiologist, and asthma or respiratory nurse specialist as appropriate.	
Discuss medications prescribed, including names, actions, dosages, scheduling, side effects and adverse reaction to report (see Corticosteroid Therapy, p. 329.)	

Nursing Interventions	Rationales
Demonstrate correct technique for using metered-dose inhaler. Observe patient's technique for self-administration. If patient has difficulty triggering inhaler, obtain and instruct in use of spacer device (see Chronic Obstructive Pulmonary Disease, p. 203.)	Spacer devices such as Aerochamber or InspirEase do not require coordination of inhalation to activate inhaler. Instructions for use come with devices and can be used for patient education.
Instruct in use of peak expiratory flow meter, establishing "personal best," using PEFR measurements to monitor and manage asthma.	A peak expiratory flow meter is a device used to monitor asthma at home and detect asymptomatic deterioration. The PEFR is the maximum flow rate that can be generated during a forced expiration with fully inflated lungs. The "personal best" result is the highest measurement obtained in a 2–3 week period during which measurements are taken at least twice a day. Ongoing monitoring guidelines are as follows: (1) 80–100% of personal best signals all clear, (2) 50–80% of personal best signals trouble and an increase in medication may be needed, or (3) below 50% of personal best indicates medical emergency and need to seek medical assistance.
Explain signs and symptoms of asthma exacerbations and home management of symptoms.	
Discuss signs and symptoms which indicate a need for medical consultation or emergency room visit. Stress the importance of early treatment.	
Discuss guidelines for premedicating to avoid onset of symptoms (before exercise, exposure to irritants, etc.).	

Nursing Interventions	Rationales
Explain factors that may contribute to infections and measures to prevent infection (pneumovax and influenza vaccines, avoiding crowds, monitoring color, character, and amount of sputum, monitoring temperature).	
Teach patient stress management and anxiety-reducing strategies. Consult social worker or psychiatric or respiratory nurse specialist as appropriate.	Psychological factors do not cause asthma. Stress and emotions may contribute to severity of an attack. Relaxation techniques have been shown to reduce anxiety and dyspnea in persons with asthma.
Teach patient pursed-lip breathing and controlled coughing using "huff" technique (see Chronic Obstructive Pulmonary Disease, Tables 19.3 and 19.6).	Pursed-lip breathing reduces air trapping and dyspnea. Forceful coughing against a closed glottis causes collapse of small airways, which exacerbates the airway obstruction.
Assist patient in identifying factors that precipitate attack. Discuss environmental measures to control allergens or irritants.	Between 75 and 85% of patients with asthma have an allergic component. Once specific triggers are identified, the patient can take measures to avoid or control them. House dust mites appear to have a major role in allergic asthma and environmental measures to control exposure is essential in reducing symptoms.

NURSING DIAGNOSIS: INEFFECTIVE MANAGEMENT OF THERAPEUTIC REGIMEN

Related To

- Health beliefs
- Lack of finances
- Psychiatric or psychosocial problems

Defining Characteristics

Frequent hospitalizations or emergency room visits with no self-management of early symptoms

Verbalizes lack of ongoing follow-up on a regular basis

Verbalizes lack of adherence to treatment regimens
Demonstrates inability to take action to avoid or control allergens or irritants
Identifies psychosocial problems that interfere with managing asthma
Verbalizes perceived barriers or lack of perceived benefits to therapeutic regimen
Verbalizes lack of perceived seriousness of disease and/or personal susceptibility to complications
Verbalizes belief that behavior has no effect on management of asthma and that external factors control illness
Verbalizes history of psychiatric disorders

Patient Outcomes

The patient will

- take action to manage early symptoms or seek medical advice early in attack.
- obtain regular follow-up.
- follow treatment regimens as prescribed.
- take action to control exposure to allergens and irritants.

Nursing Interventions	Rationales
Assess health beliefs, including perceived benefits to therapeutic regimen, perceived seriousness of illness, and perceived susceptibility to complications.	Adherence to therapeutic regimens has been correlated with health benefits. Perceived benefits, seriousness, and susceptibility positively influence adherence. Perceived barriers negatively influence adherence.
Assess patient's beliefs about effect of behavior on management of asthma.	A patient who believes external forces control health (external locus of control) rather than internal forces (internal locus of control) may not be motivated to follow therapeutic regimen.
Assess for financial difficulties, psychosocial problems, or psychiatric disorders and assist with obtaining resources. Consult social services for assistance in identifying available community resources.	Lack of finances may impact use of medications such as metered-dose inhalers, which are expensive. There is a high risk of morbidity and mortality in patients with psychiatric disorder or complex psychosocial problems.
Provide information about seriousness of asthma, potential complications, and benefits of medical regimen.	

Nursing Interventions	Rationales
Consult home health care provider for assessment of home environment.	Assessment of home may help in identifying status of the environment and contribution to patient' symptoms.

▼

DISCHARGE PLANNING/CONTINUITY OF CARE

- Assure understanding of self-management plan.
- Arrange for home respiratory equipment from vendor of patient's choice.
- Refer to a home health care agency if continued nursing care, teaching, or assistance with environmental control of allergens or irritants is needed.
- Arrange follow-up with physician for continued management postdischarge.
- Assist patient in obtaining prescriptions and establishing a plan for refilling prescriptions.
- Provide with information on asthma support groups or educational programs in the area.
- Refer to a local chapter of the American Lung Association for further information.

REFERENCES

DeVito, A. J. (1990). Dyspnea during hospitalization for acute phase of illness as recalled by patients with chronic obstructive pulmonary disease. *Heart & Lung, 19*(2), 186–191.

National Asthma Education Program—Expert Panel Report. (1991). *Executive summary: Guidelines for the diagnosis and management of asthma*, Publication No. 91-3042A. Bethesda, MD: National Institutes of Health.

Reinke, L. F. & Hoffman, L. A. (1992). Breathing space: How to teach asthma co-management. *American Journal of Nursing, 92*(10), 40–48.

Traver, G. A. & Leidy, N. K. (1989). Asthma and stress. *Journal of Advanced Medical Surgical Nursing, 1*(4), 25–34.

Wilson, S. F. & Thompson, J. M. (1990). *Respiratory disorders.* St. Louis, MO: Mosby.

▼

CHEST TUBES

Linda Wonoski, RN, MSN

Chest tubes with an attached drainage system are placed in the pleural cavity to drain fluid, blood, or air and reestablish a negative pressure that facilitates expansion of the lung. To drain air, which rises in the pleural space, the chest tube is frequently inserted in the second, third, or fourth intercostal space at the midclavicular line. To drain blood or fluid, which gravity forces to the base of the lung, the chest tube is placed in the fifth or sixth intercostal space at the midaxillary line.

ETIOLOGIES (INDICATIONS)

- Pneumothorax
- Hemothorax
- Pleural effusion
- Empyema
- Postthoracotomy
- Post–heart surgery

CLINICAL MANIFESTATIONS

- Respiratory distress
- Dyspnea
- Tachypnea
- Use of accessory muscles
- Paradoxical chest movement
- Trachea deviated to unaffected side
- Lungs: hyperresonant over air-filled area, dull over fluid filled area; breath sounds diminished or absent in affected area
- Cyanosis or pallor
- Pain
- Anxiety

CLINICAL/DIAGNOSTIC FINDINGS

- Chest x-ray reveals air and/or fluid accumulation; shift of mediastinal structures.
- Arterial blood gases (ABGs) deviate from patient's baseline but are variable depending on the degree of compromised lung function, altered breathing pattern, and ability to compensate.

▼

NURSING DIAGNOSIS: ANXIETY

Related To
- Respiratory distress
- Lack of knowledge about chest tube insertion

Defining Characteristics
Patient expresses fear about inability to breathe and chest tube insertion.
Patient asks questions and verbalizes a lack of knowledge regarding chest tube insertion procedure.

Patient Outcomes
Patient will
- describe awareness of chest tube insertion.
- verbalize a decreased level of anxiety and fear.

Nursing Interventions	Rationales
Stay with patient. Maintain calm, confident reassuring approach.	
Explain the specific reason why the chest tubes are needed (e.g., to remove air or fluid or reexpand the lung).	
Review insertion procedure with patient, including	Knowledge of what to expect can decrease anxiety.
1. type of drainage system to be used (e.g., how it looks, basic function)	
2. positioning during insertion—sitting up and bending forward or lying on unaffected side	Scapula is moved out of the way for easier insertion.

Nursing Interventions	Rationales
3. area of chest tube insertion: intercostal space used	Chest tube is placed high for air removal (second, third, or fourth intercostal space) or low for removal of fluid (fifth or sixth intercostal space).
4. local anesthetic injected at insertion site	
5. small incision made at insertion site	
6. chest tube inserted using several techniques, either a trocar or hemostat, and connected to the drainage system	
7. chest tube sutured in place and a sterile dressing applied	
8. chest tube and drainage system monitored closely for bleeding and leakage of air and fluid	
9. follow-up chest x-ray performed to confirm chest tube placement and reexpansion of the lung	

▼

NURSING DIAGNOSIS: IMPAIRED GAS EXCHANGE/ INEFFECTIVE BREATHING PATTERN

Related To decreased lung expansion

- Ventilation
- Perfusion imbalance
- Pain and fatigue

Defining Characteristics

Dyspnea
Tachypnea
Hypoxemia
Restlessness
Use of accessory muscles for breathing
Splinted or guarded respirations
Abnormal ABGs: deviate from patient's baseline
Breath sounds diminished or absent

Patient Outcomes

Patient will demonstrate

- normal rate, rhythm, and depth of respirations
- ABGs within normal limits or patient's baseline
- reexpansion of the lung
- breath sounds bilaterally equal and clear

Nursing Interventions	Rationales
Auscultate lungs and assess respiratory rate, depth, and quality. Immediately report signs of increased respiratory distress (rapid, shallow breathing, cyanosis, or pressure in the chest).	Early detection of respiratory distress may indicate a tension pneumothorax which can develop when air leaks into the pleura and cannot escape.
Monitor level of consciousness and vital signs frequently.	
Monitor ABG's and pulse oximetry.	
Administer oxygen as prescribed.	
Assess and maintain patency of closed chest drainage system:	Promotes reexpansion of the lungs by draining fluid and air from the pleural space.
1. Tape all tube connections and check periodically to ensure a closed system and patency of tubes.	An air-tight closed system is required to reexpand lung.
2. Keep chest drainage system below level of patient's chest.	Gravity will aid in drainage and prevent backflow into the chest.
3. Mark original drainage fluid level (immediately postinsertion) on the outside of the drainage system; then mark hourly/shift increments (date and time).	Drainage usually declines progressively after the first 24 hr.
4. Notify physician if drainage is greater than 100 mL/hr for two consecutive hours or if there is a sudden outpouring of bright red blood.	May indicate new bleeding requiring surgical intervention or fluid replacement.

Nursing Interventions	Rationales
5. Keep tubing free of kinks and prevent dependent loops. Do not let patient lie on tubing.	Kinking, looping, or pressure on the drainage tubing can create back pressure, possibly forcing drainage back into the pleural space or impeding removal of air or fluid.
6. Milk/squeeze tubing gently in the direction of the drainage container only if necessary to move drainage along. Do not *strip* tubing or use heavy pressure to tubing.	*Gently* milking/squeezing the tubing is generally enough to prevent it from becoming plugged with clots and fibrin. Chest tube stripping can create transient negative pressure on the pleural space possibly causing lung entrapment in the chest tube eyelets and tissue infarction. This results in less efficient air/fluid drainage.
7. Check fluid level in water seal chamber and maintain patient at level prescribed.	Water in the water seal chamber serves as a barrier which prevents atmospheric air from entering the pleural space. The greater the fluid level in the water seal chamber, the more positive pressure is required to push air out of the drainage unit, which makes breathing more difficult.
8. Monitor water seal for fluctuation (tidaling). Absence of fluctuation indicates lung reexpansion or that there is an obstruction which must be corrected (clots, kinking, or tubing).	Fluctuation of 2–6 cm during inspiration generally indicates that the chest tube and collection tube are patent.
9. Monitor for air leaks in the drainage system as indicated by constant bubbling in the water seal chamber. Report any sudden increase in bubbling; determine location of and correct any inappropriate air leak (e.g., tighten connection).	Bubbling in the water seal chamber indicates an air leak which may be present because the lung has not yet reexpanded or there may be a leak in the system before the water seal drainage, such as a loose tubing connection or air leak around the entrance site of the chest tube.

Nursing Interventions	Rationales
10. Monitor patient for development of subcutaneous emphysema.	Subcutaneous emphysema indicates air is leaking into the tissues faster than it is being removed by the tube. The physician may change the chest tube to a larger one and/or additional suction may be applied to the chest tube in an attempt to remove air more rapidly.
11. Check suction control chamber for correct fluid level.	Amount of suction being applied to the pleural space is regulated by the amount of fluid in the suction control chamber, not the amount dialed on the wall suction.
12. Keep two hemostats at the bedside. Clamp only if the closed chest drainage system is being changed to a new system, the physician ordered clamping to verify the patient's readiness to have the chest tube removed, or to locate the source of an air leak. If the system becomes accidently disconnected, reconnect it as quickly as possible, clamping is not recommended.	Clamping chest tubes is dangerous because no air or fluid can escape and a tension pneumothorax can occur.
Encourage patient to change positions frequently. Recommended positions include semi-Fowler's and lateral with a rolled towel placed under the chest tubing to protect it from the weight of the patient's body.	Promotes drainage from the chest tube. Moves abdominal contents away from the diaphragm, enhancing chest expansion and movement of the diaphragm. Promotes patient comfort and prevents the chest tube from being compressed when the patient turns that way.
Assist patient to cough, deep breath, and use the incentive spirometer every 2–4 hr.	

▼

NURSING DIAGNOSIS: PAIN

Related To pleural tissue trauma associated with the chest tubes

Defining Characteristics

Complaints of pain: around chest tubes, on moving, with coughing, and deep breathing
Hesitation to move, cough, and deep breath
Facial grimaces
Rigid posture

Patient Outcomes

Patient will
- verbalize a decrease in pain.
- increase participation in moving, coughing, and deep breathing.
- display a relaxed facial expression and body sphere.

Nursing Interventions	Rationales
Assess for pain, using a rating scale from 1–10.	
Administer prescribed analgesics at regular intervals, especially prior to coughing, turning, and/or mobility exercises.	Pain will interfere with coughing, turning, and progressive mobility. Patient may attempt rapid, shallow breathing to splint the lower chest and avoid movement of the chest tubes, which will impair ventilation.
Provide splinting to chest tube area when encouraging patient to cough and deep breath to lessen muscle pull and pain as patient coughs.	
Encourage abdominal breathing.	
Place rolled towel around chest tube to prevent pulling when assisting patient to turn or move.	
Make sure chest tubes are adequately taped to patient's chest.	

NURSING DIAGNOSIS: IMPAIRED PHYSICAL MOBILITY

Related To
- Chest tubes
- Pain
- Fatigue

Defining Characteristics
Reluctance to move
Requests for assistance to move
Limited range of motion in arm and shoulder on the side of the chest tubes
Complaints of pain with movement

Patient Outcomes
Patient will
- exhibit full range of motion
- require minimal or no assistance
- state minimal pain with movement

Nursing Interventions	Rationales
Medicate for pain 20–30 min prior to repositioning, exercise, and/or ambulation.	
Assist with passive range-of-motion exercises to the arm and shoulder on the side of the chest tubes, beginning the evening of chest tube insertion.	
Encourage active range-of-motion exercises two to three times daily beginning the first day after chest tube insertion (e.g., rotate shoulder 360°, hunch shoulder).	
Assist with repositioning every 2 hr and ambulate as ordered. Patient may ambulate with chest tubes in place as long as the water seal remains below the level of the chest.	
Promote rest periods between exercises and ambulation.	

NURSING DIAGNOSIS: KNOWLEDGE DEFICIT—CHEST TUBE REMOVAL AND HOME CARE

Related To lack of exposure to information

Defining Characteristics

Expressions of fear and lack of knowledge regarding chest tube removal and home care management

Asking questions about chest tube removal and home care management

Patient Outcomes

Patient will

- verbalize an understanding of the chest tube removal procedure.
- describe care at home.

Nursing Interventions	Rationales
Explain chest tube removal procedure: 1. Patient placed in semi-Fowler's or side position. 2. Instruct to take a deep breath and hold or perform a gentle Valsalva maneuver. Do not inhale; inspiration may result in pneumothorax. 3. Chest tube suture is clipped and chest tube quickly removed. 4. May experience burning, pain, and/or pulling on removal. Medication for pain is usually given prior to removal of tubes. 5. Pressure dressing with petroleum gauze or antibiotic ointment is placed over site and sealed with tape. 6. Rate of respirations, quality of breath sounds, and chest tube dressing are assessed frequently.	
Explain the need to continue to do coughing and deep breathing and range-of-motion exercises after discharge.	

Nursing Interventions	Rationales
Encourage to avoid exposure to smoke and air pollution. If patient smokes, explain the importance of not smoking. Provide information on smoking cessation as needed.	Irritation to the lungs can cause bronchoconstriction resulting in an irritating cough with a rapid shallow respiratory rate.
Encourage to increase activity level gradually avoiding strenuous activity or exercise until recommended by physician.	
Instruct to report the following to the physician: 1. upper respiratory infection 2. elevated temperature 3. cough 4. difficulty breathing 5. sudden sharp chest pain 6. any redness, pain, swelling, or tenderness at the puncture site	

▼

DISCHARGE PLANNING/CONTINUITY OF CARE

- Assure understanding of self-management plan.
- Arrange follow-up with physicians for continued management postdischarge.
- Assist patient in obtaining prescriptions and establishing a plan for refilling prescriptions.
- Refer patient to a home health agency if continued nursing care, teaching, or assistance with activities of daily living is needed.
- Arrange for home respiratory equipment from vendor if needed.

REFERENCES

Erickson, R. (1989). Chest drainage—Part two. *Nursing, 19*(6), 46–49.

Suddarth, D. (1991). *Manual of nursing practice* (5th ed). Philadelphia, PA: Lippincott.

Teplitz, L. (1991). Update: Are milking and stripping chest tubes necessary? *Focus on Critical Care, 18*(60), 506–511.

Thompson, J., McFarland, G., Hirsch, J., Tucker, S., & Bowers, A. (1989). *Mosby's manual of clinical nursing* (2nd ed). St. Louis, MO: Mosby.

Wilson, S. & Thompson, J. (1990). *Respiratory disorders.* St. Louis, MO: Mosby Year Book.

▼

CHRONIC OBSTRUCTIVE PULMONARY DISEASE: ACUTE EXACERBATION

Ellen M. Jovle, RN, MS

The term chronic obstructive pulmonary disease (COPD) is used to describe a group of respiratory disorders. Emphysema and chronic bronchitis are the two most common disorders. The characteristic common to these disorders is an irreversible obstruction to air flow from the lungs. Emphysema is a loss of lung elasticity resulting in permanent enlargement of the distal air spaces and destruction of the alveolar capillary membrane. Chronic bronchitis is characterized by airway inflammation resulting in excessive mucus production. Although distinct processes, it is common for a patient to have a combination of both conditions.

ETIOLOGIES

- Cigarette smoking
- Exposure to environmental or occupational pollutants
- Inherited deficiency of $alpha_1$-antitrypsin resulting in destruction of lung elastin

CLINICAL MANIFESTATIONS

Emphysema
- General appearance: pink puffer
- Weight: thin, cachectic
- Dyspnea: severe, disabling
- Respiratory rate: tachypnea
- Cough minimal
- Sputum scanty
- Cyanosis absent
- Use of accessory muscles common
- Peripheral edema absent

- Chest exam: marked increase in anterior-posterior diameter, decreased breath sounds
- Blood gases: near normal, hypoxemia late in disease course
- Chest x-ray: hyperventilation, flat diaphragm, normal heart size, presence of bullae
- Pulmonary function tests
  - total lung capacity (TLC) increased
  - residual volume increased
  - functional residual capacity (FRC) increased
  - vital capacity (VC) increased
  - forced expiratory volume in one second of expiration (FEV_1) decreased
  - FEV_1 forced vital capacity (FVC) ratio decreased by less than 70%
  - forced midexpiratory flow rate (FEV 25–75%) decreased
  - diffusion capacity for carbon monoxide (DCO) increased
  - airway resistance (R_{aw}) increased
- Hemoglobin/hematocrit: normal, elevated in advanced disease
- Electrocardiogram (ECG): atrial and ventricular arrhythmias common

Chronic Bronchitis

- General appearance: blue bloater
- Weight: tendency toward obesity
- Dyspnea: variable, exertional
- Respiratory rate normal or slightly elevated
- Cough considerable
- Sputum copious, purulent
- Cyanosis often dramatic
- Use of accessory muscles less predominant than for emphysema
- Peripheral edema present
- Chest exam: may have some degree of barrel chest, prominent ronchi, scattered rales, variable wheezing
- Blood gases: hypercapnea, hypoxemia, respiratory acidosis
- Chest x-ray: cardiac enlargment, normal or flattened diaphragm, congested lung fields, evidence of chronic inflammation
- Pulmonary function tests
  - TLC normal or slightly increased
  - residual volume increased
  - FRC normal or increased
  - VC decreased
  - FEV_1 decreased
  - FEV_1/FVC ratio decreased to below 70%
  - FEV 25–75% decreased
  - DCO normal
  - R_{aw} increased
- Hemoglobin/hematocrit increased
- Electrocardiogram: evidence of right ventricular hypertrophy, atrial and ventricular arrhythmias

Clinical Clip

NOTE: Cyanosis is not always a sensitive indication of hypoxia. The appearance of cyanosis depends on the thickness of pigment of the skin, peripheral blood flow, and amount of hemoglobin (Hg) present. Purplish color does not occur until 5 mg of the Hg/100 mL is not bound to oxygen. A patient with polycythemia may be cyanotic without being hypoxic.

OTHER PLANS OF CARE TO REFERENCE

Corticosteriod Therapy

▼

NURSING DIAGNOSIS: INEFFECTIVE BREATHING PATTERN

Related To

- Anxiety
- Respiratory muscle fatigue

Defining Characteristics

Dyspnea
Use of accessory muscles
Tachypnea
Prolonged expiration
Assumption of tripod position
Pulsus paradox
Gasping speech pattern
Paradoxical motion of abdomen
Asynchronous chest wall movement

Patient Outcomes

Patient will

- report a decrease in dyspnea.
- exhibit respiratory rate, rhythm, and depth within normal for this patient.
- use diaphragmatic and pursed-lip breathing.
- breathe using synchronous chest wall and abdominal movement.

Nursing Interventions	Rationales
Monitor respiratory status. Assessments include respiratory rate, depth, and rhythm, use of accessory muscles, chest wall, and abdominal movement, and inspiratory-to-expiratory ratio.	Rapid, shallow respirations, increased use of accessory muscles, asynchronous chest wall movement, paradoxical abdominal movement, and prolonged expiration reflect increasing respiratory difficulty. These observations may indicate respiratory muscle fatigue and impending respiratory failure.
Assess dyspnea level using a rating scale such as a modified Borg scale or visual analog scale. (See Tables 19.1 and 19.2.)	Dyspnea is a subjective sensation of breathlessness. A rating scale provides a measure which can be used to determine baseline level, detect changes with treatment or activities, and provide a consistent method of reporting.
Assess for cardiovascular indices of hypoxemia and hypercapnea: tachycardia, abnormal pulse rhythm, elevated blood pressure, and pulsus paradox.	Pulsus paradox is an exaggeration of the usual fall in systolic pressure during inspiration. A >10 mmHg drop in systolic blood pressure between inspiration and expiration is a sign of increased respiratory effort.
Assist patient into semi or high Fowler's position to maximize use of respiratory muscles. Support the arms to relieve nonventilatory work of respiratory muscles. Assist to forward-leaning position which promotes expansion of the thorax.	
Assist and encourage patient to use pursed-lip and diaphragmatic breathing.	These techniques decrease the work of breathing by preventing airway collapse on expiration and increasing effective use of the diaphragm and abdominal muscles.

▼

NURSING DIAGNOSIS: FEAR/ANXIETY

Related To

- Acute episodes of breathlessness
- Loss of control
- Threat of death

Table 19.1 • Modified Borg Scale for Rating Shortness of Breath

Numerical Rating	Amount of Shortness of Breath
0	Nothing at all
0.5	Very, very slight (just noticeable)
1	Very slight
3	Moderate
4	Somewhat severe
5	Severe
6	
7	Very severe
8	
9	Very, very severe (almost maximal)
10	Maximal

▼

Defining Characteristics

Apprehension, tension, helplessness
Distress, uncertainty
Feelings of inadequacy
Overexcitedness, jitters
Increased heart rate, palpitations, elevated blood pressure
Increased respiratory rate, increased dyspnea
Trembling
Diaphoresis
Facial tension

Table 19.2 • Visual Analog Scale for Rating Shortness of Breath

How much shortness of breath are you having right now? Please indicate by marking the line. If you are not experiencing any shortness of breath at present, circle the marker at the left end of the line.

|— —|

No shortness of breath	Shortness of breath as bad as can be

▼

Patient Outcomes

Patient will

- use pursed-lip breathing and diaphragmatic breathing during episodes of breathlessness.
- verbalize emotional response to episodes of breathlessness.
- report a decrease in frequency and severity of acute episodes of dyspnea.
- report an increased level of control.
- report decrease in fear and anxiety levels.

Nursing Interventions	Rationales
Assess for level of anxiety and reasons for fear.	Anxiety may range from mild to severe. The level of anxiety guides nursing interventions.
Assess for nonverbal cues of anxiety and fear.	During acute breathlessness patient may be unable to verbalize anxiety and fear but may reveal nonverbal responses.
During severe panic levels of anxiety: 1. Stay with the patient. 2. Acknowledge patients fear, anxiety and helplessness. 3. Demonstrate respect for the seriousness of the episode. 4. Reinforce your ability to help and attend. 5. Accept level of dyspnea for what patient says it is. 6. Do not attempt to distract patient from breathing. 7. Be aware of your own anxiety and avoid transferring to patient. 8. Avoid use of empty phrases such as "try to relax" or "try to get in control." 9. Demonstrate breathing techniques that patient can imitate rather than attempting to talk patient through technique. 10. Respect need for increase of personal space. 11. Take charge of the environment and control traffic level of activity and noise.	

Nursing Interventions	Rationales
When anxiety levels have decreased: 1. Encourage discussion of acute episode, what helped and what did not. 2. Teach patient use of anxiety/fear reducing techniques: pursed-lip breathing (see Table 19.3), diaphragmatic breathing (see Table 19.4), relaxation techniques, and calming self-talk. 3. Assist patient in identifying common antecedents to episodes of, dyspnea, strategies to prevent episodes, and effect of anxiety on breathing. 4. Encourage patient to discuss behaviors that would be helpful during breathlessness episode with family.	Learning and problem solving can only take place when anxiety level is reduced to mild or moderate level. These techniques have shown to reduce anxiety and dyspnea in patients with COPD. Family members often feel helpless and anxious. Learning how to be helpful and supportive in future episodes will assist in reducing patient's and family's anxiety.

▼

NURSING DIAGNOSIS: IMPAIRED GAS EXCHANGE

Related To low ventilation-to-perfusion ratio.

Defining Characteristics

Hypoxemia
Hypercapnea
Decreased cognitive ability
Confusion, disorientation
Drowsiness, mental fatigue, somnolence
Euphoria, unruly or combative behavior, restlessness, irritability

Patient Outcomes

The patient will demonstrate improved gas exchange, as evidenced by

- absence of neurological signs of hypoxemia and/or hypercapnea
- $PaO_2 > 60$ mmHg
- $SaO_2 > 90\%$
- $PaCO_2$ at baseline (typically less than 50 mmHg)
- arterial pH within normal range

Table 19.3 • Patient Teaching Guide: Pursed-Lip Breathing

1. Hold a tissue: one corner in each hand, about 18 inches from your mouth.
2. Breathe in slowly through your nose. Be sure to breathe through your nose to avoid gulping air.
3. Breathe out slowly through puckered (pursed) lips, as if you were going to whistle or give someone a kiss.
4. Try to make the tissue ripple and float gently, not flap.
5. Use pursed-lip breathing whenever you feel short of breath.

▼

Table 19.4 • Patient Teaching Guide: Abdominal (Diaphragmatic) Breathing

1. Lie on your back in a comfortable position (can also sit or stand).
2. Rest one hand on your abdomen just below your rib cage and rest the other hand on your chest.
3. Slowly breathe in. Focus using your abdominal muscle; the hand resting on your abdomen should rise.
4. Slowly breathe out through your mouth (can use pursed lips). The hand on your abdomen should fall.
5. The hand on your chest should be almost still.
6. Practice this type of breathing several times a day until it becomes second nature. Use it also whenever you feel short of breath.

▼

Nursing Interventions	Rationales
Monitor arterial blood gases and report results as indicated.	A deterioration in respiratory status is reflected in ABG measurements. A $PaO_2 < 50$ mmHg and $PaCO_2 > 50$ mmHg indicate respiratory failure and a need for further intervention such as intubation and mechanical ventilation.
Monitor SaO_2 by oximetry as indicated by patient's condition.	Use of oximetry is a noninvasive method to monitor SaO_2 in order to rapidly detect hypoxemia and guide therapy. The SaO_2 does not reflect $PaCO_2$ which may increase with initiation of oxygen.

Nursing Interventions	Rationales
Administer low-flow oxygen therapy generally 1–3 L/min.	Administration of excessive levels of oxygen can result in removal of hypoxic drive to breath in patients who are chronic carbon dioxide (CO_2) retainers, causing CO_2 narcosis and respiratory failure. Chronic CO_2 retention is reflected in Pa_{CO_2} levels that are elevated, a normal pH, and an elevated bicarbonate (HCO_3) level. Acute CO_2 retention is reflected by an increased Pa_{CO_2} level with a normal HCO_3 and decreased pH.
Avoid use of medications which are respiratory depressants or beta blockers.	Further depression of ventilation can lead to respiratory failure. Beta blockers can lead to bronchospasm by blocking (beta$_2$) β_2 receptor.
Administer pharmacological agents as prescribed, including	
1. inhaled beta agonist by nebulizer or metered-dose inhaler	Stimulation of β_2 receptors in the airways causes bronchodilatation. Inhaled form is preferred over oral form because of fewer systemic side effects. Beta agonists are the treatment for acute dyspnea because of rapid onset of action. Bronchodilatation is equivalent with delivery of medication by a nebulizer or metered-dose inhaler. In the patient who is in acute distress and unable to use a correct metered-dose technique, nebulization may be more effective.
2. inhaled anticholinergic agents	Anticholinergic agents are often used in combination with beta agonists for bronchodilatation.

Nursing Interventions	Rationales
3. theophylline preparations, oral or intravenous (IV); extended-release and rapid-acting forms	Use of theophylline preparations is controversial. There is a narrow therapeutic window with use of theophylline. Therapeutic levels are 10–20 µg/mL. Excessive dosages result in toxic side effects. Effects of theophylline are stimulation of mucous clearance, increase in diaphragm contractivity, stimulation of respiratory drive, and modest bronchodilatation.
4. corticosteroids, inhaled, oral or IV	Major effects in reduction is airway inflammation. Inhaled use decreases the numbers of systemic side effects.
5. antibiotics	Upper and lower respiratory infections are the most common cause of exacerbations of COPD.
Instruct patient/family on action, name, dose schedule, importance of adherence, side effects and long-term effects, of medication. (See also Corticosteroid Therapy for further interventions.)	
Instruct patient/family in correct technique for using metered-dose inhaler including sequencing of medications (beta agonist, then anticholinergics if prescribed, then steroids). (See Table 19.5.)	
Teach patient/family early signs of impaired gas exchange and when to call physician.	

Nursing Interventions	Rationales
Teach patient/family use of home oxygen therapy. Consult respiratory therapist and discharge planner to assist with instruction as needed. Include information on 1. available vendors in area and available systems (gaseous, concentrator, liquid) 2. Use and care of equipment 3. danger of excessive levels 4. safety precautions	

▼

NURSING DIAGNOSIS: INEFFECTIVE AIRWAY CLEARANCE

Related To

- Excessive and/or tenacious mucous production
- Ineffective cough
- Respiratory infection

Defining Characteristics

Abnormal breath sounds
Tachypnea, dyspnea
Uncontrolled nonproductive cough

Patient Outcomes

Patient will be able to cough effectively and expectorate secretions without excessive fatigue.

Table 19.5 • Patient Teaching Guide: Use Of Metered-Dose Inhaler

1. Shake the canister vigorously to mix the medication.
2. Tilt your head back slightly to create a straighter airway.
3. Hold the canister mouthpiece 1–1½ inches in front of your mouth. As an option, the mouthpiece can also be positioned in the mouth just inside your lips. DO NOT close your lips around the mouthpiece. Always leave your mouth open.
4. Exhale completely through pursed lips.
5. As you begin, take a slow deep breath while counting to 5, squeeze the inhaler to release the medication on the count of 2.
6. Try to H-O-L-D your breath for 5–10 s before exhaling.
7. After using steroid inhaler, rinse your mouth with water to avoid a yeast infection.

▼

Nursing Interventions	Rationales
Evaluate effectiveness of cough.	
Auscultate lungs for ronchi, crackles, or wheezing.	
Assess sputum for amount, color, consistency, and odor to detect the presence of infection.	
Maintain hydration by oral or IV fluids at 2–3 L/day, unless contraindicated.	
Provide local hydration of airways by humidification or nebulization to avoid drying of secretions.	
Administer prescribed medications, which may include	
1. bronchodilators	Bronchodilatation facilitates secretion clearance.
2. mucolytics	Effect of these drugs is to thin mucous and promote ciliary action.
3. antibiotics	
Assist and teach patient to cough and deep breathe (see Table 19.6):	
1. Position in high Fowler's positions.	
2. Perform maximal inspiration and expiration through pursed lips.	
3. Exert external pressure against abdomen in upward inward motion with pillow or arms (quad cough).	Quad cough supports use of abdominal muscles and the diaphragm during expiratory phase.
4. Huff cough forced expiratory effort with an open glottis. Say the word "huff."	Huff coughing is thought to prevent collapse of small airways, which occurs in cough with closed glottis.

Nursing Interventions	Rationales
Perform chest physiotherapy if secretions are greater than 30 mL/day. Monitor SaO_2 during treatment.	Chest physiotherapy is only of benefit if secreting greater than 30 mL/day. Hypoxia is a common adverse reaction to chest physiotherapy.
Teach patient/family techniques to avoid infections and environmental irritants, maintain adequate hydration, cough effectively, and perform chest physiotherapy.	
Instruct patient/family in need for pneumovax and influenza vaccine.	The pneumococcal vaccine provides protection from 23 of the most common organisms and is administered only once. The influenza vaccine is given every fall. These are important measures in preventing respiratory infections.
Teach patient/family to avoid cough suppressants and antihistamines.	Cough is a protective mechanism to maintain airway clearance; antihistamines dry secretions.

▼

Table 19.6 • Patient Teaching Guide: Controlled Coughing

When you feel a cough coming on, you can follow these steps:

1. Sit in a chair with your chin slightly bent toward your chest.
2. Place a pillow in your lap to help support your stomach muscles. If a pillow is not available, cross your arms over your stomach.
3. It is important to cough using small, short huffs rather than big blasts of air. It might help to say the word "huff" as you cough. Coughing forcefully can collapse small air sacs in the lungs.
4. Always keep your mouth open when you cough.
5. Take a deep, slow breath through your nose and hold it for a few seconds.
6. Cough once (to loosen mucus).
7. Cough a second time (to move mucus forward). Spit mucus into a tissue. Swallowing mucus can upset your stomach.
8. Avoid taking a big deep breath after coughing as this might cause an uncontrolled cough and drive mucus back in. Breathe in gently through your nose.

▼

NURSING DIAGNOSIS: ACTIVITY INTOLERANCE

Related To
- Fatigue
- Hypoxemia
- Physical deconditioning

Defining Characteristics

Increased dyspnea with usual activities
Inability to perform usual activities
Complaints of weakness
Decreased SaO_2 with activity/exertion
Increased respiratory rate, increased use of accessory muscles, and increased inspiratory-to-expiratory ratio with activity
Excessive increase or decrease in heart rate with activity
Decreased or failure to increase blood pressure with activity

Patient Outcomes

Patient will
- verbalize increased energy, less fatigue, and weakness with activities.
- increase activity level to baseline.
- demonstrate less dyspnea with usual activities.
- maintain SaO_2 above 88% with activity.
- demonstrate increase in blood pressure and normal increase in heart rate with activity.

Nursing Interventions	Rationales
Assess patient's response to activity, SaO_2 levels, pulse rate and rhythm, respiratory rate, and dyspnea rating.	These measures are used to determine the need for supplemental O_2 during activity.
Determine patient's baseline activity level prior to admission. How far can patient walk without stopping due to dyspnea? Have patient describe activities of an average day to establish realistic activity goals.	
Determine if causes of activity intolerance are other than pulmonary-related factors, such as depression, fear, and lack of knowledge.	

Nursing Interventions	Rationales
Perform activities for patient until he or she is able to perform them, especially those activities requiring use of upper extremities.	Upper extremity use places additional nonventilatory demands on respiratory muscles and provokes severe dyspnea. Arm endurance is shorter than leg endurance. Consequently, seemingly simple tasks such as cutting meat may be more difficult for patient with COPD than walking to and from bathroom.
Provide progressive increase in activity as tolerated.	Patients with COPD may be so afraid of dyspnea that they actually need to be "desensitized" to their dyspnea by exposing them to small levels at first beginning and increasing levels over time.
Provide upper extremity support during activities requiring use of arms.	Arm support during upper extremity activities reduces metabolic and ventilatory demand.
Provide oxygen as needed during activities based on SaO_2 measurements.	Supplement oxygen will increase tolerance for activity in patient who desaturates ($SaO_2 < 88\%$) with activity.
Administer and teach use of inhaled beta agonist 30–60 min prior to initiating activity.	Most inhaled beta agonists show peak bronchodilation 30–60 min after administration.
Encourage and teach the use of pursed-lip breathing and diaphragmatic breathing during activity. Emphasize that work is performed during exhalation. For example, when climbing stairs, step up while exhaling through pursed lips and rest to inhale before taking next step.	Inhaling before doing work ensures optimal oxygenation of tissues during the work.
Teach patient/family work simplification techniques to conserve energy, thereby decreasing oxygen requirement during activities.	

▼

NURSING DIAGNOSIS: SLEEP PATTERN DISTURBANCE

Related To

- Anxiety
- Depression
- Cough
- Dyspnea
- Stimulant effects of medications

Defining Characteristics

Complaints of insomnia, frequent awakening, inability to fall asleep
Reports of fatigue, not feeling rested
Changes in behavior or performance

Patient Outcomes

Patient will

- report improved sleep pattern.
- report feelings of being rested.

Nursing Interventions	Rationales
Identify usual sleep patterns and difficulties.	
Explore with patient causative factors of sleep disturbance such as symptoms of depression.	Antidepressants can significantly improve sleep in patients with depression.
Observe patient for signs and symptoms of sleep apnea including noisy snoring with or without apnea, morning headaches, and abnormal movement during sleep.	Sleep apnea may cause insomnia as well as nocturnal hypoxemia. A definitive diagnosis may require sleep studies.
Assess for symptoms of gastroesophageal reflux, chest pain, heartburn, regurgitation, nocturnal cough, and dyspnea.	There is a high incidence of gastroesophageal reflux disease in patients with respiratory disorders. Reflux results in bronchospasm and chronic aspiration. Theophylline preparations can exacerbate gastroesophageal reflux.
Assess SaO_2 during sleep.	Patients with COPD may not be able to tolerate decrease in tidal volume that occurs with sleep.

Nursing Interventions	Rationales
Encourage patient to verbalize emotional response to sleep disturbance.	Fear of insomnia can perpetuate sleepless cycle.
Administer O_2 therapy at night as prescribed.	The already hypoxemic COPD patient cannot tolerate any further decrease in PaO_2 levels which normally occur during sleep. Hypoxemia causes pulmonary vasoconstriction which can precipitate or exacerbate cor pulmonale.
Consult physician about scheduling evening doses of medications such as extended-release theophylline prior to 5 p.m. to minimize stimulant effects during sleep.	
Assist and instruct patient in performing bronchial hygiene measures prior to retiring.	
Identify and instruct patients in methods of relaxation.	
Avoid and teach patient to avoid respiratory depressants such as sedatives and alcohol before bedtime.	

▼

NURSING DIAGNOSIS: ALTERED NUTRITION—LESS THAN BODY REQUIREMENTS

Related To

- Work of breathing
- Depression
- Inability to prepare or procure food

Defining Characteristics

Body weight < 20% of ideal
Reports of early satiety, bloating, and/or decreased appetite
Muscle wasting, weakness
Poor skin integrity

Patient Outcomes

Patient will

- increase body weight to within 10% of ideal.
- report less dyspnea during meals.
- maintain adequate caloric and nutritional intake.

Nursing Interventions	Rationales
Monitor patient's weight and nutritional intake daily.	Metabolic demands may increase during a period of COPD exacerbation. Daily assessment detects need for dietary intervention.
Assess psychological factors such as depression that might decrease food intake.	
Monitor serum albumin, total lymphocyte count, and transferrin levels.	Protein calorie malnutrition is common among patients with COPD and is reflected in a decrease in visceral protein synthesis.
Assess dyspnea level during meals. Monitor SaO_2 during meals if indicated.	The act of eating requires energy, and patient may become hypoxemic during meals.
Survey patient's medications for drug which may contribute to anorexia. Discuss potential problems with physician.	Theophylline preparation and antibiotics are common drugs administered to COPD patients which may cause anorexia and gastrointestinal upset.
Obtain dietary consultation as soon as diagnosis is established to determine caloric requirement and devise meal plan which considers patient's preferences and dietary restrictions.	Early dietary consultation can prevent further complications from malnutrition. A direct correlation exists between nutritional status and respiratory muscle function.
Use supplemental O_2 during meal times as prescribed.	Relief of hypoxemia may reduce dyspnea.
Provide frequent small meals of softer food. Administer nutritional supplements as indicated.	Smaller meals may decrease problems with early satiety and bloating. Soft foods require less energy to chew. Supplements will provide condensed source of calories in liquid form.
Provide a high-protein, low-carbohydrate diet. Avoid gas-forming foods.	Metabolism of carbohydrates produces more carbon dioxide than metabolism of protein. Gas-forming foods may contribute to bloating and early satiety and hamper use of diaphragm.

Nursing Interventions	Rationales
Assist and teach patient to perform bronchial hygiene measures prior to meals. Administer inhaled bronchodilator if indicated.	Ensures maximum bronchodilatation during meals.
Assist patient with development of a plan to monitor adequate intake postdischarge.	
Teach patient/family: 1. importance of adequate nutrition 2. monitoring weight daily 3. use of oxygen during meals 4. use of supplements 5. bronchial hygiene measures and use of bronchodilator before meals 6. available community resources	

▼

DISCHARGE PLANNING/CONTINUITY OF CARE

- Assure patient's understanding and ability to continue care at home.
- Arrange for home oxygen supplies from vendor of patient's choice.
- Refer patient to a home health care agency if continued nursing care or assistance with activities of daily living is needed.
- Arrange follow-up with physician for continued management.
- Assist patient in obtaining prescriptions and establishing a plan for refilling prescriptions.
- Provide patients with information on support groups, smoking cessation, or pulmonary rehabilitation programs in the area.

REFERENCES

Breslin, E. H. (1992). Dyspnea-limited response in chronic obstructive pulmonary disease: Reduced unsupported arm activities. *Rehabilitation Nursing*, *17*(1), 12–20.

DeVito, A. J. (1990). Dyspnea during hospitalizations for acute phase of illness as recalled by patients with chronic obstructive pulmonary disease. *Heart & Lung*, *19*(2), 186–191.

Dougherty, S. (1988). The malnourished respiratory patient. *Critical Care Nurse*, *8*(4), 13–15, 18–22.

Gift, A. G., Moore, T. G., Soeken, K. (1992). Relaxation to reduce dyspnea and anxiety in COPD patients. *Nursing Research*, *41*(4), 242–246.

Nesse, R. E. (1992). Pharmacologic treatment of COPD. *Postgraduate Medicine* *91*(1), 71–84.

▼

PLEURAL EFFUSION

Ellen M. Jovle, RN, MS

Pleural effusion is the accumulation of excess fluid in the pleural space. Normally the space between the parietal and visceral pleurae contains less than 10 mL of serous fluid. The balance between hydrostatic and colloidal osmotic pressure maintains the rate of pleural fluid production and rate of its removal in balance. Pleural effusion occurs when the rate of fluid production exceeds the rate of its removal. Pleural effusion is rarely a primary disease. It occurs as a secondary problem when one of the following mechanisms is present: increased systemic hydrostatic pressure, as in congestive heart failure; increased capillary permeability, as with trauma or inflammation; decreased rate of removal because of lymphatic obstruction, as in malignancy; decreased colloid osmotic pressure, as in hypoalbuminemia which occurs in liver disease; and increased intrapleural negative pressure, as in atelectasis.

ETIOLOGIES

- Pulmonary infections or infarction
- Malignancies
- Rheumatoid arthritis
- Cardiac or chest surgery
- Systemic lupus erythematous
- Subphrenic infection
- Lung abscess
- Congestive heart failure
- Renal failure
- Liver failure
- Myxedema
- Chest trauma
- Atelectasis
- Peritoneal dialysis
- Pancreatitis
- Esophageal perforation

CLINICAL MANIFESTATIONS

- Dyspnea
- Dry, nonproductive cough
- Reduced chest wall movement on affected side
- Mediastinal shift toward contralateral side
- Pleuritic pain when inflammation present
- Dullness to percussion which shifts with change in position
- Decreased or absent breath sounds over affected area
- Fever present with infection and inflammation
- Tachycardia and hypotension with loss of fluid into pleural space

CLINICAL/DIAGNOSTIC FINDINGS

- Chest x-ray: Fluid accumulation of more than 200 mL is detected on usual posteroanterior and lateral chest films. Lateral decubitus films show much smaller amounts of fluid.
- Ultrasound: if chest x-rays are inconclusive.
- Blood gases: hypoxemia.
- Pleural fluid analysis: Done to diagnose cause of effusion. Common tests include stain, culture and sensitivity, cytologic examination, protein, red and white blood cell (RBC, WBC) counts, amylase, lactic dehydrogenase (LDH), specific gravity, glucose, cholesterol, triglycerides, antinuclear antibody (ANA) titers, and pH.

OTHER PLANS OF CARE TO REFERENCE

- Chest tubes
- Thoracentesis

▼

NURSING DIAGNOSIS: INEFFECTIVE BREATHING PATTERN

Related To decreased expansion of lungs due to fluid accumulation and/or pleuritic pain

Defining Characteristics

Dyspnea
Tachypnea
Shallow respirations
Decreased chest wall movement
Verbalizations of pain with coughing and deep breathing

Patient Outcomes

Patient will exhibit

- decrease in dyspnea

- respiratory rate and depth within normal limits for patient
- absence of complications of atelectasis and pneumonia
- coughing and deep breathing effectively

Nursing Interventions	**Rationales**
Assess patient's respiratory status, including rate, depth of respirations, and chest wall movement. Note respiratory effort, including use of accessory muscle and intercostal retractions.	
Auscultate lungs. Note areas of decreased/absent airflow and adventitious breath sounds.	Decreased airflow occurs in areas compressed by effusion. Adventitious sounds detect areas of atelectasis or retained secretions.
Assess for pain.	Splinting or guarding of affected area decreases effectiveness of breathing pattern and may prevent patient from coughing and deep breathing.
Elevate head of bed and assist patient in changing positions frequently.	
Administer analgesic as prescribed. Monitor effect on respirations.	Analgesics may depress respirations.
Assist patient in cough and deep-breathing exercises. Splint chest when performing exercises.	Facilitates lung expansions. Splinting chest reduces pain.
Maintain patency of chest tubes, if present (see Chest Tubes, p. 193.)	Promotes removal of fluid from pleural space and expansion of lung.
Teach patient importance of regular coughing and deep breathing. Demonstrate effective techniques. Encourage use of blow bottles or incentive spirometry.	
Instruct patient/family in signs of pleural effusion and symptoms to report if pleural effusion is a recurrent problem.	

▼

NURSING DIAGNOSIS: IMPAIRED GAS EXCHANGE

Related To

- Low ventilation to perfusion rates
- Intrapulmonary shunting
- Hypoventilation

Defining Characteristics

Dyspnea
Hypoxemia
Decreased or absent breath sounds over effusion
Tachycardia
Restlessness/changes in mentation

Patient Outcomes

Patient will demonstrate

- absence of signs and symptoms of hypoxemia
- normal breath sounds
- arterial blood gases within patients normal limits

Nursing Interventions	Rationales
Monitor arterial blood gases and arterial oxygen saturation (SaO_2) using oximetry.	Hypoxemia may be present due to areas of decreased or absent alveolar ventilation. Carbon dioxide levels may also be elevated if hypoventilation is the primary etiology.
Observe for signs and symptoms of hypoxemia. Assess mental status. Monitor heart rate and rhythm, and assess color of skin, mucous membranes, and nail beds.	
Monitor hemoglobin and hematocrit.	Determines amount of hemoglobin present to carry oxygen to the tissues. Hematocrit detects blood loss into pleural space.
Maintain decreased level of activity. Pace activities as patient tolerates. Monitor response to activity including respiratory rate, heart rate, blood pressure, and SaO_2.	Reduces oxygen demands and detects need for supplemental oxygen with activity.

Nursing Interventions	Rationales
Administer oxygen as prescribed.	Corrects hypoxemia due to low ventilation to perfusion ratio.
Anticipate possible thoracentesis or chest tube insertion as treatment methods. Explain procedure to patient. Assist physician and patient with procedure.	

NURSING DIAGNOSIS: HIGH RISK FOR DECREASED CARDIAC OUTPUT

Risk Factors

- Hypovolemia secondary to loss of blood or fluid into the pleural space
- Rapid reperfusion of pulmonary blood vessels when too much fluid is pulled out of pleural space too rapidly

Patient Outcomes

Patient will demonstrate

- normal pulses and blood pressure
- normal urine output
- normal breath sounds
- normal skin color and temperature
- normal mentation

Nursing Interventions	Rationales
Monitor blood pressure, heart rate, peripheral pulses, skin color and temperature, mental status, and urinary output.	
Monitor quantity, color, and characteristics of chest tube drainage.	
Clamp chest tube, as ordered, to avoid pulmonary edema.	Lung tissue and pulmonary blood vessels have been compressed with large pleural effusion. To ensure gradual reperfusion, the chest tube may be clamped after 1 L of fluid is drained and repeated according to patient's condition and physician preference.

Nursing Interventions	Rationales
Anticipate need for fluid volume replacement if signs and symptoms of hypovolemia are present.	

▼

NURSING DIAGNOSIS: FEAR/ANXIETY

Related To
- Change in health status
- Uncertainty of diagnosis and outcome
- Insufficient knowledge of diagnostic and therapeutic procedures

Defining Characteristics
Expressed concern about health status
Expressed fearfulness, uncertainty, apprehension
Increased muscle tension
Inability to relax
Signs and symptoms of insomnia
Sympathetic stimulation

Patient Outcomes
The patient and family will
- acknowledge and discuss fears and anxiety.
- appear relaxed.
- verbalize understanding of disease process and diagnostic and therapeutic procedures.

Nursing Interventions	Rationales
Observe physical responses indicating anxiety and fear.	
Assess current level of understanding of diagnosis, treatment plan, and potential outcomes.	
Encourage expression and discussion of fear and anxiety and assist patient/family in identifying source of anxiety. Acknowledge and validate patient's anxiety and fears.	

Nursing Interventions	Rationales
Accept patient's use of anxiety-reducing behaviors such as acting out, withdrawal, and somatizing. Do not reinforce behaviors. Understand and help patient to identify feelings and meaning behind behavior.	These are mechanisms the patient is using to cope with the situation and perceived threat.
Provide opportunity for questions. Assist patient/family in asking questions of physicians.	
Explain anticipated procedures and treatment including the purpose, process, and sensations patient will experience. Reinforce physician explanations of procedure and treatments.	
Involve patient and family in planning of care.	May decrease feeling of powerlessness and loss of control.
Assist patient and family in assessing effectiveness of current coping behavior, exploring other behaviors that may be more effective. NOTE: Other diagnosis will need to be individualized depending on the cause of the pleural effusion and medical treatments.	

DISCHARGE PLANNING/CONTINUITY OF CARE

- Assure patient understanding and ability to perform self-care at home.
- Arrange medical follow-up.
- Assist in obtaining prescriptions.
- Refer to home health care agency if ongoing nursing care is required.
- Arrange hospice care as appropriate.
- Provide information on cancer, arthritis, or lupus community resources or support groups.

REFERENCES

Connor, P., Berg, P., Flaherty, N., Klem, L., Lawton, R., & Tremblay, M. (1989). Two stages of care for pleural effusion. *RN, 52*(2), 30–34.

Light, R. W. (1992). Pleural diseases. *Disease-a-Month, 28*(5), 263–331.
Lutz, M. M. (1991). Getting the facts on pleural effusion. *Nursing 91, 21*(3), 32S–32T.
Wilson, S. F. & Thompson, J. M. (1990). *Respiratory disorders.* St. Louis, MO: Mosby.

▼

PNEUMONIA

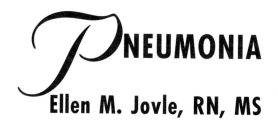

Ellen M. Jovle, RN, MS

Pneumonia is an inflammatory process affecting the lung parenchyma. Pneumonia is the most common lethal infection in the United States, ranking sixth among all disease categories as cause of death. Types of pneumonia include lobar, which is consolidation of an entire lobe; bronchopneumonia, which is patchy distribution of consolidation around and involving bronchi; and interstitial pneumonia, which is involvement of alveoli walls. Pneumonia occurs when the respiratory defense mechanisms are impaired or are overwhelmed by the duration of exposure or the virulence of the infectious agent.

ETIOLOGIES (see Table 21.1)

- Bacteria: Most common cause of community-acquired pneumonias is gram-positive bacteria; gram-negative bacteria account for most hospital-acquired pneumonias
- Viruses: influenza, adenovirus, parainfluenza, respiratory and syncytial viruses
- Mycoplasma organisms: most common cause of atypical pneumonia
- Fungi: histoplasmosis, coccidioidomycosis, or blastomycosis
- Protozoa: *Pneumocystis carinii*

CLINICAL MANIFESTATIONS

- Fever, chills, headache, malaise
- Tachypnea
- Dyspnea
- Pleuritic chest pain
- Cough productive of abnormal amounts of sputum with change in color or odor
- Tachycardia
- Abnormal breath sounds such as crackles, pleural friction rub, or decreased sounds over area of consolidation

Table 21.1 • Factors Contributing to Development of Pneumonia

Loss of cough reflex
- Nasogastric tube
- Stroke
- Neuromuscular disease
- Anesthesia
- Sedation
- Conditions affecting level of consciousness

Impairment of mucociliary escalator mechanism
- Air pollution
- Cigarette smoking
- Normal changes of aging

Loss of nasopharyngeal defense mechanism
- Tracheal intubation
- Altered oropharyngeal flora

Altered resistance
- Malnutrition
- Alcoholism
- Debilitating illnesses
- Immunosuppression

▼

CLINICAL/DIAGNOSTIC FINDINGS

- Chest x-ray: presence of consolidation
- Sputum showing causative organism. Sputum is obtained by deep cough, intubation, transtracheal aspiration, bronchoscopy, or open lung biopsy.
- Elevated white blood cell count
- Arterial blood gases: hypoxemia
- Positive blood cultures if bacteremia present

Clinical Clip

Organisms reach the lung by aspiration of gastric contents or from naso- or oropharynx inhalation of microbes present in the air and by spread of organism from a primary infection elsewhere in the body.

▼

NURSING DIAGNOSIS: INEFFECTIVE AIRWAY CLEARANCE

Related To
- Pain
- Fatigue
- Increased sputum production

Defining Characteristics

Abnormal breath sounds
Dyspnea
Cough
Changes in rate or depth of respiration

Patient Outcomes

The patient will demonstrate

- normal breath sounds
- absence of dyspnea
- respiratory rate within patient's normal
- effective cough with expectoration of sputum

Nursing Interventions	Rationales
Assess patient's respiratory status, including rate and depth of respiration, presence of dyspnea, chest wall movement, use of accessory muscles, presence and effectiveness of cough, and quantity and quality of sputum.	
Auscultate lungs. Note areas of decreased or absent air movement and adventitious breath sounds.	Decreased airflow occurs in areas of consolidation. Adventitious sounds indicate accumulation of fluid, secretions, and airway constriction.
Assess for pain which may cause an avoidance of coughing and deep breathing.	
Assist patient to cough effectively by 1. administering analgesic before coughing 2. splinting the chest when coughing 3. elevating head of bed 4. encouraging deep inspiration and forceful abdominal contraction with cough	
Encourage use of blow bottles or incentive spirometer.	

Nursing Interventions	Rationales
Maintain hydration by oral or intravenous fluids. Intake of 2–3 L is optimum unless contraindicated.	Water is a natural expectorant. Patients with cardiac or renal disease may require a fluid restriction.
Maintain local hydration of airways by humidification or nebulization to avoid drying of secretions.	
Administer prescribed medications, which may include 1. bronchodilators to facilitate secretion clearance 2. mucolytics to thin mucus and promote ciliary action 3. antimicrobials to reduce infection	
Perform chest physiotherapy if secretions are greater than 30 mL/day. Monitor arterial oxygen saturation (SaO_2) using oximetry during treatment.	Hypoxemia may be a complication of chest physiotherapy.
Teach patient/family coughing and deep-breathing exercises and explain rationale. Discuss importance of adequate fluid intake.	

▼

NURSING DIAGNOSIS: IMPAIRED GAS EXCHANGE

Related To

- Low ventilation and perfusion ratio
- Intrapulmonary shunting
- Hypoventilation

Defining Characteristics

Hypercapnea
Restlessness/mentation changes
Irritability

Patient Outcomes

The patient will demonstrate

- absence of signs and symptoms of hypoxemia

- normal breath sounds
- normal mentation
- arterial blood gases within patient's normal limits

Nursing Interventions	Rationales
Observe patient for signs and symptoms of hypoxemia, including tachycardia, abnormal pulse rhythm, elevated blood pressure, mental status changes, and cyanosis.	
Monitor arterial blood gases or arterial oxygen saturation (SaO_2) using oximetry. Report changes from baseline values.	Hypoxemia may be present due to areas of decreased or absent alveolar ventilation. Arterial carbon dioxide ($PaCO_2$) may also be elevated if hypoventilation is present.
Administer oxygen as prescribed to correct hypoxia.	
Maintain bed rest during acute phase. Progressively increase activities as patient tolerates, monitoring patient's response to activity (respiratory rate, dyspnea level, SaO_2, heart rate, blood pressure).	Progressive activity reduces deconditioning. Monitoring response to activity detects hypoxia and need for supplemental oxygen.
Position patient to maintain ventilation and perfusion to nonaffected lung tissue. Monitor effect of position changes on arterial blood gases (ABGs) or pulse oximetry.	Hypoxemia may occur if affected lung is in a dependent position.
Reduce elevated temperature with antipyretics, tepid sponging, or hypothermia blankets.	High fever increases metabolic demands and oxygen consumption.

▼

NURSING DIAGNOSIS: HIGH RISK FOR INFECTION

Risk Factors

- Reduced host defenses
- Increased virulence of organism

Patient Outcomes

Patient will exhibit resolution of lung infection without dissemination of infection to other areas of the body.

Nursing Interventions	Rationales
Monitor for signs and symptoms of pleural effusion (see Pleural Effusion).	
Monitor for signs and symptoms of bacteremia and septic shock:	
1. early stage: bounding pulse, warm, flushed, dry skin, polyuria, hyperthermia, tachycardia	The early phase of septic shock ("warm" septic shock") is characterized by a high cardiac output in an initial response of the body to the increased metabolic demands. The key to recovery is early recognition and institution of prompt therapy.
2. sustained ("cold") septic shock: hypotension, cold, clammy skin, decreased level of consciousness, weak, rapid pulse, and oliguria.	Sustained septic shock results in decreased cardiac output. There is a less favorable outcome in this stage of septic shock.

▼

NURSING DIAGNOSIS: ALTERED NUTRITION—LESS THAN BODY REQUIREMENTS

Related To

- Anorexia
- Dyspnea
- Fatigue
- Increased metabolic rate secondary to infection

Defining Characteristics

Body weight <20% of ideal
Muscle wasting, weakness
Poor skin integrity
Aversion to eating
Loss of weight with adequate food intake

Patient Outcomes

The patient will

- increase or maintain body weight to within 10% of ideal.

- maintain adequate caloric intake.
- exhibit normal serum albumin, total lymphocyte count, and transferrin levels.

Nursing Interventions	Rationales
Evaluate nutritional status by assessing height and weight and caloric intake.	
Monitor serum albumin, total lymphocyte count, and transferrin levels.	Protein calorie malnutrition is reflected by a decrease in visceral protein synthesis.
Identify factors affecting intake such as food choices, dyspnea, unpleasant environment, decreased appetite, depression, and fatigue.	
Auscultate bowel sounds. Observe for abdominal distention.	Paralytic ileus can result from inactivity and debilitated condition. Air swallowing may cause abdominal distention.
Identify prescribed medications which may contribute to anorexia and/or gastrointestinal (GI) upset and discuss with physician.	Antibiotics are common drugs which cause anorexia and GI upset.
Provide oxygen during meal times as prescribed.	
Assist with oral hygiene prior to meals.	
Reduce negative environmental stimuli.	
Obtain dietary consultation if initial interventions are not effective. Administer nutritional supplements as indicated.	Supplements provide a condensed form of calories in liquid form.
Teach patient/family: 1. importance of adequate nutrition in recovery 2. measures to maintain nutritional status 3. available community resources 4. use of supplements	

▼

NURSING DIAGNOSIS: KNOWLEDGE DEFICIT—TREATMENT PLAN

Related To lack of prior exposure to information

Defining Characteristics

Requesting information

Patient Outcomes

Patient will be able to

- describe disease process.
- state how to prevent future infections.
- state how to prevent transmission.
- discuss treatment regimen after discharge.

Nursing Interventions	Rationales
Assess current level of knowledge, readiness, and ability to learn and retain information.	Patient's inability to perform self-care may necessitate a discharge referral for ongoing assistance.
Review pathophysiology of pneumonia, as appropriate.	
Review techniques for coughing and deep-breathing exercises and encourage continued use.	
Emphasize importance of continuing full course of antibiotic therapy to prevent relapse.	
Teach importance of using tissue when coughing, properly disposing of tissue, and frequent hand washing to prevent transmission of infection. Advise against contact with persons who are at high risk for infection.	
Encourage patient to balance rest and activity and maintain adequate nutrition and fluid intake to promote healing.	

Nursing Interventions	**Rationales**
Review importance of smoking cessation if appropriate.	Smoking decreases body's defense against infection.
Instruct patient/family to report dyspnea, weight loss, fever, chills, persistent productive cough, chest pain, and ongoing fatigue.	
Encourage patient to obtain pneumococcal and influenza vaccines.	The pneumoccocal vaccine provides protection from 23 of the most common pneumococcal organisms and is administered only once. Yearly influenza vaccines in the fall are recommended.

▼

DISCHARGE PLANNING/CONTINUITY OF CARE

- Assure patient understanding and ability to continue care at home.
- Assist in arranging medical follow-up.
- Assist in obtaining prescriptions and establishing plan for refilling prescriptions.
- Refer to a home health care agency if ongoing nursing care is required.
- Refer to public health department for vaccinations.
- Refer to smoking cessation programs in the area, if appropriate.

REFERENCES

Markowitz, S. M. (1990). Pneumococcal pneumonia. *Postgraduate Medicine, 88*(7), 33–47.

Messner, R. & Zink, K. (1992). Nosocomial pneumonia—Combating a hospital menace. *RN, 55*(6), 48–52.

Ramsey, K. M. (1990). Viral pneumonias. *Postgraduate Medicine, 88*(7), 49–56.

Stogner, S. W. & Anderson, W. (1990). Mycoplasmal pneumonia. *Postgraduate Medicine, 88*(7), 61–69.

Wilson, S. F. & Thompson, J. M. (1990). *Respiratory disorders.* St. Louis, MO: Mosby.

▼

TRACHEOSTOMY

Linda Wonoski, RN, MSN

A tracheostomy is used to provide long-term ventilatory support, to facilitate suctioning of trachobronchial secretions, and to bypass a respiratory obstruction. The tube is inserted into the trachea through an incision made at the level of the second or third tracheal ring, totally bypassing the upper airway.

ETIOLOGIES (INDICATIONS)

- Upper airway obstruction (tumor, foreign body, laryngeal spasm)
- Burns
- Infections
- Surgical edema
- Traumatic injuries (head, neck, chest wall)
- Neurological disorders
- Acute respiratory failure
- Pulmonary disorders

CLINICAL MANIFESTATIONS

- Dyspnea
- Tachypnea
- Increased work of breathing
- Decreased breath sounds
- Anxiety
- Tachycardia
- Partial airway obstruction with increasing respiratory distress: gurgling, snoring, stridorous ventilations
- Complete airway obstruction
  - conscious person: no breath sounds, signs of severe respiratory distress progressing to respiratory arrest, unable to speak
  - unconscious person: ventilation attempts that produce no chest movement, no expiratory air passing from the individual's airway

CLINICAL/DIAGNOSTIC FINDINGS

- Arterial blood gases that deviate from patient's baseline
- Abnormal chest x-ray

OTHER PLANS OF CARE TO REFERENCE

Nutrition support plans of care

▼

NURSING DIAGNOSIS: ANXIETY REGARDING RESPIRATORY DISTRESS AND KNOWLEDGE DEFICIT REGARDING NEED FOR TRACHEOSTOMY

Related To new experience

Defining Characteristics

Expression of anxiety about inability to breathe effectively
Asking many questions about tracheostomy

Patient Outcomes

Patient will

- state a decreased level of anxiety.
- verbalize an understanding of a tracheostomy.

Nursing Interventions	Rationales
Assess anxiety level and readiness to learn.	
Provide written and audiovisual teaching materials to supplement teaching.	
Review patient's individual reason for the tracheostomy and its particular purpose.	
Demonstrate and encourage handling of the tube and suctioning equipment.	

Nursing Interventions	Rationales
Review insertion procedure:	
1. surgical/sterile procedure after consent is obtained	Infection of the lower airway is a serious potential problem. Establishment of an artificial airway bypasses the normal defense mechanisms that prevent bacterial contamination of the lower airway.
2. positioning: supine with head extended to bring the trachea forward	Below this level the end of the tracheostomy tube can erode the innominate or right common carotid arteries and hemorrhage can occur.
3. medicated as prescribed	
4. incision made at the level of the second or third tracheal ring	
5. tracheostomy tube inserted and cuff inflated	Cuff is inflated with air to fill the space between the outside of the tube and trachea.
6. tracheostomy tube secured with ties to minimize chance of dislodgment	
7. chest x-ray obtained to confirm proper placement	
Explain that frequent assessments are made after insertion.	
Inform that an extra tube, obturator, and hemostat are kept at bedside at all times in case the tube is dislodged and reinsertion of a new tube is necessary.	
Explain that frequent suctioning is done often to remove secretions.	

Nursing Interventions	Rationales
Explain the inability to speak after insertion. Discuss and plan for an alternative form of communication.	Tracheostomy tubes are inserted below the vocal cords, blocking normal airflow and impairing the patient's ability to speak. Often the patient can speak when the cuff is not fully inflated. However, speech is still difficult since air must be forced around the tube and up through the larynx.

▼

NURSING DIAGNOSIS: INEFFECTIVE AIRWAY CLEARANCE

Related To
- Tracheostomy tube
- Thick secretions
- Fatigue

Defining Characteristics
Tachypnea
Increased work of breathing: use of accessory muscles
Pallor, cyanosis
Dyspnea
Adventitious breath sounds (rales, rhonchi)
Ineffective cough, inability to manage secretions

Patient Outcomes
The patient will
- experience a patent airway.
- demonstrate clear and equal breath sounds bilaterally.
- demonstrate normal rate, rhythm, and depth of respirations.
- demonstrate ability to cough out/manage secretions.

Nursing Interventions	Rationales
Assess respiratory rate, depth, and quality; auscultate lungs every 2–4 hr and prn.	
Encourage patient to deep breathe and cough out secretions every 2–4 hr and prn.	

Nursing Interventions	Rationales
Suction patient as often as necessary from every 5–10 min immediately after insertion to every 3–4 hr.	
1. Explain suctioning procedure to patient.	
2. Wear goggles, gown, gloves, and mask while suctioning.	
3. Use sterile technique throughout procedure.	
4. Use a catheter that is no greater than half the diameter of the tracheostomy tube to minimize hypoxia and occlusion of the cannula.	Hypoxemia created during suctioning can induce cardiac ectopy and bradycardia.
5. Before beginning suctioning, hyperoxygenate ("bag") the patient with 100% oxygen using an ambu bag connected to oxygen. Give patient five breaths.	Suctioning on insertion would unnecessarily decrease oxygen in the airway. Failure to rotate the catheter may result in damage to the tracheal mucosa.
6. Lubricate suction catheter with water. Do not apply suction while inserting. Insert 8–12 inches, gently twisting catheter while suctioning and removing.	Suctioning removes oxygen as well as secretions and may cause vagal stimulation including ectopy and bradycardia.
7. Limit suction time to 5–10 s.	The catheter obstructs the trachea and the patient must exert extra pressure to cough around it.
8. Remove the catheter if the patient starts coughing.	
9. Oxygenate the patient after suctioning by giving five breaths with the ambu bag connected to oxygen.	Instilling saline during inspiration prevents it from being blown back out of the tube. Bagging stimulates cough and distributes saline to loosen secretions.
10. If secretions are tenacious, instill 3 to 5 ml of sterile saline into the tracheostomy tube on inspiration, oxygenate with the ambu bag and then suction.	Repeated suctioning of a patient in a short time prediposes to hypoxia and is tiring and traumatic to the patient.

Nursing Interventions	Rationales
11. Continue to make suction passes, "bagging" the patient between passes, until the patient's airway is clear of secretions. Suction passes should be limited to four during each suctioning episode.	
12. Suction the patient's oral and nasal pharnyx with the catheter after suctioning the trachea.	The oral and nasal pharynx are not sterile environments. Suctioning through the tracheostomy tube after suctioning these would predispose the patient to infection.
Administer humidified oxygen as prescribed.	Humidification is necessary because the normal mechanisms of warming, moistening, and filtering the air are bypassed when an altered airway is present. Without humidification there is a greater incidence of obstruction caused by drying of secretions.
Clean inner cannula with hydrogen peroxide and saline every 4 hr and prn to maintain a patent airway by minimizing the drying and crusting of secretions on the inner cannula.	
Maintain adequate hydration of 2–3 L/day, if not contraindicated by patient's condition.	

▼

NURSING DIAGNOSIS: HIGH RISK FOR IMPAIRED GAS EXCHANGE

Risk Factors

- Tracheostomy
- Tracheal secretions
- Possible tracheostomy leak
- Plugging and decannulation process

Patient Outcomes

Patient will exhibit

- a patent tracheostomy tube/airway
- minimal secretions
- only minimal cuff leak on exhalation

Nursing Interventions	Rationales
Assess for changes in mental status, including increasing lethargy, confusion, restlessness, and irritability, every 2–4 hr and prn.	May indicate hypoxemia and/or hypercapnea and need for suctioning.
Place patient in semi- to high Fowler's position to promote full-lung expansion.	
Suction as needed when abnormal breath sounds are present and/or patient is unable to handle secretions.	
Ensure that tracheostomy ties are secured at all times to prevent tube from falling out or becoming dislocated, creating a hypoxic event.	
Keep a replacement tracheostomy tube of the same size and type, obturator, and hemostat at the bedside at all times. In case of accidental extubation, the tracheal opening should be held open with the hemostat. This will allow the patient to breathe until the replacement tube is inserted. Insert the new tube with the obturator in place which has a tapered end to provide a smooth system for entering the trachea.	
If the patient has a cuffed tracheostomy, check cuff for inflation and/or leak every shift and prn: 1. Assess amount of air leakage around cuff by listening over the cuff area with a stethoscope for a crowing sound. 2. Explain the procedure to patient.	Assures optimal sealing of the airway.

Nursing Interventions	Rationales
3. Suction the trachea and then the oral and nasal pharynx to remove the secretions around the cuff which could be aspirated into the lung when the cuff is deflated.	
4. Deflate the cuff slowly. With a new sterile catheter suction through the tracheostomy.	
5. Continually monitor patient's tolerance of the cuff deflation (e.g., respiration, color, heart rate). Provide manual ventilation, if necessary, with ambu bag.	
6. Reinflate cuff. Place stethoscope over cuff area. Slowly inflate cuff with air until no leak is heard. Aspirate about 0.1 mL of air to create a small air leak. Document amount of air injected.	The objective is to place the minimal volume of air in the cuff that will allow optimal sealing of the airway. Air leakage will be heard on exhalation. Minimal leak technique is used to avoid overinflation of the cuff which could create ischemic damage to the tracheal mucosa.

Nursing Interventions	Rationales
To wean patient from tube and eventual tube removal: 1. Suction the tracheostomy tube. 2. Remove the inner cannula. 3. Deflate the cuff. 4. Insert the decannulation cannula ("plug"). 5. Monitor the patient for any symptoms of distress. If respiratory distress occurs, remove the decannulation cannula and insert the inner cannula. 6. Continue to plug the tracheostomy tube intermittently and increase the length of time of occlusion as the patient tolerates. 7. Following tracheostomy removal, apply dressing or steri strips to approximate wound edges, check and cleanse wound site daily, and observe for signs of infection.	The tube should be removed when it is firmly established that the patient can breathe adequately through the respiratory tract and effectively manage secretions.

▼

NURSING DIAGNOSIS: HIGH RISK FOR INFECTION

Risk Factors
- Tracheostomy incision
- Suctioning
- Stagnated secretions

Patient Outcomes
Patient will exhibit
- a tracheostomy incision normal in appearance with no redness, warmth, or tenderness
- normal temperature and white blood cell (WBC) count
- no abnormal drainage around the tracheostomy site

Nursing Interventions	Rationales
Assess vital signs and temperature every 4 hr.	

Nursing Interventions	Rationales
Assess WBC count and differential for elevation.	The usual response to an infection, especially to a pulmonary infection, is to mobilize increased numbers of WBCs from the bone marrow and other storage areas.
Assess tracheostomy incision (stoma) for redness, warmth, tenderness, and exudate.	
Suction prn using sterile technique.	
Provide routine tracheostomy care every shift and as needed: 1. Explain procedure to patient. 2. Wear goggles, mask, gown, and gloves during procedure to protect from potential contamination. 3. Suction trachea and oral and nasal pharynx prior to tracheostomy. 4. With clean gloves, remove soiled tracheostomy dressing. 5. Remove inner cannula and clean it in a hydrogen peroxide and saline solution. Rinse in saline. Inspect for patency and reinsert. 6. Replace tracheostomy ties if soiled. Tie tapes at side of neck in a square knot, alternate knot from side to side to prevent irritation, and rotate pressure sites and time at which tapes are changed. Tape should be tight enough to keep tube securely in the stoma but loose enough to permit one finger between the tape and neck.	

Nursing Interventions	Rationales
7. Using sterile technique, clean tracheostomy incision with a hydrogen peroxide and saline solution using gauze sponges and sterile cotton swabs, loosen and remove any crust, repeat cleaning with saline-only solution, and apply sterile tracheostomy dressing.	

▼

NURSING DIAGNOSIS: HIGH RISK FOR ALTERED NUTRITION—LESS THAN BODY REQUIREMENTS

Risk Factors
- Anorexia
- Fatigue
- Inability to ingest food due to the tracheostomy tube

Patient Outcomes
Patient will
- maintain or increase weight.
- demonstrate adequate caloric intake for disease/metabolic state.
- demonstrate serum albumin within normal limits.
- continue to regain strength.

Nursing Interventions	Rationales
Assess daily intake of parenteral, enteral, and oral feeding and output.	
Weigh daily.	
Monitor serum albumin levels.	
If patient is receiving enteral tube feedings, monitor closely for tube placement in stomach and presence of any residual before each tube feeding (see Nutrition Support: Enteral Nutrition, see p. 15.)	If patient is unable to tolerate oral feeding and/or needs supplemental calories, enteral feeding may be utilized.

Nursing Interventions	Rationales
Monitor oral intake: Assess likes and dislikes, provide small frequent meals, and consult with dietitian about high-calorie supplements. If patient has a cuffed tracheostomy tube, make sure cuff is inflated while eating to prevent aspiration. Elevate head of bed while eating. Provide attractive clean environment at meals. Provide mouth care before meals.	The patient with a tracheostomy tube is usually able to swallow and have normal oral intake. Patient may experience loss of taste because of decreased sense of smell.
If there is a question of aspiration, methylene blue can be mixed with the enteral feeding or colored gelatin can be given to the patient. If the dye or color of gelatin does not appear in the tracheal secretions, it is safe to proceed with feeding.	
Provide for adequate rest periods between meals.	

▼

NURSING DIAGNOSIS: IMPAIRED VERBAL COMMUNICATION

Related To tracheostomy

Defining Characteristics

Weak or absent voice
Gesturing to make needs known
Difficulty in making self understood
Anxiety
Frustration

Patient Outcomes

Patient will

- communicate needs using alternative methods of communication.
- exhibit decreased signs of anxiety and frustration.

Nursing Interventions	Rationales
Assess patient's ability to speak.	Cuffed tracheostomy tubes prevent the air that is moved during inhalation and exhalation from passing over the larynx and vocal cords, blocking adequate phonation. With uncuffed tubes the patient's voice intensity may be affected.
Assess patient's and family's understanding of his or her inability to verbally communicate. Clarify information as needed.	
Speak to the patient in a normal manner and tone.	Although the patient cannot talk, he or she usually can hear. If you use overly simplistic language or talk too loud, you may frustrate the patient even more.
Provide patient with alternative forms of communication. Identify which form is best for the patient, including pad and pencil, magic slate, and a communication board with pictures or alphabet.	A magic slate ensures privacy because what is written can be erased. If writing is difficult, a communication board with common needs and equipment on it can be utilized by the patient.
To avoid damage to vocal cords, caution patient not to routinely nod or shake head in response to questions.	
Allow patient ample time to respond in writing. Avoid asking two questions at once.	Writing takes longer than speaking. Anticipating and interrupting the patient trying to communicate in writing can cause further frustration for the patient, and he or she may attempt to communicate less often.
Provide the call light within easy reach at all times and let the patient know it will be answered immediately. Devise a system for marking the intercom to alert the staff that the patient is unable to talk.	

Nursing Interventions	Rationales
If patient has a fenestrated tracheostomy tube, discuss with physician the possibility of plugging it for short periods for communication purposes.	The fenestrated tracheostomy tube has an opening at the upper curve of its outer cannula. If you remove the inner cannula and plug the tube with a tracheostomy plug or with the patient's finger, air will be forced up through the tube and the patient will be able to make short statements.

▼

NURSING DIAGNOSIS: KNOWLEDGE DEFICIT ABOUT SELF-CARE AT HOME

Related To lack of exposure to this information

Defining Characteristics

Verbalizing lack of knowledge regarding tracheostomy care, suctioning, when to call physician, resources available for support

Patient Outcomes

Patient/caregiver will

- state when to call the physician.
- demonstrate use and care of the suction equipment.
- state how to obtain supplies.
- list health care resources available.
- demonstrate cleaning and how to replace the tracheostomy tube.
- describe prevention of environmental irritants.

Nursing Interventions	Rationales
Assess patient/caregiver understanding of the tracheostomy and review information as necessary (e.g., anatomy and physiology, purpose).	

Nursing Interventions	Rationales
Review and demonstrate tracheostomy care, including 1. suctioning 2. tracheostomy tube care 3. skin care 4. replacing tracheostomy ties 5. care of equipment: suction machine, collection bottle, connecting tubing, suction catheters (making sure patient/family knows where to purchase these supplies) 6. inflation and deflation of cuff, if cuffed tracheostomy tube	
Observe patient's and/or caregiver's ability to perform all airway and tracheostomy site care independently before discharge. Arrange a home health care referral for assistance as needed.	
Instruct to 1. prevent environmental irritants from entering the tracheostomy airway by wearing a scarf or shirt with a closed collar that covers the opening, yet is of porous material thin enough to allow airflow. 2. keep products such as powders, aerosol sprays, after shave, shaving cream, soap, and so on, away from the tracheostomy. 3. keep excessive water from entering the tracheostomy tube (may bathe and shower as long as the spray and water are kept away from the stoma). 4. maintain proper humidification of the environment using room humidifier and pans of water near heat sources and drinking 2–3 quarts of liquid daily, unless physician has restricted intake.	

Nursing Interventions	Rationales
Review potential problems that should be reported to the physician, including 1. unexplained dyspnea 2. severe coughing 3. bleeding around tracheostomy site 4. hemoptysis 5. change in color or consistency of secretions to yellow, green, brown, foul smelling, thick, and difficult to remove 6. temperature of 101 °F or more	
Review signs that require immediate attention: 1. inability to pass a suction catheter down the tracheostomy tube 2. tracheostomy tube accidentally dislodged or plugged (making sure patient has an extra tracheostomy tube and instructing patient/caregiver on technique of replacing it) 3. pulsing of the tracheostomy tube.	These may be life-threatening situations. There is danger of a tube eroding into the innominate artery if pulsing of the tube is seen.
Review resources available and make appropriate contacts. 1. Visiting nurse 2. American Cancer Society 3. American Lung Association 4. community- or hospital-based tracheostomy support groups	

▼

DISCHARGE PLANNING/CONTINUITY OF CARE

- Assure understanding of self-management plan.
- Assure understanding of what should be reported to the physician.
- Arrange follow-up with physician for continued management postdischarge.
- Provide information on how to obtain tracheostomy and suctioning supplies.

- Arrange visiting nurse follow-up if continued assistance with tracheostomy care is needed.
- Provide with information on local support groups and educational programs.
- Refer to the local chapter of the American Cancer Association and/or the American Lung Association.

REFERENCES

Mapp, S. (1988). Trach care: Are you aware of all the dangers? *Nursing, 18*(7), 34–45.

Martin, C. (1989). Management of the altered airway in the head and neck cancer patient. *Seminars in Oncology Nursing, 5*(3), 182–190.

Shapiro, B., Kacmarek, R., Cane, R., Peruzzi, W., & Hamptman, D. (1991). *Clinical application of respiratory care* (4th ed). St. Louis, MO: Mosby.

Wilson, E. & Malley, N. (1990). Discharge planning for the patient with a new tracheostomy. *Critical Care Nurse, 10*(7), 73–79.

▼

Common Gastrointestinal/ Digestive Conditions and Procedures

▼

CHOLECYSTITIS/ CHOLELITHIASIS

Deborah R. Johnson, RN, MS, CNSN

Cholecystitis refers to the acute or chronic inflammation of the gallbladder. Cholelithiasis, or gallstones, is associated with acute cholecystitis in up to 90% of the cases. The stones may become lodged in the neck of the gallbladder, cystic duct, or common bile duct. The actual cause of gallstones is unknown, but cholelithiasis develops when the balance between cholesterol, bile salts, and calcium is altered, causing these substances to precipitate out and form sediments. A higher incidence of cholecystitis with cholelithiasis is seen in the following populations: multiparous women, the obese, the middle aged, those with sedentary life-styles, and those with a familial tendency. Cholecystitis can also occur without gallstones; this is referred to as an acalculous cholecystitis. Potential complications of cholecystitis/cholelithiasis are abscess, fistula formation, peritonitis, pancreatitis, cholangitis, and/or bleeding.

ETIOLOGIES

- Gallstone formation
- Bacterial invasion of the gallbladder, usually by *Escherichia coli*, streptococci, salmonella
- Chemical irritants
- Biliary surgery
- Adhesions
- Neoplasm
- Anesthesia
- Extensive fasting
- Prolonged usage of total parenteral nutrition (TPN)

CLINICAL MANIFESTATIONS

- Pain: moderate to severe, colicy, abrupt in onset; may or may not be associated with a heavy meal ingestion; localizes to right upper quadrant (RUQ) epigastric area; radiates to midtorso, scapular area (phrenic nerve irritation)

- Biliary colic: excruciating pain associated with tachycardia, diaphoresis, and prostration
- Abdominal guarding and rigidity
- Indigestion, nausea, vomiting
- Positive Murphy's sign: tenderness elicited at tip of ninth costal margin during inspiration
- Jaundice

CLINICAL/DIAGNOSTIC FINDINGS

- Gallbladder ultrasound: thickening of gallbladder wall and presence of gallstones
- Oral cholecystogram or intravenous (IV) cholangiogram: indicates presence of gallstones, nonfunctional gallbladder with ductal system deficits
- Endoscopic retrograde cholangiopancreatography (ERCP) may demonstrate presence of gallstone(s)
- Abdominal x-ray may indicate gallstones
- Elevated white blood cell (WBC) count
- Elevated serum amylase
- Elevated lactic dehydrogenase (LDH) and alkaline phosphatase
- Elevated liver function tests (SGOT, SGPT, direct and indirect bilirubin)
- Elevated clotting studies (potential)

OTHER PLANS OF CARE TO REFERENCE

- Pancreatitis
- Hepatitis
- Cirrhosis and Esophageal Varices

▼

NURSING DIAGNOSIS: PAIN

Related To

- Inflammation and distention of gallbladder
- Obstruction
- Spasm of bile duct

Defining Characteristics

Guarding behavior of abdomen, reluctance to move
Rubbing right shoulder
Facial grimacing, moaning, crying
Diaphoresis

Blood pressure, pulse changes
Communication of pain descriptors

Patient Outcomes

The patient will
- verbalize pain relief
- increase participation in activities
- display relaxed facial expressions
- have stable vital signs

Nursing Interventions	Rationales
Assess for 1. verbal complaints of pain with specific attention to severity, location, and type of pain 2. nonverbal pain cues 3. factors that alleviate or aggravate pain	
When the gallbladder diagnosis is confirmed, assure the patient that it is not a heart attack.	The symptoms of cholecystitis and cholelithiasis often mimic those of a myocardial infarction.
Implement measures to reduce pain:	
1. Maintain nothing by mouth (NPO) status as prescribed.	NPO reduces stimulation of gallbladder contraction and decreases pain.
2. Insert nasogastric tube, assure patency, and maintain suction as prescribed.	Stomach decompression reduces stimulation of gallbladder contraction and decreases pain.
3. When oral intake is resumed, maintain dietary fat restrictions.	Fat intake stimulates gallbladder contraction to release bile and increases pain.
Monitor for therapeutic effects of prescribed antibiotics.	Prevention or treatment of gallbladder infection reduces gallbladder inflammation and subsequent pain.
Monitor for therapeutic effects of prescribed narcotic analgesics.	Certain narcotics such as morphine sulfate may precipitate increased spasming at sphincter of Oddi, hence increasing abdominal pain.

Nursing Interventions	Rationales
Provide nonpharmacological interventions to reduce pain, that is, position changes and back rubs, and maintain an environment conducive to rest.	
Prepare for endoscopic ductal stone removal or cholecystectomy if indicated.	

▼

NURSING DIAGNOSIS: PAIN

Related To

- Gas accumulation associated with fat intolerance
- Impaired fat digestion due to obstructed bile flow

Defining Characteristics

Abdominal guarding
Increase in abdominal girth
Reluctance to move
Eructation
Restlessness
Facial grimacing
Verbal communication of pain descriptors

Patient Outcomes

The patient will

- verbalize pain relief
- demonstrate decreased abdominal distention
- display relaxed facial expression
- increase participation in activities

Nursing Interventions	Rationales
Assess for verbal complaints of gas pain, abdominal distention, and indigestion.	
Assess for nonverbal cues of gas pain, abdominal fullness, and indigestion.	

Nursing Interventions	Rationales
Assist with frequent position changes and ambulation as tolerated.	Activity increases flatus expulsion, reducing gastrointestinal (GI) accumulation, decreasing gas pain, abdominal distention, and fullness.
Instruct to avoid sucking on hard candy, gum chewing, and smoking.	Reduce air swallowing to decrease GI gas accumulation.
When oral intake is allowed:	
1. Maintain dietary fat restrictions, for example, butter, whole milk, ice cream, fried foods, and pork.	A diet high in fat stimulates the gallbladder to contract, in an attempt to release the bile necessary to digest the fat. This action increases abdominal pain.
2. Avoid gas-producing foods/fluids, for example, carbonated beverages, cabbage, onions, and baked beans.	Reduces additional GI gas accumulation in attempts to decrease gas pain, abdominal distention, and dyspepsia.
Consult dietitian to assist with dietary modifications as needed.	

▼

NURSING DIAGNOSIS: KNOWLEDGE DEFICIT—ABOUT SELF-CARE MANAGEMENT

Related To
- New diagnosis
- No previous exposure to information

Defining Characteristics
Verbalizes a lack of knowledge
Asking questions
Inaccurate follow-through of instructions

Patient Outcomes
The patient will
- describe a plan for known risk factor modification
- state dietary modifications
- verbalize when to call the physician
- demonstrate accurate follow-through of instruction

Nursing Interventions	Rationales
Identify and educate about realistic known risk factor modifications to eliminate or decrease the incidence of gallbladder attacks: 1. weight loss program 2. low-fat menu planning 3. exercise program participation	
Explain the purpose of a moderate/low-fat diet to prevent further gallbladder attacks: 1. Obtain dietary consult if assistance is needed with meal planning to incorporate dietary fat modifications and/or weight loss. 2. Avoid food/fluids high in fat.	
Explain the purpose, rationale, side effects, and necessity of taking the following medications as prescribed:	
1. antibiotics	Reduce gallbladder inflammation, prevent gallbladder infection, and decrease pain.
2. fat-soluble vitamins (e.g., A, D, E, K)	If bile is not present to assist with absorption of vitamin K (fat-soluble vitamin), bleeding tendencies can occur.
3. bile salts	Supplemental bile salts are administered to facilitate digestion and fat-soluble vitamin absorption.
4. cholestyramine	Binds with excess bile salts in the intestine and reduces itching and diarrhea often seen with chronic biliary stasis.

Nursing Interventions	Rationales
Instruct to report the following conditions to nurse/physician: 1. persistent nausea, vomiting, gas 2. increased abdominal distention 3. persistent abdominal pain, spasm 4. recurrent elevated temperature 5. excessive bruising 6. yellow coloring of eyes and skin, dark urine, itchy skin, clay-colored stools.	Indicates obstructed bile flow.
Answer questions, clarify information, and address concerns if surgical intervention (cholecystectomy) is a potential treatment option.	

DISCHARGE PLANNING/CONTINUITY OF CARE

- Assure patient/family understands self-care management plan, for example, medications, dietary modifications, and when to call the physician.
- Provide patient/family with appropriate individualized written patient education materials to use as a reference.
- Refer to a home care agency if continued nursing care, teaching, or assistance with self-care management is needed.
- Arrange for follow-up visits with dietitian, nurse, and/or physician for continued management after discharge, if needed.
- Assist patient with obtaining prescriptions and establishing a plan for refilling prescriptions.
- Collaborate with dietitian to provide information on community self-help weight loss programs as needed, or requested.

REFERENCES

Beck, M. & Evans, N. (1993). *SGNA—Gastroenterology nursing: A core curriculum.* St. Louis, MO: Mosby.

Doughty, D. B. & Jackson, D. B. (1993). *Gastrointestinal disorders.* St. Louis, MO: Mosby.

Lewis, S. M. & Collier, I. C. (1992). *Medical-surgical nursing: Assessment and management of clinical problems* (3rd ed). St. Louis, MO: Mosby.

CIRRHOSIS AND ESOPHAGEAL VARICES

Lynn Schoengrund, RN, MS

Cirrhosis is a progressive disease characterized by extensive degeneration and destruction of liver cells. It has an insidious and prolonged course resulting in death if undetected or without liver transplantation. Cirrhosis disturbs carbohydrate and protein metabolism; production and breakdown of red and white blood cells (RBCs, WBCs) and platelets, and production of coagulation factors. Jaundice results from the loss of function as well as compression of the bile ducts. Three progressions of cirrhosis that may be life threatening are portal hypertension with esophageal varices, ascites with peripheral edema, and portal-systemic encephalopathy. Bleeding from varices is a medical emergency with a very high mortality rate. Ascites is the accumulation of serous fluid in the abdominal or peritoneal cavity and is manifested by abdominal distention. Portal-systemic encephalopathy (PSE) results when blood enters the systemic circulation without liver detoxification, resulting in neurological changes ranging from decreased mental responsiveness from disorientation to coma.

ETIOLOGIES

- Alcoholic cirrhosis
- Viral or toxic hepatitis with necrotic cirrhosis
- Chronic biliary obstruction
- Chronic biliary infection
- Long-standing right-sided heart failure

CLINICAL MANIFESTATIONS

- Anorexia, dyspepsia, flatulence, nausea, vomiting
- Jaundice
- Skin lesions; spider angiomas on face, upper trunk, and shoulders

- Ascites
- Easy bruising or bleeding tendencies

CLINICAL/DIAGNOSTIC FINDINGS

- Elevated liver enzymes [serum glutamic oxaloacetic and pyruvic transaminases, lactic dehydrogenase (SGOT, SGPT, LDH)]
- Elevated serum and urine bilirubin
- Prolonged prothrombin time
- Pathology identified on liver biopsy

NURSING DIAGNOSIS: SENSORY/PERCEPTUAL ALTERATIONS

Related To toxic metabolites in the brain secondary to decreased liver function

Defining Characteristics

Euphoria
Apathy
Irritability
Memory loss
Confusion
Agitation
Impaired judgment
Disorientation

Patient Outcomes

- The patient is oriented to time, place, and person.
- The patient's anxiety and irritability are decreased.
- The patient's environment is protective.
- Serum albumin levels are within normal limits.

Nursing Interventions	Rationales
Assess environment for safety and stimuli. Adjust environment to decrease stimuli, for example, noise, lights, and interruptions, and assure safety.	A quiet environment will decrease opportunities for misinterpretations of the environment resulting in patient anxiety and fear.
Assess patient's neurological status, including mentation, orientation to time, place and person, and thought patterns, regularly. Calmly reorient and listen to patient, providing a reassuring presence when the patient becomes anxious.	Increased production of ammonia with cirrhosis causes neurological changes. Medical management aimed at decreasing production of ammonia may control progression of symptoms.

Nursing Interventions	Rationales
Encourage fluids if unrestricted. Give laxatives and enemas as prescribed. Administer lactulose and/or neomycin as prescribed.	Increased gastrointestinal action will decrease production of ammonia by decreasing bacterial action on feces. Lactulose will decrease the production of ammonia. Neomycin decreases available bacteria to act on feces.
If patient's activities are unsafe (getting out of bed, pulling at tubes, etc.) arrange for increased observation and support, for example, provide a sitter or bed alarm or move closer to nurse's area.	
Avoid physical restraint unless other means fail.	

▼

NURSING DIAGNOSIS: INEFFECTIVE BREATHING PATTERN

Related To

- Reduced lung volume
- Pressure on diaphragm from ascites

Defining Characteristics

Rapid shallow respirations
Cyanosis
Abnormal blood gases
Shortness of breath
Orthopnea

Patient Outcomes

- Patient will be able to breathe easily with comfort.
- Signs of hypoxia are absent.

Nursing Interventions	Rationales
Elevate head of bed. Support arms and chest with pillows.	Use gravity to move fluid away from lungs and diaphragm.
Monitor rate of fluid accumulation by measuring abdominal girth, daily, for comparison.	Rapid fluid accumulation may need to be treated with paracentesis.

Nursing Interventions	Rationales
Encourage position changes, ambulation, and deep breathing to maintain lung expansion.	
If paracentesis is required, explain procedure to patient. Assist physician and support patient throughout procedure.	

NURSING DIAGNOSIS: ALTERED NUTRITION—LESS THAN BODY REQUIREMENTS

Related To

- Anorexia
- Nausea and vomiting
- Feelings of fullness

Defining Characteristics

Poor food intake
Weight loss
Hypoalbuminemia

Patient Outcomes

- Nutrition is balanced and adequate.
- The patient's weight is maintained.
- Nausea and vomiting are decreased.
- Serum albumin levels are within normal limits.

Nursing Interventions	Rationales
Assess nutritional status by measuring caloric intake, intake and output, daily weights, and serum albumin levels. Consult with the dietitian, if available.	Prevention of catabolism can occur if intervention is early.
Provide small, frequent high-calorie meals. A low-protein diet may be recommended for patients with impending hepatic coma or portal systemic encephalopathy (PSE), a high-protein diet for those without ascites or impending coma.	There is controversy on the amount of protein recommended at various stages of the disease process. Pressure of fluid in ascites prevents tolerance of larger meals.

Nursing Interventions	Rationales
Meet patient requests for food choices. Encourage eating whenever possible to decrease effects of starvation.	Individualizing meals will increase compliance. Starvation effects will increase ammonia levels as cells break down for energy.

▼

NURSING DIAGNOSIS: HIGH RISK FOR IMPAIRED SKIN INTEGRITY

Risk Factors

- Itching
- Scratching
- Skin dryness
- Cracks in skin
- Difficulty moving due to edema and ascites
- Bilirubin deposition in skin

Patient Outcomes

- Skin remains intact.
- Itching is relieved or tolerated.

Nursing Interventions	Rationales
Inspect skin over entire body, daily, for pressure areas, breakdown, and edema.	Breakdown may occur quickly and in unusual areas due to edema and salt deposition.
Avoid use of tape, dressings, or linen that may irritate the skin.	Puritis is a common symptom. Any irritation of skin can lead quickly to skin breakdown.
Use skin moisturizers and other means of treatment to increase patient comfort, such as therapeutic baths (oatmeal, etc.) and showers. Consult skin care specialist, if available.	

▼

NURSING DIAGNOSIS: ACTIVITY INTOLERANCE

Related To

- Anemia
- Fatigue
- Ascites

- Dyspnea
- Edema

Defining Characteristics

Subjective reports of fatigue
Increased pulse rate on activity
Diaphoresis with small amount of exertion
Difficulty in performing physical tasks

Patient Outcomes

Patient is able to perform activities without fatigue, diaphoresis, or increased pulse rate.

Nursing Interventions	Rationales
Develop a schedule with activities spaced between scheduled rest to prevent exhaustion.	
Perform active range-of-motion exercises regularly and encourage patient to do passive range-of-motion while in bed or chair.	Lack of activity increases activity intolerance as muscles become debilitated.
Encourage the patient to increase activities to gradually build tolerance.	
Consult with physical or exercise therapists to develop a plan to build tolerance.	

▼

NURSING DIAGNOSIS: HIGH RISK FOR INFECTION

Risk Factors

- Leukopenia
- Multiple invasive procedures
- Inadequate secondary defense
- Chronic disease

Patient Outcome

Patient is free from infection.

Nursing Interventions	Rationales
Use universal precautions (body substance isolation) and aseptic technique in all procedures.	
Assess for signs and symptoms of local or systemic infection, including fever; presence of redness, swelling, or drainage at wounds or catheter sites; cough; changes in respiratory assessment; and urgency of, frequency of, or foul-smelling urine.	Risk for infection is increased with invasive procedures.
Report all signs of infection and anticipate use of antibodies.	

▼

NURSING DIAGNOSIS: HIGH RISK FOR INJURY

Risk Factors

- Lack of clotting ability
- Easy bleeding and bruising
- Esophageal varices

Patient Outcomes

Patient exhibits no injury related to bleeding or bruising of skin or rupture of esophageal varices.

Nursing Interventions	Rationales
Avoid injury by providing padded side rails.	
Teach the patient to protect skin and mucous membrane from trauma, for example, use caution with toothbrushes, electric razor for shaving, straining at stool, and blowing nose.	Patients may be unaware of how daily actions may precipitate bleeding.

Nursing Interventions	Rationales
Assess for signs and symptoms of bleeding, including stool, urine, expectorations, vomitus, for color change, hypotension, rapid pulse, pallor, and cool, clammy skin. Monitor hemoglobin and hematocrit.	
If symptoms of upper gastrointestinal (GI) bleeding occur, *immediately* prepare for treatment of bleeding esophageal varices:	This is a medical emergency. Transfer to the intensive care unit may be required to meet needs for care and monitoring.
1. Monitor vital signs and rate of bleeding. Measure all vomitus.	
2. Anticipate placement of gastric and esophageal balloons and nasogastric tube.	
3. Explain procedures to patient and obtain his or her cooperation.	
4. Maintain esophageal tamponade by keeping tube in place with gastric and esophageal balloons inflated and gastric suction operational. Maintain airway by suctioning and oral mucosa by frequent oral hygiene.	Esophageal tamponade puts direct pressure of gastric tube with inflatable balloons in the esophagus and stomach. The oral gastric tube often irritates the oral mucosa and makes cleaning of oral secretions difficult for patients.
5. Administer intravenous vasopressor medication as prescribed, titrated to maintain blood pressure in prescribed ranges while stopping bleeding.	Vasopressors may act directly on varices to cause vasoconstriction. Vasoconstriction of varices must be accomplished without causing hypertension.
6. Replace blood and fluids as prescribed and indicated by rate of bleeding. Maintain constant communication with the physician.	

Nursing Interventions	Rationales
7. Assess respiratory status frequently for distress, increased breathing effort, adventitious breath sounds, and changes in arterial blood gases.	Inflated balloons may impair normal respiratory ability, and rapid loss of blood may result in decreased oxygen level.
8. If inflated esophageal balloon migrates to upper airway, the airway may become blocked. Deflate the balloon immediately and remove the tube. Keep the scissors at the bedside to facilitate rapid deflation.	
9. Observe frequently for airway obstruction. Suction oral and pharyngeal areas as needed. Elevate head of bed. Assure availability of call light to patient.	
10. Provide frequent oral hygiene while tubes are in place.	
11. Assist the patient to tolerate tubes by using relaxation, distraction, and antianxiety medication as needed.	

▼

NURSING DIAGNOSIS: ANTICIPATORY GRIEVING

Related To to poor prognosis of cirrhosis

Defining Characteristics

Expressions of grief, guilt, anger, sorrow

Patient Outcomes

The patient will

- discuss feelings and concerns
- request and use supportive counseling as needed

Nursing Interventions	Rationales
Provide a consistent nurse-patient relationship. Assess patient's perception of stage of illness.	The nurse's positive responses to patient expressions may assist with the grieving process.
Encourage discussion of feelings. Listen with an accepting attitude, validating patient's concerns.	
Help patient develop realistic short-term goals.	
Support patient's discussion of death and dying. Answer questions honestly.	
Refer to counseling and/or pastoral care if accepted by the patient.	

▼

DISCHARGE PLANNING/CONTINUITY OF CARE

- Assure patient's understanding of self-management plan, including avoiding alcohol, eating an adequate diet, activity, and symptoms to report.
- Refer to a home health care agency if continued assistance with care or monitoring is indicated.
- Coordinate referral to a hospice or psychosocial support services if the patient needs assistance with coping.
- Arrange continuing medical follow-up.
- Assist patient in obtaining prescriptions, discussing a medication schedule and a plan for refilling prescriptions.

REFERENCES

Lewis, S. M. & Collier, I. C. (1992). *Medical surgical nursing.* St. Louis, MO: Mosby.

Patrick, M. L., Woods, S. J., Crawer, R. F., Rokoshy, J. S., & Boraine, P. (1991). *Medical surgical nursing pathophysiological concepts.* Philadelphia, PA: Lippincott.

Porth, C. M. (1990). *Pathophysiology—Concepts of altered health stakes.* Philadelphia, PA: Lippincott.

Rhoads, J. (1990). Cirrhosis of the liver. *Emergency Medicine Services, 19*(3), 44–47.

▼

DIVERTICULAR DISEASE

Deborah R. Johnson, RN, MS, CNSN

Diverticulosis is the presence of abnormal outpouchings or herniations in the intestinal wall, known as diverticula. These outpouchings are due to high pressures in the intestinal lumen. They can occur in any part of the intestine but most frequently occur in the sigmoid colon. Diverticulitis, or inflammation of one or more diverticula, results when the diverticulum perforates with local abscess formation. A perforated diverticulum can progress to generalized peritonitis.

ETIOLOGIES

- No known cause
- Associated with dietary fiber deficiencies
- Old age
- Constipation

CLINICAL MANIFESTATIONS

- Majority of patients asymptomatic
- Crampy abdominal pain located in left lower quadrant, usually relieved by flatus or a bowel movement
- Alternating constipation/diarrhea
- Diverticulitis: abdominal pain, localized over area of involved colon; tender left lower quadrant mass may be palpated; fever, chills

CLINICAL/DIAGNOSTIC FINDINGS

- Barium enema demonstrates presence of diverticulum, shortening, narrowing, or other intestinal deformities. Should not be done on patients with acute diverticulitis because of possible perforation.

- Computerized tomography (CT) scan/ultrasound may demonstrate abscess or mass.
- Sigmoid or colonoscopy demonstrates diverticula (should not be done on patient with acute diverticulitis because of possible perforation).
- Stool may be positive for occult blood.
- White blood cell (WBC) count may be elevated with left shift.
- Intravenous pyelogram may be done to rule out left ureter mass or colonic vesical fistula.
- Urinalysis may indicate a few red blood cells if left ureter is affected.

▼

NURSING DIAGNOSIS: KNOWLEDGE DEFICIT—REGARDING SELF-CARE

Related To lack of exposure to information or misunderstanding

Defining Characteristics

Asking questions
Inaccurate follow-through of instructions

Patient Outcomes

The patient will
- state dietary modifications.
- state plan for weight loss program.
- describe ways to foster a regular predictable bowel elimination pattern.
- describe ways to minimize intra-abdominal pressure

Nursing Interventions	Rationales
Assess current stool pattern and usual bowel elimination habits.	
Explain that uncomplicated diverticular disease is primarily treated by a high-fiber diet and bulk laxatives.	When diverticula form, the colon's smooth muscle wall thickens; lack of dietary fiber slows transit time, and hence stool and bacteria are retained in the colon. This forms a hardened mass, causing inflammation and small perforations. More free water is absorbed from the stool, making it more difficult to pass through the lumen.

Nursing Interventions	Rationales
Assess therapeutic effectiveness of high-fiber diet, stool softeners, mineral oil, and bulk laxatives as prescribed.	Avoiding constipation minimizes the potential complications of diverticular disease.
Increase fluid intake, if not contraindicated, when a high-fiber diet is prescribed.	Minimizes the potential for dehydration.
Collaborate with dietitian to assist with high-fiber dietary modifications, weight loss, meal planning, or additional dietary restrictions as prescribed. For acute exacerbation use low residual diet until stable.	
Avoid factors that increase abdominal pressure: 1. straining at stool 2. vomiting 3. bending, lifting 4. wearing tight restrictive clothing 5. obesity (encourage weight loss).	Factors that increase abdominal pressure may precipitate a diverticular attack.

▼

NURSING DIAGNOSIS: HIGH RISK FOR INFECTION

Risk Factors

- Inadequate primary defenses, for example, ruptured/perforated diverticulum with significant abscess formation or peritonitis
- Inadequate secondary defenses, for example, potentially decreased hemoglobin levels related to blood loss, age, or poor nutritional status

Patient Outcomes

Patient demonstrates no signs of abdominal abscess or peritonitis, as evidenced by

- afebrile state
- WBC count within normal limits
- stable vital signs
- soft, nondistended abdomen
- normal bowel sounds
- no verbal complaints of severe abdominal pain

Nursing Interventions	Rationales
Assess for sudden abdominal pain, rigid tense abdomen, abdominal rebound tenderness, diminished or absent bowel sounds, elevated temperature, tachycardia, tachypnea, and decreased blood pressure and report significant findings to physician.	These are signs and symptoms of peritonitis.
Monitor WBC results and report any increased levels to physician.	
If signs/symptoms of peritonitis occur: 1. Withhold all food and oral fluids as prescribed. 2. Insert nasogastric tube and maintain suction as prescribed. 3. Monitor for therapeutic effects of prescribed antibiotics.	This prevents further contamination of peritoneal cavity.
Monitor for therapeutic effects of prescribed intravenous fluids (colloid and crystalloid) if administered.	Prevent or treat shock, sepsis that occurs with massive infection, abscess or perforation when fluids, protein, and electrolytes leak into the peritoneal cavity.
Prepare patient for possible surgical intervention, for example, exploratory laparotomy, bowel resection, or diversion as indicated to drain the abscess or repair the perforation.	
Provide emotional support to patient and family.	

▼

DISCHARGE PLANNING/CONTINUITY OF CARE

- Assure patient/family understands self-care management plan, for example, dietary modifications, bowel routine, medications, and when to call the physician.
- Refer to a home care agency if continued nursing care, teaching, or assistance with self-care management is needed.

- Arrange for follow-up with physician, dietitian, or nurse as needed for continued management after discharge.
- Assist with obtaining prescriptions and establishing a plan for refilling prescriptions.

REFERENCES

Beck, M. & Evans, N. (1993). *SGNA—Gastroenterology nursing: A core curriculum.* St. Louis, MO: Mosby Year Book.

Coellen, D. (1989). Understanding diverticular disease. *Journal of Enterostomal Therapy, 16*(4), 176–180, 1684.

Doughty, D. B. & Jackson, D. B. (1993). *Gastrointestinal disorders.* St. Louis, MO: Mosby Year Book.

Lewis, S. M. & Collier, I.C. (1992). *Medical-surgical nursing: Assessment and management of clinical problems* (3rd ed). St. Louis, MO: Mosby Year Book.

▼

HIATAL HERNIA: MEDICAL MANAGEMENT

Deborah R. Johnson, RN, MS, CNSN

Hiatal hernia is also referred to as an esophageal or diaphragmatic hernia. A hiatal hernia is a herniation of a portion of the stomach into the esophagus/thoracic cavity through an opening (hiatus) in the diaphragm. Hiatal hernias are classified into two types.

Type I, a sliding hiatal hernia, is the most common. The esophagogastric junction is above the hiatus of the diaphragm. A part of the stomach slides through the hiatal opening in the diaphragm. This part of the stomach slides up into the chest cavity when the patient is supine and moves back down into the abdominal cavity when the patient is upright. Esophagitis and gastric reflux are common complications.

Type II, paraesophageal or rolling hernia, occurs when the esophagogastric junction remains in the normal position but the greater curvature of the stomach and the fundus roll up beside the esophagus through the diaphragm forming a pocket alongside the esophagus (peritoneal hernia sack). Type II hernias can be large enough to accept almost the entire stomach. These hernias are more frequently associated with strangulation.

ETIOLOGIES

- Structural changes that weaken the muscular collar of the diaphragm around the esophagogastric opening
- Increased intra-abdominal pressure: pregnancy, obesity, tumors, ascites, prolonged heavy lifting, intensive physical exertion
- Increased age, trauma, poor nutrition, and congenital weakness

CLINICAL MANIFESTATIONS

- Heartburn (pyrosis) from reflux due to irritation of the esophagus by gastric acids. Typically no symptoms occur until the lower esophageal sphincter (LES) becomes incompetent. When LES pressure is decreased, reflux occurs.

- Pain after large meals, alcohol, and smoking
- Regurgitation of stomach contents
- Dysphagia, eructation, bloating
- Painful swallowing
- Shortness of breath, tachycardia, retrosternal pain, substernal chest pain radiating to back, shoulder, or arm, unrelieved by lying down

CLINICAL/DIAGNOSTIC FINDINGS

- Barium swallow: hernia appearing as an outpouching
- Endoscopy: determines LES incompetence and gastric reflux
- Chest x-ray: shows shadow behind heart if hernia is large

▼

NURSING DIAGNOSIS: IMPAIRED SWALLOWING

Related To

- Esophageal irritation
- Muscle spasm associated with gastric reflux

Defining Characteristics

Coughing, choking
Observed difficulty swallowing

Patient Outcomes

Patient will

- verbalize improvement with swallowing.
- demonstrate strategies to improve swallowing.

Nursing Interventions	Rationales
Assess for signs and symptoms of impaired swallowing to determine patient's individual baseline.	
Assess for factors that appear to aggravate or alleviate swallowing problems.	

Nursing Interventions	Rationales
Implement measures to ease the passage of food/fluids through the esophagus and instruct accordingly: 1. Sit in high Fowler's position during all meals and snacks. 2. Encourage to drink fluids with meals. 3. Encourage to swallow frequently when eating. 4. Moisten dry foods with gravy or sauces. 5. Consult with dietitian to select foods that are nutritious and easy to swallow.	
Implement measures to prevent additional increased abdominal pressure and/or reflux of gastric contents and instruct patient accordingly. (See Altered Nutrition, first two interventions.)	Preventing additional increased abdominal pressure and/or gastric reflux minimizes esophageal irritation and hence facilitates swallowing.

▼

NURSING DIAGNOSIS: ALTERED NUTRITION—LESS THAN BODY REQUIREMENTS

Related To

- Gastroesophageal reflux
- Heartburn
- Pain

Defining Characteristics

Weight loss
Pain with food ingestion
Aversion to eating
Abdominal cramping
Lack of interest in food

Patient Outcomes

Patient will

- relate less trouble with gastroesophageal reflux.
- verbalize less pain and heartburn.
- demonstrate strategies to decrease gastroesophageal reflux.
- maintain weight.
- ingest nutrients in adequate and balanced amounts.

Nursing Interventions	Rationales
Implement measures to prevent additional increases in abdominal pressure that may potentiate gastroesophageal reflux and instruct accordingly: 1. Avoid coughing and straining to evacuate stool. 2. Position items the patient may need within easy reach to avoid excessive twisting or bending at the waist. 3. Avoid snug clothing around abdomen/waist. 4. Avoid activities that increase air swallowing: chewing gum, smoking, drinking through a straw, sucking on hard candy. 5. Provide small, more frequent meals. 6. Avoid gas-producing foods/beverages. 7. Consult dietitian to assist with dietary modifications or weight reduction if necessary.	
Implement measures to prevent reflux of gastric contents and instruct accordingly: 1. Eat in an upright position and avoid lying down for 2–3 hr after eating. 2. Elevate head of bed 6–10 inches at all times.	
3. Avoid chocolate, peppermint, coffee, alcohol, and fatty foods.	These substances decrease LES pressure and increase reflux. Fatty foods stimulate the release of cholecystokinin, which decreases LES pressure.
4. Stop smoking.	Smoking immediately decreases LES pressure.

Nursing Interventions	Rationales
5. Monitor for therapeutic effects of medications: • cholinergics • gastrointestinal stimulants	Cholinergics directly increase LES pressure and decrease reflux. Gastrointestinal stimulants hasten gastric emptying and increase LES pressure.
Implement actions to reduce esophageal mucosal irritation if reflux occurs and instruct accordingly: 1. Provide bland diet as ordered.	
2. Drink water after meals or reflux episodes.	Cleanses the esophagus.
3. Administer any prescribed ulcerogenic medications with meals or snacks. Common ones include aspirin, corticosteroids, and ibuprofen.	
4. Monitor for therapeutic effects of prescribed medications: • histamine 2 (H_2) blockers (e.g., ranitidine, cimetidine) • antisecretory compounds (e.g., omeprazole) • antacids, acid-protective agents	Histamine 2 blockers and antisecretory compounds suppress and/or block gastric acid secretion, hence reducing stomach acid. Acid-protective agents are mucosal barrier fortifiers providing a cryoprotective coating, and antacids neutralize or buffer hydrochloric acid.

▼

DISCHARGE PLANNING/CONTINUITY OF CARE

- Assure patient/family understands the self-care management plan, for example, medications, activity, dietary restrictions, and when to notify the physician.
- Refer to a home care agency if continued nursing care, teaching, or assistance with self-care management plan is needed.
- Arrange for follow-up with physician or nurse for continued management postdischarge as needed.
- Assist with obtaining prescriptions and establish a plan for refilling prescriptions.
- Provide with information about smoking cessation groups, local self-help weight reduction educational programs, or recovery programs if

alcohol problems are suspected or acknowledged. Initiate a referral as indicated.

- Anticipate potential need to clarify information, alleviate fears, and dispel myths if conservative medical measures are not effective to treat the hiatal hernia and the patient requires surgical intervention (Nissen Fundoplication) for correction of the hiatal hernia.

REFERENCES

Beck, M. & Evans, N. (1993). *SGNA—Gastroenterology nursing: A core curriculum.* St. Louis, MO: Mosby Year Book.

Doughty, D. B. & Jackson, D. B. (1993). *Gastrointestinal disorders.* St. Louis, MO: Mosby Year Book.

Kennedy-Caldwell, C. & Guenter, P. A. (1988). *Nutrition support nursing core curriculum* (2nd ed). Silver Spring, MD: American Society for Parenteral and Enteral Nutrition.

Lewis, S. M. & Collier, I. C. (1992). *Medical-surgical nursing: Assessment and management of clinical problems* (3rd ed). St. Louis, MO: Mosby Year Book.

Massoni, M. (1990). Nurses' GI handbook. *Nursing, 20*(11), 65–80.

▼

INFLAMMATORY BOWEL DISEASE: CROHN'S DISEASE AND ULCERATIVE COLITIS

Deborah R. Johnson, RN, MS, CNSN

Crohn's disease and ulcerative colitis are the most common forms of inflammatory bowel disease (IBD). Crohn's disease is a chronic inflammatory bowel disease that involves the entire thickness of the bowel wall. It can begin anywhere in the intestinal tract, but the terminal ileum is most frequently involved. Patients with Crohn's disease often develop bowel fistulas and/or anorectal fissures, abscesses, and intestinal obstruction. Ulcerative colitis is a chronic inflammatory bowel disease that involves the mucosa and submucosa of the bowel wall. It typically starts in the rectum and proceeds in a continuous manner toward the cecum. The small intestine usually has minimal involvement. Patients with ulcerative colitis have a higher incidence of rectal bleeding toxic mega colon, perforation, and a greater predisposition for colon cancer.

ETIOLOGIES

The cause of both ulcerative colitis and Crohn's disease is unknown.

CLINICAL MANIFESTATIONS

- Crohn's disease
  - 5–6 soft, loose stools per day
  - abdominal cramping
  - right lower quadrant pain
  - low-grade fever
- Ulcerative colitis
  - 10–20 liquid, bloody stools per day
  - mild abdominal cramping
  - intermittent low-grade fever

- fatigue
- anorexia
- weight loss

CLINICAL/DIAGNOSTIC FINDINGS

- Ulcerative colitis
  - barium enema: Shows ulceration of mucosa, shortening of the bowel, pseudopolyps
  - sigmoidoscopy: submucosal inflammation and edema
  - colonoscopy: hyperemia, mucosal friability, ulcerations, pseudopolyps
  - blood work: decreased hematocrit, decreased hemoglobin, decreased serum albumin, guaiac positive stools, biopsy revealing inflammatory changes
- Crohn's disease
  - barium enema: shows asymmetric disease, skip lesions, ulcerations, fissures, stricture fistulas
  - sigmoidoscopy: perirectal fissures, fistulas, abscesses
  - colonoscopy: skip lesions, cobblestone mucosa
  - blood work: decreased hematocrit, decreased hemoglobin, decreased serum albumin, guaiac positive stools

OTHER PLANS OF CARE TO REFERENCE

Nutrition Support: Enteral Nutrition
Nutrition Support: Total Parenteral Nutrition
Corticosteroid Therapy

▼

NURSING DIAGNOSIS: DIARRHEA

Related To
- Irritated bowel
- Inflammation
- Intestinal hyperactivity

Defining Characteristics
Abdominal pain
Cramping
Increased frequency of stools and bowel sounds
Loose liquid stools
Urgency

Patient Outcomes

Patient will

- have less frequent bowel movements.
- have more formed stools.
- experience an absence of or a decrease in abdominal pain, cramping, and urgency associated with evacuation.

Nursing Interventions	**Rationales**
Assess usual bowel elimination pattern: 1. frequency, consistency, odor, and amount of stools 2. diarrhea in relationship to pain, eating, stress, activity 3. urgency to expel stool 4. flatus 5. Note signs of blood and/or steatorrhea.	In IBD, the colon fails to reabsorb water and electrolytes, the rectum loses capacity to retain a fluid load, and the small intestine may not absorb water, bile, or lactose. All these factors contribute to diarrhea.
Promote actions to facilitate bowel rest: 1. Maintain nothing by mouth (NPO) status or specific fluid/food restrictions as prescribed. 2. Promote physical and emotional rest.	Bowel rest assists with reducing inflammation and hyperactivity of the bowel to help control diarrhea.
Discourage smoking and caffeine.	Nicotine and caffeine stimulate the gastrointestinal tract.
Collaborate with dietitian to instruct about avoidance of poorly digested foods/fluids that act as irritants to an inflamed bowel: 1. dairy products 2. high fat, high residue, high caffeine, known gas-producing foods	Minimizes inflammation and hyperactivity of the bowel in order to control diarrhea. Many patients with Crohn's disease may have a lactose intolerance related to lactase deficiency.
Provide small frequent meals.	
Introduce/add any new foods one at a time.	
Monitor for therapeutic effects of the following medications, as prescribed: 1. corticosteriods	Reduce inflammation.

Nursing Interventions	Rationales
2. sulfasalazine	Primarily anti-inflammatory in action but may also provide some antibacterial effects.
3. immunosuppressive agents	Reduce inflammation associated with an immune response.
4. anticholinergic agents and opiate or opiatelike agents	Decrease intestinal spasms and motility. The use of these agents may be controversial because of their tendency to cause toxic megacolon, a serious IBD complication.
5. cholestyramine	Bind bile salts. Diarrhea may occur due to intestinal irritation of excessive bile salts or bile salt malabsorption related to IBD of terminal ileum.
6. bulk-forming agents (e.g., psyllium derivatives, methylcellulose)	Absorb water in the bowel and produce a soft formed stool.
7. absorbent and protectant agents (e.g., pectin, kaolin)	Absorb bacteria and toxins; also coat the intestinal mucosa.
Provide information about stress management techniques.	Stress may precipitate diarrhea exacerbation.

▼

NURSING DIAGNOSIS: ALTERED NUTRITION—LESS THAN BODY REQUIREMENTS

Related To

- Decreased nutrient intake
- Increased nutritional loss through diarrhea
- Decreased absorption of nutrients by inflamed intestine

Defining Characteristics

Nausea, vomiting, cramping
Weight loss, poor muscle tone
Weakness, lethargy
Aversion to eating
Abdominal pain
Abdominal cramping, diarrhea, and/or steatorrhea
Hyperactive bowel sounds

Patient Outcomes

Patient will

- demonstrate progressive weight gain.
- tolerate a balanced diet.
- establish a predictable bowel elimination pattern; stools are soft and formed.
- display adequate energy to perform activities of daily living.

Nursing Interventions	Rationales
Assess patient to determine causes of inadequate intake, for example, pain, nausea, diarrhea, and cramping associated with food intake.	
Assist in identifying irritating foods.	
Consult dietitian, if available, to assist with dietary restrictions, guidelines, and menu planning as needed.	
Weigh at least every other day and report weight changes to dietitian or physician.	
Provide nutritional supplements as prescribed.	
Assess laboratory values indicative of nutritional status, specific to IBD:	
1. hemoglobin/hematocrit and serum iron	Anemia is common with IBD.
2. serum folate and vitamin B_{12}	Deficiencies often exist because IBD adversely affects the absorption of these substances and sulfasalazine impairs folate absorption.
Assess for appropriateness of initiating enteral or parenteral nutrition if intolerance to oral intake persists.	Patients with IBD frequently have increased protein and calorie requirements because of the catabolic effects of chronic inflammation, superimposed infections, and/or corticosteroid therapy.

▼

NURSING DIAGNOSIS: PAIN

Related To

- Abdominal cramping
- Intestinal inflammation
- Ulceration of intestinal wall

Defining Characteristics

Communicating of pain descriptors
Guarding behavior
Narrowed focus
Behaviors indicative of pain (moaning, crying, restlessness)
Diaphoresis
Pulse, blood pressure, and respiratory rate change

Patient Outcomes

Patient experiences decreased abdominal pain, as evidenced by

- verbalization of pain relief
- increased participation in activities
- relaxed facial expressions
- stable vital signs

Nursing Interventions	Rationales
Assess for verbal complaints of abdominal pain with specific attention to severity, location, and type of pain.	
Assess for nonverbal cues for pain.	
Assess for factors that alleviate or aggravate pain.	
Implement measures to reduce inflammation and hyperactivity of the bowel.	Abdominal pain and cramping are reduced when bowel inflammation and hyperactivity are decreased.
Administer narcotic analgesics cautiously.	Narcotic analgesics slow gastrointestinal motility and may cause a serious bowel obstruction.

Nursing Interventions	Rationales
Provide or assist with nonpharmacological measures for pain relief, for example, back rubs, position changes, restful environment, quiet music, relaxation techniques, or other activities helpful to the patient.	

▼

NURSING DIAGNOSIS: HIGH RISK FOR FLUID VOLUME DEFICIT

Risk Factors

- Diarrhea
- Intestinal bleeding

Patient Outcomes

Patient will demonstrate no signs of active bleeding, as evidenced by

- normalizing hemoglobin and hematocrit levels
- balanced intake and output (I&O)
- absence of blood in stool
- absence of frank rectal bleeding
- vital signs within normal limits
- no change in mental status
- normal bowel sounds and no evidence of abdominal pain or distention
- warm, dry, skin with usual color
- palpable peripheral pulses

Nursing Interventions	Rationales
Assure patient has at least one patent, large-bore (18-gauge or larger) intravenous access site available.	Allows rapid infusion of blood products and volume expanders as needed.
Assess diarrhea stools for amount, frequency, consistency, and presence of frank or occult blood. Notify physician of significant findings.	

Nursing Interventions	Rationales
Assess for decreases in blood pressure, orthostatic blood pressure changes; increased resting pulse rate; diminished peripheral pulses; cool, pale cyanotic skin; urine output less than 30 mL/hr; rapid labored respirations; restlessness; agitation; or change in mental status. Report significant findings to physician.	These are signs/symptoms of hypovolemia.
Monitor hemoglobin, hematocrit, and red blood cell counts. Report declining values to physician.	
If signs and symptoms of hypovolemia occur: 1. Monitor vital signs frequently. 2. Administer oxygen. 3. Place patient in Trendelenburg position, if not contraindicated. 4. Administer blood products and/or volume expanders as prescribed. Monitor for transfusion reactions. 5. Increase rate of intravenous crystalloid solution as prescribed.	
Prepare patient for transfer to an intensive care setting if closer observation and more invasive interventions are needed.	
Prepare patient for surgical intervention, for example, bowel resection and total or partial colectomy, as prescribed, if indicated to control bleeding.	
Provide emotional support to patient and family.	

▼

NURSING DIAGNOSIS: HIGH RISK FOR INFECTION

Risk Factors

- Corticosteroid therapy
- Bowel perforation with peritonitis
- Bowel obstruction
- Toxic megacolon

Patient Outcomes

Patient demonstrates no evidence of infection, as evidenced by

- afebrile state
- white blood cell (WBC) count within normal limits
- normal bowel sounds
- stable vital signs
- soft nondistended abdomen
- no complaints of sudden severe abdominal pain

Nursing Interventions	Rationales
Closely monitor vital signs, body temperature, bowel sounds, presence or absence of abdominal distention, breath sounds, presence or absence of sputum production, and character, odor, and amount of urine output.	Patients with IBD are susceptible to many types of opportunistic infections. Close observation is necessary because patients may not demonstrate the typically dramatic rise in body temperature and/or WBC count due to medication-related immunosuppression and chronicity of illness.
Utilize careful aseptic technique with any invasive procedures or necessary interventions.	
Monitor for increases in WBC levels and report findings to the physician.	
Assess for sudden severe abdominal pain, rigid tense abdomen, abdominal rebound tenderness, diminished or absent bowel sounds, elevated temperature, tachycardia, tachypnea, and decreased blood pressure and report significant findings to physician.	These are signs and symptoms of perforation or peritonitis.

Nursing Interventions	Rationales
Assess for vomiting. Note type of vomitus, abdominal distention, and any change in bowel sounds.	These are potential signs and symptoms of bowel obstruction. With bowel obstruction, vomitus initially contains gastric juices and bile and eventually contains fecal material. Bowel sounds are initially high pitched and hyperactive with a mechanical obstruction and absent with paralytic ileus.
Monitor abdominal x-ray results. Report findings of colonic dilation and/or complete or partial bowel obstruction.	Colonic dilation may indicate toxic megacolon.
Assess for severe abdominal pain, tenderness, and distention associated with hypoactive, absent bowel sounds with tympanic percussion, sudden decreases in diarrhea, febrile response, and elevated WBC count.	May indicate toxic megacolon and the risk of bowel perforation increases when toxic megacolon develops.
Administer narcotic analgesics and anticholinergics cautiously.	These medications decrease gastric motility and can precipitate or worsen a bowel obstruction/toxic megacolon situation.
Monitor serum potassium levels and notify physician if decreased levels are apparent.	Hypokalemia must be prevented or quickly corrected because low potassium levels slow gastric motility.
If signs and symptoms of toxic megacolon, bowel obstruction, and/or peritonitis occur, prepare to	
1. withhold all food and fluid.	Prevents further contamination of peritoneal cavity, prevents pressure in obstructed intestine, and decreases risk of aspiration during anesthesia induction if surgery is necessary.
2. insert nasogastric tube and maintain suction.	
3. monitor for therapeutic effects of prescribed antibiotics.	

Nursing Interventions	Rationales
4. monitor for therapeutic effects of intravenous fluids (colloid and crystalloid) as prescribed.	Prevents or treats shock that can occur when fluids, protein, and electrolytes leak into the peritoneal cavity with peritonitis associated with perforation. Maintains adequate intravascular volume when hypovolemia occurs due to third-spacing from increased intraluminal pressure seen in bowel obstruction or toxic megacolon.
Prepare patient for surgical intervention if indicated to correct bowel obstruction, prevent/treat toxic megacolon, or repair perforation.	
Provide emotional support to patient and family.	

▼

NURSING DIAGNOSIS: HIGH RISK FOR IMPAIRED SKIN INTEGRITY

Risk Factors
- Poor nutritional status
- Corticosteroid usage
- Diarrhea
- Potential enterocutaneous fistula formation
- Potential rectal or rectal-vaginal fistula formation

Patient Outcomes
- Areas of skin breakdown heal completely or significantly improve.
- Skin remains intact by utilizing preventative measures.

Nursing Interventions	Rationales
Assess fluid and nutrient intake. Collaborate with dietitian as needed.	Adequate hydration and nutrients are necessary to prevent skin breakdown and heal existing areas of breakdown.

Nursing Interventions	Rationales
Assess perianal area for evidence of fistulas, fissures, or abscesses.	Fistula formation is very common in Crohn's disease. Fistulas, fissures, and walled-off abscesses can cause severe skin care management problems for the patient.
Assess perianal area for irritation from chronic diarrhea.	
Assess enterocutaneous fistulas for type and amount of drainage.	
Protect the perianal skin of patients with chronic diarrhea using preventative measures: 1. Use soft toilet tissue after each bowel movement. 2. Cleanse perianal area with mild soap and warm water or a commercial gentle cleansing product after each bowel movement. 3. Apply a protective ointment or creme to clean, dry perianal skin (e.g., Triple care, Sween creme, Desitin, Vaseline).	
Provide treatment for perianal fissures as prescribed for example, sitz baths and skin cleansing routines.	
Protect skin from erosive, caustic fistula drainage with ostomy appliance pouching techniques. Collaborate with enterostomal therapist if available.	
Prepare patient for surgical intervention, for example, fistulectomy, incision, and drainage, as prescribed, to correct/treat the fistula or abscess.	
Provide emotional support to patient and family.	

NURSING DIAGNOSIS: KNOWLEDGE DEFICIT—ABOUT MEDICATION THERAPY

Related To lack of exposure to information

Defining Characteristics

Verbalizing a lack of knowledge
Demonstrates inaccurate follow-through of instructions

Patient Outcomes

The patient will

- demonstrate an understanding of medication therapy used to prevent/minimize IBD exacerbations.
- demonstrate accurate follow-through with plan of care while hospitalized.

Nursing Interventions	Rationales
Explain the rationale for, side effects of, and the importance of taking medications as prescribed.	
Provide written materials about medications for patient/family reference and consult with pharmacist, if available, to assist with teaching, follow-up, and reinforcement of medication information.	
Reinforce the need to inform physician/nurse of any other medications being taken and avoid ingesting any over-the-counter medications before checking with a health care professional.	
If it is necessary for patient to take corticosteroids, instruct in the following: 1. Take medications exactly as prescribed; usually the daily dose or a larger dose is taken in the morning.	This simulates the body's normal pattern of steroid secretion.

Nursing Interventions	Rationales
2. Avoid discontinuing medication suddenly or on own accord. Adjust dosage only as prescribed by physician. Notify physician if unable to tolerate oral medication.	Serious complications (e.g., acute adrenal insufficiency) occur if long-term or high-dose therapy is abruptly discontinued.
3. Take medications with food or milk.	This reduces gastric irritation often caused by corticosteroids.
4. Explain side effects of corticosteroids: slight weight gain, swelling, facial rounding, increased appetite, and potential mood changes. Provide reference on recognizing Cushingoid symptoms.	
5. Report the following side effects to physician: more than 5 lb weight gain in a week, marked swelling in the extremities, tarry stools, coffee ground or bloody emesis, extreme emotional and behavioral changes, insomnia, and severe headaches.	
6. Avoid contact with large crowds or people with known infections.	Corticosteroids lower resistance to infection.
7. Instruct patient to carry a medical alert card indicating use of corticosteroids.	This alerts health care professionals not familiar with patient's medical condition that in case of a medical emergency the patient may need supplemental glucocorticoids during stress.
If it is necessary for patient to take sulfasalazine, instruct in the following:	
1. Drink at least 8–10 glasses of liquid per day if not contraindicated.	This reduces risk of kidney stone formation.
2. Avoid exposure to excessive sunlight and ultraviolet light.	This prevents photosensitivity reaction.

Nursing Interventions	Rationales
3. Anticipate urine may be orange-yellow color.	
4. Notify physician of the following: fever, unusual fatigue, continuous headache, or aching joints, unusual bleeding, bruising, rash, marked decline in urine output.	

NURSING DIAGNOSIS: HIGH RISK FOR INEFFECTIVE INDIVIDUAL COPING

Risk Factors

- Effect of disease on life-style
- Chronicity of condition
- Need for repeated hospitalizations
- Inadequate support systems
- Fear of needing an ostomy

Patient Outcomes

Patient demonstrates healthy coping behaviors, as evidenced by

- verbalization of ability to cope with inflammatory bowel disease and its effects.
- utilization of appropriate problem-solving techniques.
- willingness to participate in treatment plan and self-care activities.
- identification of stressors.
- recognition and utilization of available support systems.

Nursing Interventions	Rationales
Assess effectiveness of current coping strategies, for example, ability to express feelings, willingness to participate in cares, and treatment plan.	
Assess for cues that may indicate ineffective coping, for example, verbalization of such, sleep pattern disturbances, inability to concentrate, or inability to problem solve.	

Nursing Interventions	Rationales
Utilize interventions to promote effective coping: 1. Provide continuity and consistency with caregivers and inform patient when changes will be made. 2. Encourage maximum participation in plan of care, allowing choices and options. 3. Assist patient/family with ways to adjust personal/family goals rather than abandoning them. 4. Make arrangements with another individual (with or without an ostomy) who is better adjusted to IBD to visit with the patient experiencing difficulty if such a service is available and agreeable to all parties involved.	 1. Consistency and continuity promote trust. Do not want patient to interpret changes as rejection. 2. Conveys respect and enables patient to maintain sense of control.
Provide with information about national/local support groups, for example, the National Foundation for Ileitis and Colitis and/or the United Ostomy Association. Initiate a referral as needed or as requested.	
Recognize own limitations and biases and refer to additional counseling resources as needed, for example, an enterostomal therapist, social worker, or psychologist/psychiatrist.	
Acknowledge and reinforce those behaviors that indicate positive adaptation to changes and stressors.	
Encourage the continued emotional support and concern from significant others.	

▼

DISCHARGE PLANNING/CONTINUITY OF CARE

- Assure that patient/family understands self-care management plan, for example, medications, dietary modifications, skin care treatment regimes, and when to notify the physician.
- Refer patient to a home care agency if continued nursing care, teaching, or assistance with self-care management plan is needed.
- Arrange for follow-up with physician, nurse, enterostomal therapist, and/or dietitian for continued management after discharge.
- Assist patient with obtaining prescriptions and establishing a plan for refilling prescriptions.
- Provide patient/family with information regarding available community resources that can assist in coping with IBD, for example, colitis support groups, ostomy support groups, and counseling services. Initiate a referral if indicated.
- Provide patient/family with information on and resources for stress reduction, biofeedback, vocational rehabilitation, and/or massage. Initiate a referral if indicated.

REFERENCES

Cooke, D. M. (1991). Inflammatory bowel disease: Primary health care management of ulcerative colitis and Crohn's disease. *Nurse Practitioner, 16*(18), 27–39.

Crohn's and Colitis Foundation of America 444 Park Avenue South, New York. (Resource for Patient Education.)Tel: (212) 685–3440 or 1–(800)-343–3637.

Doughty, D. B. & Jackson, D. B. (1993). *Gastrointestinal Disorders.* St. Louis, MO: Mosby Year Book.

Lewis, S. M. & Collier, T. C. (1992). *Medical-surgical nursing: Assessment and management of clinical problems* (3rd ed). St. Louis, MO: Mosby Year Book.

▼

PANCREATITIS

Deborah R. Johnson, RN, MS, CNSN

Pancreatitis is the inflammation of the pancreas. There are two classifications of pancreatitis, acute and chronic. In acute pancreatitis the most common pathogenic mechanism is believed to be autodigestion of the pancreas. The etiological factors cause injury to the pancreatic cells, or activation of pancreatic enzymes in the pancreas, instead of in the intestines. The structure and function of the pancreas is usually restored when inflammation subsides. The degree of inflammation varies from mild edema to severe hemorrhage necrosis. In chronic pancreatitis changes in pancreatic structure, tissue, and functions are permanent. There is a progressive destruction of the pancreas with fibrotic replacement of pancreatic tissue. Enzyme action is markedly decreased or absent. Potential complications of pancreatitis include the development of pancreatic phlegmon, pseudocyst, and abscess; chronic pancreatitis can induce permanent alterations in blood glucose control.

ETIOLOGIES

- Alcoholism
- Biliary tract disease: gallstones
- Trauma (blunt, surgical, penetrating)
- Metabolic disorders: renal failure, hyperlipidemia, hyperparathyroidism
- Pancreatic carcinoma
- Medications: estrogens, oral contraceptives, corticosteroids, thiazide diuretics
- Pregnancy
- Infections: mononucleosis, viral hepatitis, mycoplasma, mumps

CLINICAL MANIFESTATIONS

- Mild pancreatitis: Mid epigastric or left upper quadrant pain with radiation to the back, aggravated by food and/or alcohol intake, unrelieved by vomiting

- Severe pancreatitis
  - excruciating pain
  - severe nausea, abdominal rigidity
  - diminished bowel sounds or ileus
  - left pleural effusion
  - malaise, mottled skin, low-grade fever, tachycardia, hypovolemia, jaundice, bluish flank discoloration (Grey Turner's spots or signs), bluish periumbilical discoloration (Cullen's sign), and fulminating hemorrhagic pancreatitis that may lead to diabetic ketoacidosis, massive hemorrhage, shock, coma, and death

CLINICAL/DIAGNOSTIC FINDINGS

- Elevated amylase levels in serum, urine, ascites, or pleural fluid
- Elevated serum lipase levels
- Elevated serum triglycerides
- Elevated serum glucose
- Elevated white blood cell count
- Elevated lactic dehydrogenase (LDH), serum glutamic oxaloacetic/pyruvic transaminase (SGOT, SGPT), and alkaline phosphatase
- Stool specimens positive for fat (steatorrhea)
- Hypoalbuminemia
- Hypocalcemia
- Chest x-ray may show left pleural effusion.
- Abdominal x-rays may show calcification of pancreas, dilated large, and small bowel.
- Upper gastrointestinal (GI) series shows evidence of delayed gastric emptying and duodenal enlargement related to edema at the head of the pancreas.
- Computerized tomography (CT) scan may reveal pancreatic inflammation, pseudocyst, abscess, or obstruction of biliary tract.
- Ultrasound may demonstrate diffuse pancreatic enlargement, abscess, or pseudocyst formation.
- Endoscopic retrograde cholangiopancreatography (ERCP) may reveal pancreatic duct abnormalities.

  (NOTE: ERCP is usually contraindicated during acute pancreatitis.)

OTHER PLANS OF CARE TO REFERENCE

- Pain Management: Patient-Controlled Analgesia
- Nutrition Support: Enteral Nutrition
- Nutrition Support: Total Parenteral Nutrition

▼

NURSING DIAGNOSIS: PAIN

Related To
- Inflammation and distention of the pancreas
- Peritoneal irritation
- Obstruction and/or spasms of pancreatic and biliary duct

Defining Characteristics

Communication of pain descriptors, guarding behavior
Narrowed focus (withdrawal from social contact)
Altered time perception
Impaired thought process
Behaviors indicative of pain (moaning, crying, restlessness)
Diaphoresis
Pulse, blood pressure, and respiratory rate changes

Patient Outcomes

- Patient displays behaviors demonstrating an absence of pain or the presence of pain that is less intense and tolerable.
- Patient reports
  - diminished pain in epigastric area, back, flank, and left upper quadrant.
  - satisfaction with pain control

Nursing Interventions	Rationales
Anticipate patient will have nothing by mouth (NPO).	
Insert nasogastric tube and maintain suction as prescribed.	Prevents gastric contents from entering the duodenum and stimulating the pancreas. It is important to reduce or suppress pancreatic enzyme activity to decrease pancreatic stimulation and hence pancreatic inflammation. This will foster pancreatic rest.
Administer medications as prescribed and monitor for therapeutic effects:	
1. antacids	Neutralizes gastric secretions. Hydrochloric acid (HCl) can stimulate pancreatic secretions, which can cause further pancreatic inflammation and injury.

Nursing Interventions	Rationales
2. histamine 2 receptor antagonists, for example, ranitidine (Zantac)	Reduce output of HCl. Hydrochloric acid stimulates pancreatic activity. Goal is to foster rest of the pancreas.
3. antispasmodics	Decrease vagal stimulation, motility, and pancreatic outflow.
4. analgesics: meperidine (Demerol) is preferred over other opiates	Meperidine causes less smooth-muscle duct spasms (e.g., sphincter of Oddi), hence decreases potential for additional pancreatic inflammation.
Minimize patient's exposure to the odor and sight of food until oral intake is allowed.	The odor and smell of food stimulates pancreatic enzyme secretion.
Provide or assist with nonpharmacological measures for pain relief: backrubs, position changes, side lying with knees flexed, restful environment, quiet music, guided imagery, or other activities helpful to the patient.	

▼

NURSING DIAGNOSIS: ALTERED NUTRITION—LESS THAN BODY REQUIREMENTS

Related To

- Anorexia
- Nausea
- Vomiting
- Impaired digestion of fats, proteins, and carbohydrates from the obstructed outflow of pancreatic enzymes resulting in decreased nutrient utilization

Defining Characteristics

Weight loss, weight below normal for patient's age, sex, height, and activity level.
Weakness, fatigue
Abdominal pain
Hypocalcemia
Steatorrhea

Patient Outcomes

Patient will

- demonstrate progressive weight gain.
- tolerate a balanced diet.
- display adequate energy to perform activities of daily living.

Nursing Interventions	Rationales
Assess for causes of inadequate intake, for example, pain, nausea, food, or fluid restrictions.	
Monitor for bowel sounds.	
Consult with dietitian if available.	Assist with monitoring food tolerances, menu planning, and dietary education.
Implement measures to improve or maintain nutritional status.	
1. Effectively reduce abdominal pain, nausea, and vomiting.	
2. Provide oral care before and after meals.	
3. If oral intake is allowed, provide small portions of appealing foods.	
4. Collaborate with dietitian, if available, to assure diet is bland, free of stimulants (caffeine), and low fat, high protein, and high carbohydrate.	These dietary modifications will optimize pancreatic rest to facilitate healing.
5. Monitor for therapeutic effects of fat-soluble vitamins and pancreatic enzymes as prescribed.	Pancreatic enzyme replacement therapy and fat-soluble vitamin supplementation are sometimes necessary to aid in digestion if the pancreas loses its exocrine function.
6. Administer total parenteral nutrition (TPN) as prescribed if oral intake is not allowed or patient is intolerant of oral feeding.	Administering TPN reduces pancreatic enzyme activity and facilitates pancreatic rest.
Correct persistent hyperglycemia with insulin administration as prescribed.	Pancreatic insufficiency can be characterized by loss of endocrine function, resulting in diabetes mellitus.

Nursing Interventions	Rationales
Weigh patient daily at the same time with the same clothing and using the same scale.	
Observe patient's stools for color, consistency, amount, frequency, and presence of fat (steatorrhea).	Steatorrhea can occur in pancreatitis and is an indicator of fat malabsorption.
Assess for signs and symptoms of hypocalcemia (Chvostek's, Trousseau sign). Note serum calcium level.	The pancreatic enzyme lipase is not released into the intestinal tract to digest fat. Hence calcium binds with the free fats and is excreted in the stool. Hyocalcemia can occur.

NURSING DIAGNOSIS: IMPAIRED GAS EXCHANGE

Related To
- Pain
- Irritation near diaphragm
- Pleural effusion
- Ineffective cough

Defining Characteristics
Confusion, sommolence, restlessness, irritability
Inability to move secretions, hypercapnea, hypoxia

Patient Outcomes
- Patient is free of respiratory infection, as evidenced by
  - clear chest x-ray
  - negative sputum culture
- Patient is afebrile.
- Breath sounds are clear.
- Patient demonstrates no signs or symptoms of hypoxia.

Nursing Interventions	Rationales
Auscultate lung fields at least every shift; more frequently as needed.	
Observe for fever or changes in respiratory assessment, for example, dyspnea and tachypnea.	

Nursing Interventions	Rationales
Place patient in semi-Fowler's position to promote deeper respirations.	
Assist patient to cough, turn, and deep breathe every 1–2 hr while awake.	
Implement measures to control pain.	

NURSING DIAGNOSIS: HIGH RISK FOR INFECTION

Risk Factors

- Pancreatic pseudocyst formation
- Pancreatic abscess formation due to inflamed or necrotic pancreatic tissue
- Rupture or perforation of pseudocyst or abscess

Patient Outcomes

Patient demonstrates no pancreatic infectious process, as evidenced by

- normalizing white blood cell (WBC) count
- normal CT scan
- lack of febrile episodes
- no increase in abdominal pain

Nursing Interventions	Rationales
Anticipate, monitor, and assess for signs/symptoms of pancreatic pseudocyst formation: 1. Amylase levels remain elevated. 2. Blood glucose levels are elevated from patient baseline. 3. Patient experiences increased abdominal pain. 4. Patient experiences persistent nausea, vomiting and anorexia. 5. A palpable epigastric mass may be found on physical exam. Prepare the patient for a drainage procedure if the pancreatic pseudocyst does not spontaneously resolve.	A pseudocyst is a cavity continuous with or surrounding the outside of the pancreas. It is filled with necrotic products and liquid secretions such as plasma, inflammatory exudates, and pancreatic enzymes. As liquids escape from the pseudocyst, the serosal surfaces next to the pancreas become inflamed and subsequently form granulation tissue leading to encapsulation of the exudate. The cysts can perforate, causing peritonitis or rupture into the stomach or duodenum. There is a 15% mortality associated with pancreatic pseudocysts.

Nursing Interventions	Rationales
Anticipate, monitor, and assess for signs/symptoms of pancreatic abscess formation: 1. high fever 2. leukocytosis 3. hyperglycemia 4. upper abdominal pain 5. apparent abdominal mass Prepare the patient for prompt surgical drainage if pancreatic abscess is suspected.	A pancreatic abscess is a large fluid-filled cavity within the pancreas resulting from extensive pancreatic necrosis. It may become infected and perforate into adjacent organs. There is 100% mortality if the abscess is not surgically drained. Multiple drainage procedures are often needed.

NURSING DIAGNOSIS: HIGH RISK FOR FLUID VOLUME DEFICIT

Risk Factors

- Restricted oral intake, vomiting, and nasal gastric tube drainage
- Third-space fluid shifts associated with increased vascular permeability from the inflammatory response and increased activation of kinin peptides, stimulated by the pancreatic enzyme, trypsin.
- Blood loss/hemorrhage related to the activation of elastase, a pancreatic enzyme that destroys and dissolves blood vessel wall fibers

Patient Outcomes

Patient's fluid volume status is adequate and balanced, as evidenced by

- stable weight
- moist mucous membranes
- warm, dry skin with normal turgor
- normal pulse and blood pressure
- normal level of consciousness
- no signs of shock
- normal electrolyte levels
- normal hemoglobin and hematocrit levels
- clear yellow urine output in at least 30 mL/hr amounts

Nursing Interventions	Rationales
Monitor vital signs and note postural changes in blood pressure.	
Monitor cardiac rate and rhythm.	
Monitor and record accurate intake and output (I&O).	

Nursing Interventions	Rationales
Weigh patient daily and record.	
Monitor electrolyte levels for abnormalities, especially sodium, potassium, chloride, and calcium.	
Monitor hemoglobin and hematocrit levels.	
Monitor serum or capillary blood glucose levels.	
Assess mucous membranes and skin turgor for signs of dehydration.	
Assess for presence of peripheral edema, ascites, dyspnea, diminished breath sounds, absent breath sounds, or crackles.	
Assess level of consciousness.	
Assess for presence of blue, green, and/or brown discoloration on abdomen, flanks (Grey Turner's sign) or periumbilical area (Cullen's sign).	Intravascular damage from the pancreatic enzyme trypsin may cause areas of discoloration in the abdominal wall. Ecchymosis at the flank or periumbilical area results from seepage of blood-stained pancreatic exudate and may be present in hemorrhagic pancreatitis.
Maintain patent intravenous line(s) for the administration of any necessary colloid or crystalloid products.	

▼

DISCHARGE PLANNING/CONTINUITY OF CARE

- Encourage alcohol abstinence to prevent further pain, extension of the inflammation, and pancreatic insufficiency.
- Provide with information on local self-help or recovery programs if alcohol dependency is suspected or acknowledged.
- Provide patient/family with dietary information to plan bland, low-fat, high-protein, high-carbohydrate meals that will minimize pancreatic stimulation and enzyme release.

- Teach patient/family to recognize and report symptoms of diabetes mellitus and steatorrhea.
- Assist in obtaining prescriptions and establish a plan for refilling prescriptions.
- Assure that patient/family understands the proper dosage and timing of pancreatic enzyme therapy to optimize digestion of nutrients.
- Assure that patient will notify the physician of acute abdominal pain or symptoms of biliary tract disease such as clay-colored stools, jaundice, or dark urine.
- Refer to a home health agency if continued nursing care, teaching, or assistance with blood glucose management (oral hypoglycemics, insulin injections, or blood glucose monitoring) is needed.
- Arrange for follow-up with nurse, dietitian, and/or physician for continued management postdischarge.

REFERENCES

Alspach, J. G. (1991). *AACN—Core curriculum critical care nursing* (4th ed). Philadelphia, PA: Saunders.

Doughty, D. B. & Jackson, D. B. (1993). *Gastrointestinal Disorders.* St. Louis, MO: Mosby Year Book.

Krumberger, J. M. (1993). Acute pancreatitis. *Critical Care Nursing Clinics of North America, 5*(1), 185–202.

Lewis, S. M. & Collier, I. C. (1992). *Medical surgical nursing: Assessment and managment of clinical problems* (3rd ed). St. Louis, MO: Mosby Year Book.

Smith, A. (1991). When the pancreas self-destructs. *American Journal of Nursing, 9*, 38–48.

▼

PEPTIC ULCER DISEASE

Deborah R. Johnson, RN, MS, CNSN

A peptic ulcer occurs when there is a mucosal break along any part of the gastrointestinal (GI) tract that comes in contact with hydrochloric (HCl) acid and pepsin. Acid production, vasodilatation, and increased capillary permeability occur due to histamine release. Complications from peptic ulcer disease (PUD) include bleeding, perforation, obstruction, penetration resulting in fistula formation, and intractability. The types of peptic ulcers include duodenal, gastric, and stress ulcers. *Duodenal* is the most common type of peptic ulcer. It is characterized by high gastric acid secretion. Duodenal ulcers account for a greater percentage of upper GI bleeding when compared to gastric ulcers. *Gastric ulcers* typically occur in the lesser curvature of the stomach near the pylorus; gastritis often surrounds the area of ulceration. These ulcers have an increased incidence of malignancy when compared to duodenal ulcers. *Stress ulcers* also referred to as a Curling's ulcer, are caused by a form of erosive gastritis associated with severe body trauma. The body of the stomach experiences transient ischemia, and multiple superficial gastric mucosal erosions result.

ETIOLOGIES

- Medication usage: aspirin, nonsteroidal anti-inflammatory drugs (NSAIDs), corticosteroids
- Gastritis
- Cigarette usage
- Alcohol usage
- Life-style, perceived stressors
- Dietary intake: alcohol, caffeine, other irritants
- Chemo/radiation therapy
- Familial tendencies

CLINICAL MANIFESTATIONS

- Aching, burning, cramplike, gnawing pain possibly radiating to the back

- Relationship of pain to eating, with discomfort relieved by eating food, or taking antacids, and pain occurring after meals
- Heartburn, epigastric distress
- Nausea, vomiting, early satiety

CLINICAL/DIAGNOSTIC FINDINGS

- Fiberoptic endoscopy demonstrates presence and location of ulcer.
- Urine, stool, and/or emesis are positive for blood.
- Liver enzyme studies are elevated in patients with liver disturbances (cirrhosis).
- Serum amylase elevated if posterior penetration of the pancreas is suspected from a perforated ulcer.
- Gastric analysis is abnormal.
- Upper gastrointestinal (GI) barium contrast study identifies interruptions in GI mucosa.
- Exfoliative cytology studies distinguish between a benign and a malignant ulcer.
- Chest x-ray shows free air under diaphragm with perforated ulcers.

OTHER PLANS OF CARE TO REFERENCE

Cirrhosis and Esophageal Varices

▼

NURSING DIAGNOSIS: PAIN

Related To
- Ingestion of gastric irritants
- Increased gastric secretion
- Decreased gastric mucosal protection

Defining Characteristics

Guarding behavior, moaning, crying, restlessness
Diaphoresis
Blood pressure and pulse changes
Pupillary dilation
Burning or cramplike epigastric and abdominal discomfort
Onset of gastric ulcer pain, occurring 1–2 hr after meals with occasional relief after food or liquids ingested
Onset of duodenal ulcer pain, occurring 2–4 hr after meals, may be associated with nausea and vomiting, with pain relief after antacids and food

Patient Outcomes

The patient will

- not demonstrate guarding behavior, moaning, crying, diaphoresis, blood pressure, pulse changes, or pupillary dilatation.
- verbalize satisfactory pain control.

Nursing Interventions	Rationales
Assess for nonverbal signs of pain, for example, restlessness, diaphoresis, guarding behavior, blood pressure, or pulse changes.	
Assess for verbal complaints of pain and sequence of the pain experience, noting location, intensity, and duration of pain.	
Assess for any specific factors thought to alleviate or aggravate pain.	
Implement measures that will promote healing of the ulcerated area and/or prevent further irritation of the ulcerated area:	
1. Insert a nasogastric tube and maintain suction as prescribed.	Removes gastric secretions.
2. Monitor for therapeutic effectiveness of the following prescribed medications, if administered:	
• antacids	Neutralize or buffer hydrochloric acid.
• histamine 2 (H_2) blockers, for example, rantidine.	Block gastric acid secretion.
• anticholinergics	Decrease gastric acid secretion.
• prostaglandin analogues, for example, misoprostol (Cytotec)	Inhibit gastric acid secretion and contribute to mucosal barrier.
• mucosal barrier fortifiers, for example, sucralfate, Pepto Bismol	Provide cytoprotective coating over ulcerated area to prevent further damage and are effective against the organism helicobacter pylori.

Nursing Interventions	Rationales
• antisecretory compounds, for example, Omeprazole	Suppress gastric acid secretion.
Implement measures that will reduce the stimulation of hydrochloric acid and pepsin secretion:	
1. Reduce patient's fear, stress, and anxiety.	These emotions stimulate hydrochloric acid production.
2. Provide bland diet using small frequent feedings and snacks.	Bland diet will not irritate the stomach; food in the stomach neutralizes gastric acidity.
3. Avoid caffeine products, for example, tea, cola, coffee, and chocolate.	Caffeine stimulates gastric acid secretion.
Encourage patient to stop smoking.	Tobacco enhances reflux of duodenal contents to the antrum of the stomach. Smoking may cause a decrease in pancreatic bicarbonate secretion. This creates a more acidic environment.
Encourage patient to avoid alcohol.	Alcohol is source of GI irritation and interferes with tissue repair.
Avoid the use of known ulcerogenic drugs if possible.	
1. aspirin and other related NSAIDs.	Alter and/or destroy the protective GI mucosal barrier by inhibiting the synthesis of prostaglandins and mucus.
2. corticosteroids	Decrease the rate of GI mucous cell renewal, hence decreasing protective effectiveness.
Evaluate effectiveness of interventions.	
Prepare patient for surgical intervention as indicated (e.g., vagotomy) if conservative medical management is deemed ineffective.	

▼

NURSING DIAGNOSIS: HIGH RISK FOR FLUID VOLUME DEFICIT

Risk Factors

- Bleeding peptic ulcer
- Erosion of granulation tissue at base of ulcer during healing
- Erosion of the ulcer through a major blood vessel
- Excessive vomiting
- Gastric outlet obstruction (extensive peristaltic activity that creates hypertrophy, dilation and atony of the stomach wall; fibrous scar tissue with edema, inflammation and pylorospasm).

Patient Outcomes

Patient will

- demonstrate no signs of active GI bleeding.
- maintain normal oral intake.
- demonstrate no signs of gastric outlet obstruction, as evidenced by
  - a soft, nondistended epigastric area
  - no complaints of epigastric fullness
  - absence of nausea, vomiting, and foul breath odor

Nursing Interventions	Rationales
Assure patient has at least one patent large-bore (18 gauge or larger) intravenous access site available.	Allows rapid infusion of blood products/volume expanders if needed.
Maintain nasogastric tube to suction and assure patency.	
Assess and report signs and symptoms of GI hemorrhage: hematemesis, melena, complaints of epigastric fullness, or increased epigastric pain.	

Nursing Interventions	Rationales
Assess and report signs and symptoms of hypovolemia: 1. decreased blood pressure, orthostatic blood pressure changes, increased resting pulse rate, diminished peripheral pulses 2. cool, pale, cyanotic skin 3. urine output < 30 mL/hour 4. rapid, labored respirations 5. restlessness, agitation, or change in mental status	
Monitor hemoglobin, hematocrit, and red blood cell (RBC) levels. Report declining values to physician.	
If signs and symptoms of hypovolemia occur: 1. Monitor vital signs frequently. 2. Administer oxygen as prescribed. 3. Place patient in Trendelenburg position if not contraindicated. 4. Administer blood products/volume expanders as prescribed. Monitor for transfusion reactions. 5. Assist with iced saline or ice water gastric lavage, endoscopic laser, photocoagulation, endoscopic electrocoagulation, heat probe, elective arterial embolization, and/or intra-arterial administration of vasopressin as prescribed.	These are measures to control bleeding; however gastric lavage is controversial.
Assess and report signs and symptoms of gastric outlet obstruction: 1. epigastric distention, complaints of epigastric fullness, nausea and vomiting	

Nursing Interventions	**Rationales**
2. vomitus of food particles ingested hours or days before	
3. fetid breath	Breath and vomitus often have an offensive odor if contents have been dormant in stomach for some time.
If signs/symptoms of gastric outlet obstruction occur and patient has persistent symptomatic vomiting: 1. Withhold all food and oral fluids. 2. Insert a nasogastric tube and maintain suction as prescribed. 3. Monitor for therapeutic effects of intravenous fluid volume and electrolyte replacement.	
Prepare patient for transfer to an intensive care unit if closer observation and more invasive interventions are needed.	
Prepare patient for surgical intervention, if indicated, to control bleeding or to correct gastric outlet obstruction.	Vagotomy with antral resection, pyloroplasty, or partial gastrectomy may be indicated to control bleeding or gastric outlet obstruction.
Provide emotional support to patient and family.	

▼

NURSING DIAGNOSIS: HIGH RISK FOR INFECTION

Risk Factors

- Inadequate primary defenses: Perforated ulcer is a result of broken skin and traumatized tissue.
- Inadequate secondary defenses: decreased hemoglobin levels related to blood loss, suppressed inflammatory response, immunosuppression from corticosteroid use
- Advanced age
- Ulcerogenic substance use

Patient Outcomes

Patient demonstrates no evidence of infection, as evidenced by

- afebrile status
- white blood cell (WBC) count within normal limits
- normal bowel sounds
- stable vital signs
- soft, nondistended abdomen
- no complaints of sudden severe abdominal pain.

Nursing Interventions	Rationales
Assess for sudden severe upper abdominal pain, right shoulder pain or pain at midback, abdominal tenderness, and report significant findings to physician.	The referred shoulder pain results from phrenic nerve stimulation.
Assess for rigid, tense abdomen, abdominal rebound tenderness, diminished or absent bowel sounds, elevated temperature, tachycardia, tachypnea, and decreased blood pressure and report significant findings to physician.	Signs and symptoms of perforation/peritonitis.
Monitor increases in WBC levels and report findings to physician.	
If signs/symptoms of perforation/peritonitis occur:	
1. Withhold all food and oral fluids as prescribed.	Prevents further contamination of peritoneal cavity.
2. Insert nasogastric tube and maintain suction as prescribed.	
3. Place patient on bedrest in semi-Fowler's position.	May assist with localizing GI contents in the pelvis rather than under the diaphragm.
4. Monitor for therapeutic effects of antibiotics as prescribed.	
5. Monitor for therapeutic effects of intravenous fluids (colloid and crystalloid) as prescribed.	Prevents or treats shock that can occur when fluids, protein, and electrolytes leak into the peritoneal cavity.

Nursing Interventions	Rationales
Prepare patient for transfer to an intensive care setting if closer observation and more invasive interventions are needed.	
Prepare patient for surgical intervention, if indicated, to repair perforation.	
Provide emotional support to patient and family.	

▼

NURSING DIAGNOSIS: KNOWLEDGE DEFICIT—ABOUT MEDICATION THERAPY AND PREVENTION

Related To lack of exposure to information

Defining Characteristics

Verbalizing a lack of knowledge
Inaccurate follow-through of instructions

Patient Outcomes

The patient will

- demonstrate an understanding of medication therapy, strategies to promote healing of the existing ulcer, and/or prevention of ulcer recurrence.
- demonstrate accurate follow-through with plan of care while hospitalized.

Nursing Interventions	Rationales
Explain the rationale for, side effects of, and importance of taking medications as prescribed.	
Provide written materials about medications for patient/family reference and consult with pharmacist, if available, to assist with teaching, follow-up, and reinforcement of medication information.	

Nursing Interventions	Rationales
For long-term antacid therapy, instruct the following:	
1. Take antacids after meals as prescribed.	Neutralizing effects of antacids on an empty stomach last only 20–30 min. Antacids taken after a meal can neutralize stomach acid for 3–4 hr.
2. Avoid use of flavored antacids.	Mint may hasten gastric emptying.
3. Use liquid antacid preparations. If tablets are preferred, chew tablets thoroughly and follow with a glass of water.	Assures antacids optimally coat the GI tract and not stay adhered to teeth, lips, and gums.
4. Lie down for an hour after meals.	Delays gastric emptying and enhances antacid effectiveness.
5. Alternate aluminum-containing antacids and magnesium-containing antacids.	Aluminum preparations cause constipation and magnesium preparations cause diarrhea.
6. Contact physician/nurse if diarrhea/constipation is persistent problem.	
7. Inform physician/nurse of any other medications being taken. Discuss potential specific medication interactions with pharmacist or physician.	Antacids alter the absorption of many other medications.

Nursing Interventions	Rationales
Instruct on strategies to prevent recurrence of peptic ulcers and/or promote healing of existing ulcer: 1. Continue to take medication as prescribed even if pain free. 2. Consult/collaborate with a dietitian to teach: • bland diet • avoidance of caffeine, alcohol, ingestion of foods known to irritate gastric mucosal directly (spicy foods, fresh fruit, raw vegetables) 3. Avoid ingesting any over-the-counter medications before checking with a physician, as they may contain ulcerogenic substances. 4. Avoid all products containing aspirin or aspirin like compounds (ibuprofen) unless prescribed by physician. 5. Stop smoking. 6. Avoid stressful situations and learn to participate in stress reduction exercises and relaxation techniques.	

DISCHARGE PLANNING/CONTINUITY OF CARE

- Assure patient/family understands self-care management plan, for example, medications, dietary restrictions, and when to notify the physician.
- Refer patient to a home care agency if continued nursing care, teaching, or assistance with self-care management plan is needed.
- Arrange to follow-up with physician or nurse for continued management postdischarge.
- Assist patient with obtaining prescriptions and establishing a plan for refilling prescriptions.
- Provide patient with information on smoking cessation groups or other appropriate educational programs in the area. Initiate a referral if indicated.

- Provide patient with information on local self-help or recovery programs if alcohol dependency is suspected or acknowledged. Initiate a referral if indicated.
- Provide patient with information on and resources for stress reduction, biofeedback, guided imagery, counseling, vocational rehabilitation, and/or massage. Initiate a referral if indicated.

REFERENCES

Alspach, J. G. (1991). *AACN—Core curriculum, critical care nursing*, (4th ed). Philadelphia, PA: Saunders.

Doughty, D. B. & Jackson, D. B. (1993). *Gastrointestinal Disorders.* St. Louis, MO: Mosby Year Book.

Kennedy-Caldwell, C. & Guenter, P. A. (1988). *Nutrition support nursing and core curriculum*, (2nd ed). Silver Springs, MD: American Society for Parenteral and Enteral Nutrition.

Lewis, S. M. & I. C. Collier (1992). *Medical-surgical nursing: Assessment and management of clinical problems* (3rd ed). St. Louis, MO: Mosby Year Book.

Wardell, T. L. (1991). Assessing and managing a gastric ulcer. *Nursing, 21*(3), 34–41.

▼

Common Endocrine Conditions and Therapies

CORTICOSTEROID THERAPY

Ellen M. Jovle, RN, MS

Corticosteroids are produced by the adrenal cortex and include several hormones: glucocorticoids, mineralocorticoids, androgens, estrogens, and progesterones. Synthetic corticosteroids include glucocorticoids and mineralcorticoids. Glucocorticoids are medications used to treat adrenocorticol disorders, produce immunosuppression, and reduce inflammation (Table 29.1). When used on a long-term basis, glucocorticoids suppress the hypothalamic-pituitary-adrenal (HPA) axis. Glucocorticoids have effects on carbohydrate, fat, and protein metabolism and also have mineralcorticoid activity, which regulates electrolyte and water balance. Examples of common steroids are cortisone acetate, dexamethasone, hydrocortisone, prednisolone, prednisone, and methylprednisolone.

CLINICAL MANIFESTATIONS/DIAGNOSTIC FINDINGS

N/A

ETIOLOGIES

N/A

OTHER PLANS OF CARE TO REFERENCE

- Diabetes Mellitus: Initiating Insulin
- Peptic Ulcer Disease
- Thrombophlebitis/Deep-Vein Thrombosis
- Stroke/Cerebral Vascular Accident

▼

NURSING DIAGNOSIS: HIGH RISK FOR INFECTION

Risk Factors

- Immune system depression
- Environmental exposure
- Invasive techniques

- Malnutrition
- Chronic disease
- Stress

Table 29.1 • Major Uses Of Glucocorticoids

Treatment of Addison's disease
Treatment of hypercalcemia as a result of breast cancer, multiple myeloma, sarcoidosis, or vitamin D intoxication.
Suppression of allergic reactions
Immunosuppression in organ and tissue transplants
Relief of cerebral edema as a result of brain tumors or neurosurgery
Emergency treatment of shock
To decrease airway inflammation in asthma and COPD
A conjunctive treatment of leukemias, lymphomas, and myelomas
Relief of inflammation in autoimmune diseases such as rheumatoid arthritis, systemic lupus erythematosus, dermatomyositis, ulcerative colitis, vasculitis, myasthenia gravis, and nephrotic syndrome

▼

Patient Outcomes

Patient will remain free of infection, as evidenced by absence of signs and symptoms of infection.

Nursing Interventions	Rationales
Monitor and report signs and symptoms of infection, including temperature, diaphoresis, chills, mental status changes, purulent drainage, pain, and fatigue.	Steroid therapy can mask the usual signs of infection such as temperature elevation. Infections may present with subtle changes.
Monitor white blood cell (WBC) count and differential.	Elevated WBCs with shift to left may indicate infection.

Nursing Interventions	Rationales
Prevent transmission of organisms by 1. meticulous hand washing 2. maintaining closed sterile drainage systems 3. meticulous care of intravascular lines following hospital protocol 4. assessing the continued need for invasive lines and catheters 5. providing personal hygiene 6. limiting exposure to individuals (visitors, staff, or other patient) with known or exposure to infections 7. avoiding unnecessary diagnostic or therapeutic invasive procedures	
Maintain patient's defense against infection by 1. encouraging adequate nutrition 2. maintaining skin integrity 3. encouraging respiratory hygiene 4. encouraging stress management	
Teach patient and family risk factors for infection, precautions to prevent infection, signs and symptoms of infection, and importance of early recognition and reporting.	

▼

NURSING DIAGNOSIS: HIGH RISK FOR INJURY WITH HIGH-DOSE AND/OR LONG-TERM USE OF STEROIDS

Risk Factors

- Adrenal insufficiency secondary to suppression of HPA axis
- Increased lipogenesis
- Protein catabolism
- Insulin resistance
- Increased gluconeogenesis
- Gastrointestinal irritation
- Hypercoagulopathy
- Potassium and calcium loss

Patient Outcomes

Patient will exhibit no/minimal signs and symptoms of

- adrenal insufficiency
- peptic ulcer disease
- diabetes
- osteoporosis
- thromboembolism
- hypokalemia
- hypocalcemia

Nursing Interventions	Rationales
Monitor for signs and symptoms of adrenal insufficiency, including fatigue, weight loss, vomiting, diarrhea, abdominal pain, hypotension, dehydration, tachycardia, and shock. Alert physician if symptoms occur.	Adrenal insufficiency may occur when steroids are withdrawn or tapered due to suppression of HPA axis. Adrenal insufficiency may also occur during periods of stress such as surgery or trauma.
Monitor for signs and symptoms of hyperglycemia: polyuria, polyphagia, polydypsia, and elevated blood glucose.	Steroids promote gluconeogenesis resulting in hyperglycemia.
If patient develops hyperglycemia, implement plans of care for diabetes mellitus.	
Monitor for signs and symptoms of gastrointestinal irritation and bleeding: gastric pain, positive stool guaiac test, and hematemesis.	Steroids stimulate secretion of gastric acid, thereby causing gastric irritation and ulceration.
If signs and symptoms of gastrointestinal bleeding occur, notify physician and implement plan of care for peptic ulcer disease.	
Administer oral steroid medications with food or milk to reduce gastric irritation.	
Monitor patient for signs and symptoms of thromboembolism, deep-vein thrombosis (DVT), pulmonary emboli, or cerebrovascular accident (CVA).	Steroids stimulate production of red blood cells, which increases blood viscosity and the risk of thrombus formation.

Nursing Interventions	Rationales
If signs and symptoms of thromboembolism develop, notify physician. Implement appropriate nursing plan of care for thrombophlebitis or stroke.	
Monitor for signs and symptoms of hypokalemia, muscular weakness, nausea, vomiting, electrocardiographic changes, and decreased serum potassium level.	Steroids increase potassium excretion.
If signs and symptoms of hypokalemia occur, notify physician and anticipate potassium replacement.	
Monitor for signs and symptoms of osteoporosis: pain, kyphosis, and evidence of pathological fractures.	Steroids increase calcium and phosphorous excretion, which leads to a reduction of bone density.

▼

NURSING DIAGNOSIS: HIGH RISK FOR FLUID VOLUME EXCESS

Risk Factors

- Increase sodium reabsorption
- Compromised regulatory mechanism

Patient Outcomes

Patient will maintain normal fluid balance, as evidenced by

- absence of edema
- blood pressure reading within patient's baseline
- absence of weight gain

Nursing Interventions	Rationales
Monitor fluid status by measuring daily weight, intake and output, blood pressure, and presence of edema.	
Assess and review sodium and fluid intake (food, oral and IV fluids and medication). Compare to fluid output.	

Nursing Interventions	Rationales
Teach patient and family: 1. importance of monitoring daily weight 2. sodium-restricted diet as appropriate 3. signs and symptoms of fluid volume excess 4. importance of early recognition and early reporting of symptoms	

▼

NURSING DIAGNOSIS: HIGH RISK FOR IMPAIRED SKIN INTEGRITY

Risk Factors

- Nutritional deficit
- Edema
- Immobility
- Protein tissue wasting
- Capillary fragility

Patient Outcomes

The patient will maintain skin integrity, as evidenced by absence of skin breakdown or irritation.

Nursing Interventions	Rationales
Inspect skin frequently; note areas of erythema, blanching, warmth, maceration, or excoriation.	
Initiate appropriate protective measures, including 1. keeping skin surfaces clean and dry 2. using pressure relief measures 3. reducing shear and friction forces 4. promoting optimal circulation	These measures are critical nursing interventions in the prevention of pressure ulcers. (See Prevention and Care of Pressure Ulcers.)

Nursing Interventions	Rationales
Implement strategies to reduce dependent edema. 1. Elevate legs. 2. Avoid pressure under knee. 3. Encourage passive/active exercise.	Areas of edema may be especially vulnerable to breakdown.
Maintain adequate nutrition.	
Teach patient/family: 1. importance of good skin hygiene 2. protecting skin from trauma 3. importance of adequate nutrition	

▼

NURSING DIAGNOSIS: HIGH RISK FOR ALTERED NUTRITION—MORE THAN BODY REQUIREMENTS

Risk Factors

- Altered fat, protein, and carbohydrate metabolism
- Increased appetite

Patient Outcomes

Patient will maintain body weight within normal limits.

Nursing Interventions	Rationales
Monitor daily weight. Note increases.	
Assess daily intake. Note caloric and fat intake.	
Discuss patient's usual activity and exercise pattern. Assist patient in establishing progressive exercise program.	
Assist patient in identifying personal and environmental factors which contribute to excessive intake.	

Nursing Interventions	Rationales
Assist patient in determining appropriate caloric intake and daily dietary plan. Consult dietitian as appropriate.	
Discuss techniques to decrease excessive intake, such as 1. setting down utensils between bites 2. serving food on smaller plates 3. eating only one designated place 4. eating slowly and chewing food thoroughly 5. eating only when sitting down 6. avoiding other activities when eating 7. never eating from another person's plate 8. eating low-calorie snacks 9. substituting diet soda or water for high-calorie drinks 10. decreasing intake of calorie-dense or high-fat food	Techniques that modify behavior will assist in success with weight maintenance or loss.
Instruct patient and family on 1. health hazards associated with obesity 2. effects of steroids on metabolism and appetite 3. realistic weight loss goals 4. calorie-restricted diet (if appropriate) 5. behavior modification techniques to decrease excessive intake 6. role of exercise in maintaining/reducing weight 7. beginning exercise program 8. exercise guidelines	

▼

NURSING DIAGNOSIS: HIGH RISK FOR BODY IMAGE DISTURBANCE

Risk Factors

- Cushingoid appearance
- Weight gain

Patient Outcomes

Patient will

- identify factors contributing to altered body image.
- express improved perception of body image.

Nursing Interventions	Rationales
Assess meaning of changes in appearance to patient.	Identifies if patient response to changes in appearance are negative or affecting feelings about self.
Identify behavioral cues which indicate inability to accept image changes, including 1. verbalizing negative feelings of self or appearance. 2. avoiding looking at self 3. exhibiting self-destructive behavior 4. neglecting personal grooming 5. refusing to discuss changes 6. withdrawing from social contacts	
Discuss effect of steroids on appearance.	
Discuss individualized strategies with patient and family that maintain acceptance of appearance and minimize negative response, such as 1. maintaining social contacts 2. personal grooming 3. importance of expression of feelings 4. avoiding negative self-talk and negative criticism	

▼

NURSING DIAGNOSIS: KNOWLEDGE DEFICIT—REGARDING USE OF STEROIDS MEDICATION

Related To lack of exposure to information

Defining Characteristics

Verbalized lack of knowledge about use of steroid medication

Patient Outcomes

Patient will

- identify signs and symptoms of adrenal insufficiency.
- identify correct schedule of medication.
- identify signs and symptoms of complications.
- state measures to reduce complications of steroid therapy.
- describe when to contact health care professionals.
- verbalize intention to wear Medic-Alert ID.

Nursing Interventions	Rationales
Assess current knowledge base, readiness and ability to learn and preferred learning style, and barriers to learning.	
Provide written material for home use in addition to verbal explanations.	
Instruct patient in use of steroids, including 1. purpose and actions 2. dosages 3. schedule of tapering dosages or alternate-day dosing	Abruptly discontinuing steroids may cause adrenal insufficiency.
4. not to discontinue taking steroids without physician's instruction	(Identify importance of communicating steroid use to other health professionals who may provide care.)
5. administering daily dose in the morning	Timing of dosage with body's endogenous secretion decreases suppression of HPA axis.
6. administering steroid with food or milk	Decrease gastric irritation.

Nursing Interventions	Rationales
Teach patient and family signs and symptoms of serious complications (see Table 29.2).	
Discuss prevention of complications: 1. regular eye exams 2. ongoing follow-up for early detection of elevated blood sugar, electrolyte imbalance, and high blood pressure 3. infection control measures 4. weight control measures 5. need for salt restriction and potassium supplementation. 6. protection of skin 7. calcium supplementation to decrease risk of osteoporosis 8. regular exercise to control weight and minimize osteoporosis and muscle atrophy	

▼

Table 29.2 • Possible Adverse Effects of Long-term Glucocorticoid Therapy

Hyperglycemia
Hypertension
Osteoporosis
Peptic ulcer disease
Thromboembolism
Hypokalemia
Atherosclerosis acceleration
Cataract formation
Glaucoma
Sodium and fluid retention
Depression
Mood changes
Insomnia
Impaired wound healing
Thinning of skin, easy bruising
Muscle weakness and weight gain
Susceptibility to infection
Cushingoid appearance (moonface, acne, hirsutism, buffalo humps)

▼

DISCHARGE PLANNING/CONTINUITY OF CARE

- Assure patient's understanding and ability to take medications as prescribed at home.
- Arrange follow-up for continued management.
- Assist patient in obtaining prescriptions and establishing plan for refilling prescriptions.
- Refer patient to a home health care agency if continued nursing care is needed.

REFERENCES

Cook, D. M. (1992). Safe use of glucocorticoids. *Postgraduate Medicine, 91*(3), 145–154.

Lewis, S. M. & Collier, I. C. (1992). *Medical-surgical nursing*. St. Louis, MO: Mosby Year Book.

Porth, C. M. (1990). *Pathophysiology—Concepts of altered health states.* Philadelphia, PA: Lippincott.

▼

DIABETES MELLITUS: EFFECTS OF HOSPITALIZATION AND SURGERY

Bonnie Allbaugh, RN, MS, CDE

Diabetes mellitus is the absence or insufficient secretion of insulin by the beta cells of the pancreas, resulting in abnormal carbohydrate, protein, and fat metabolism. Diabetes is classified into two types: Type I, insulin-dependent diabetes mellitus (IDDM), and Type II, non-insulin-dependent diabetes mellitus (NIDDM). (See Table 30.1.). Impaired glucose tolerance (IGT) is a form of prediabetes characterized by intermittent, mild hyperglycemia, which if untreated could become frank diabetes. Hospitalization and surgery present particular concerns for a person with diabetes due to the required changes in eating patterns and routine and the normal physiological effects of surgery. Fasting for tests, procedures, and surgery as well as the reduced physical activity during hospitalization have a major effect on the patient's normal blood sugar control. The effects of the admitting diagnosis and/or the physiological effects of surgery also adversely affect blood sugar control. The physiological stress of surgery causes release of the catecholamines, epinephrine, and norepinephrine. Epinephrine release results in hyperglycemia since it decreases the uptake of glucose by muscles, inhibits endogenous insulin release, and causes glycogen, stored in the liver, to break down into glucose. The metabolic and hemodynamic stresses may also potentiate long-term complications of diabetes, including cardiovascular disease, renal failure, and neuropathy.

ETIOLOGIES

- Witholding or delaying food
- Reduced physical activity
- Physiological stress of surgery
- Presence of illness, inflammation, and infection
- Presence of complications of diabetes

Table 30.1 • Type I and Type II Diabetes Compared

Type I (IDDM), 10–15%	Type II (NIDDM), 85–90%
Usual onset before 30 years	Usual onset after 40 years
Onset sudden	Onset gradual
Severe symptoms	No or mild symptoms
Thin	Usually overweight
Must use insulin	Some use insulin; some use oral hypoglycemics
Diet and exercise needed	Diet and exercise needed
Weak hereditary	Strong hereditary
Ketones	No ketones

CLINICAL MANIFESTATIONS

- Wide variation in blood sugar values
- Hypoglycemia
- Hyperglycemia
- Slow healing process
- Decreased renal function
- Increased neuropathy symptoms (pain, tingling, especially in legs)
- Abnormal cardiac function

CLINICAL/DIAGNOSTIC FINDINGS

- Blood glucose <60 mg/dL or >180 mg/dL
- Elevated blood urea nitrogen (BUN) and creatinine
- Elevated blood pressure

OTHER PLANS OF CARE TO REFERENCE

- Diabetes Mellitus: Initiation of Insulin Therapy
- Diabetic Ketoacidosis and Hyperosmolar Hyperglycemic Nonketotic Syndrome

NURSING DIAGNOSIS: ALTERED NUTRITION—LESS THAN BODY REQUIREMENTS

Related To

- Delaying/witholding food for diagnostic/therapeutic procedures
- Hyperglycemia
- Decreased insulin sensitivity

Defining Characteristics

- Weight loss
- Reported inadequate food intake
- Hypoglycemia
- Possible ketosis if Type I

Patient Outcomes

The patient will

- have the required intake of protein, carbohydrate, and fats.
- maintain prehospital weight.
- maintain blood sugar in own normal range.

Nursing Interventions	Rationales
Identify usual meal pattern including times and size of meals and snacks. Try to maintain or return to the patient's usual pattern as soon as possible.	If patient is in good diabetes control before admission, maintaining usual patterns of eating will prevent unexpected hypoglycemia or hyperglycemia.
Assess usual food intake and consult with dietitian, if available, to review any needed changes.	Hospitalization is a good time to update patient on new information and recommendations on the diabetic diet. Current recommendations include high complex carbohydrate (60%), moderate protein (25–30%), low fat (10–15%), low salt, and high fiber. The American Diabetes Association (ADA) diet follows the same recommendations as the American Heart Association and American Cancer Society diets.
When food and fluids must be held for a short time (1–2 hr), do not give prescribed insulin (especially regular insulin) or oral hypoglycemics until the patient is able to eat.	Regular insulin begins its hypoglycemic action within 30 min of injection. Intermediate-acting insulins (NPH, UL) begin to work within 1–2 hr.
When food and fluids are withheld for long periods of time, such as preoperatively, discuss a plan with the physician , for adjustment in insulin or oral hypoglycemic dosing and intravenous fluids.	

Nursing Interventions	Rationales
Consider selecting one of the following alternative insulin regimens for patients using insulin:	
1. glucose-insulin infusion regimen, which is an an insulin drip of rapid-acting insulin in normal saline at 0.5 U/mL, infused by infusion pump, with a 5% dextrose (D_5W) solution given to balance glucose levels.	This is recommended for patients having lengthy procedures when allowed nothing by mouth (NPO) for 2 days or more.
2. dividing the total dose of intermediate-acting insulin and rapid-acting insulin into four equal doses of regular insulin and giving an insulin dose every 6 hrs with a D_5W solution infusing	This is recommended for short procedures and 1 or 2 days of NPO or when total parenteral nutrition (TPN) or continuous enteral feeding is being used.
3. withholding morning rapid-acting insulin and giving one half the intermediate-acting insulin	This method, while frequently used for 1-day surgery, may lead to unpredictable glycemic excursions due to the variable absorption times of intermediate-acting insulin.
Consider selecting one of the following alternatives for patients with Type II diabetes who use oral hypoglycemics:	
1. Withhold doses until able to eat and give rapid-acting human insulin subcutaneously based upon blood sugar value.	This is acceptable for short procedures or periods of NPO of 1–2 days. If long-acting oral agent was being used, such as chlorpropamide (Diabinese), it should be discontinued 36–72 hr before surgery due to its long half-life. Second-generation oral agents, glyburide and glipizide, can be discontinued the morning of surgery.

Nursing Interventions	Rationales
2. Temporarily discontinue oral hypoglycemics and begin human insulin using a prescribed sliding scale of regular insulin.	This is recommended for long procedures and 2 or more days of NPO. Human insulin is recommended for short-term therapy. Since it is the least immunogenic insulin, it decreases the possibility of future insulin resistance and/or allergy.
Monitor blood sugar using a bedside meter at a frequency appropriate to the insulin therapy: 1. hourly if on insulin drip 2. every 6 hr if NPO and receiving insulin every 6 hr 3. before meals (AC) and at bedtime (HS) if eating 4. Two-hour postprandial may be requested when intermittent tube feedings are being given.	
Assure accuracy of meter test results by using a sufficient drop of blood and a clean meter and following procedures recommended by the meter company and your institution or agency.	Accuracy is dependent upon the sample size, clean, dust-free meter, and proficiency of the tester. The Clinical Laboratories Improvement Act (CLIA) is a federal mandate which requires quarterly quality control testing and tester certification.
Test for urinary ketones every 8–12 hr for patients with IDDM whose blood sugars are less than 200 mg/dL on average. If blood sugar is over 250 mg/dL and/or the patient exhibits signs and symptoms of diabetic ketoacidosis, test ketones every 4 hr or with each void. (See Diabetic Ketoacidosis, p. 359.)	
Do not withhold insulin when the patient has a normal or low blood sugar. If it is low, consult the physician for a dose adjustment.	Withholding insulin will result in a dramatic rise in blood glucose level. The dosage should be aimed at maintaining a normal range of blood sugar.

Nursing Interventions	Rationales
If a sliding scale is prescribed, consult with the physician to establish scheduled doses of insulin as soon as possible to be used with or instead of the sliding scale. Return to usual insulin regimen as soon as patient is eating normally.	The sliding scale "chases" the blood glucose rather than preventing elevated blood glucose. A scheduled dose with an additional sliding scale results in less extremes in blood sugar.

▼

NURSING DIAGNOSIS: HIGH RISK FOR INJURY

Risk Factors

- NPO or delayed meals
- Excess insulin dose
- Hypoglycemia
- Hypoglycemia symptom unawareness
- Dehydration
- Renal insufficiency

Patient Outcomes

The patient will

- recognize, report, and receive appropriate treatment for hypoglycemia.
- have a balanced intake and output.
- prevent low levels of blood glucose if hypoglycemia unawareness is present.
- have BUN and creatinine that are unchanged from prehospital levels.

Nursing Interventions	Rationales
Regularly assess for signs of hypoglycemia. Early signs include "a funny feeling," shakiness, headache, light-headedness, hunger, weakness, and sweating. Late signs include numbness and tingling of the lips and tongue, vision changes, inability to concentrate, disorientation, confusion, mood changes, irritability, and paleness.	Early signs typically occur when the blood sugar is dropping slowly below normal. Late signs usually occur as the blood sugar drops greatly below normal but can be initial signs if the blood sugar drops very rapidly.

Nursing Interventions	Rationales
Anticipate times when the patient is most at risk for hypoglycemia, for example, when food is delayed, snack or meals is skipped, or NPO, at the peak action times of the insulins used and during or after scheduled physical therapy or stress tests. At high-risk times, check blood sugar as well as assess for signs and symptoms of hypoglycemia.	Patients with long-term diabetes may no longer be able to sense early or any signs of hypoglycemia.
If patient is receiving narcotics, recovering from anesthesia, or in pain, assess for increased heart rate, decreased blood pressure, and irritability as signs of hypoglycemia. Check blood sugar to verify.	
Prevent hypoglycemia by always scheduling tests/procedures requiring NPO early in the morning and consult with physician regarding adjustment of insulin dose using options described in previous diagnosis.	
Schedule physical therapy, exercise, or stress tests ½–1 hr after meals to prevent hypoglycemia.	
Treat hypoglycemia immediately following a standard for treatment. (See Tables 32.1 and 32.2, p. 367 and p. 370.) Institutions may have their own standard or protocol for treatment.	The goal of treatment is to bring the blood sugar to normal and eliminate the hypoglycemia symptoms. Overtreating hypoglycemia is common but should be avoided. It results in rapidly fluctuating blood sugars. Following a standard for treatment reduces the frequency of overtreatment.

Nursing Interventions	Rationales
Monitor and protect renal function: 1. Maintain a balanced intake and output. 2. Report hypertension and monitor until adequately treated. 3. Monitor urine albumin, BUN, creatinine, and potassium, especially if renal function is challenged (e.g., tests using iodine-based contrast medium). 4. Assure adequate hydration before dye/contrast studies.	Renal function may begin to decline after 10 years of IDDM.

▼

NURSING DIAGNOSIS: HIGH RISK FOR INFECTION/ALTERED TISSUE PERFUSION

Risk Factors

- Hyperglycemia
- Peripheral vascular disease
- Peripheral neuropathy

Patient Outcomes

The patient will

- demonstrate normal healing of surgical wounds.
- maintain normal skin integrity.
- have palpable peripheral pulses.

Nursing Interventions	Rationales
Assess and report hyperglycemia which does not normalize with current treatment.	Hyperglycemia is associated with several problems, including decreased effectiveness of leukocytes, increased risk of platelet aggregation, and increased rigidity of red blood cells, which decreases circulation through the small vessels, depriving them of oxygen and nutrients.

Nursing Interventions	Rationales
Observe for signs of inflammation and infection. Also observe for hyperglycemia.	An increase in blood sugar may be an early sign of developing inflammation or infection.
Provide meticulous wound care.	
Assess for and promote adequate circulation in extremities by 1. encouraging active and passive range of motion 2. assisting with early ambulation 3. assuring antiemboli stockings properly applied	Diabetes increases the risk of thrombophlebitis and deep-vein thrombosis.
Protect feet and legs of patients with peripheral neuropathy by observing position and skin condition. (See Prevention and Care of Pressure Ulcers, see p. 576.)	

▼

NURSING DIAGNOSIS: HIGH RISK FOR DECREASED CARDIAC OUTPUT

Risk Factors

- Hypercholesteremia
- Autonomic neuropathy
- Hypertension
- History of coronary artery disease
- Impaired renal function

Patient Outcomes

- Blood pressure will be in normal range.
- Elevated cholesterol panel will be recognized and treated.
- Intake and output will be adequate and balanced.

Nursing Interventions	Rationales
Montior blood pressure and assess effectiveness of antihypertensive medication.	
Check orthostatic blood pressure to assess for autonomic neuropathy.	

Nursing Interventions	Rationales
Monitor cholesterol panel and consult with physician regarding possible long-term treatment measures: 1. Consult dietitian and instruct on low-cholesterol diet. 2. Encourage patient to monitor and control blood sugar to reduce triglycerides. 2. Encourage patient to begin a prescribed therapeutic exercise program to increase "good cholesterol": high-density lipoprotein (HDL).	
Assess pulse for regularity. If monitored, observe for arrhythmias. Investigate and report any complaints of chest pain, shortness of breath, or change on the electrocardiogram (ECG).	Diabetes increases the risk of myocardial infarction (MI), and patients may experience myocardial damage without pain, "the silent MI."

▼

NURSING DIAGNOSIS: HIGH RISK FOR INEFFECTIVE MANAGEMENT OF THERAPEUTIC REGIMEN

Risk Factors

- Complex treatment regimen
- Chronic illness requiring constant management
- Difficult life changes
- Economic difficulties
- Personal/family conflicts
- Knowledge deficit
- Denial
- Psychosocial issues

Patient Outcomes

The patient will

- identify components of the regimen which are most difficult.
- agree to follow a modified treatment regimen.
- describe signs and symptoms, prevention, and correction of hypoglycemia and hyperglycemia.
- obtain regular follow-up.

Nursing Interventions	Rationales
Assess understanding and usual practices in self-management of diabetes, recognizing and respecting the current knowledge and efforts the patient has used.	Patients with a long history of diabetes may have developed unique and successful ways to manage their diabetes. However, they may not have had an opportunity to receive recent information on diabetes. Hospitalization provides an opportunity for an update.
Monitor the level of glycosylated hemoglobin (hemoglobin A_{1C}) to indicate level of control over the previous 3 months. Discuss the A_{1C} result and possible factors affecting it with the patient.	The hemoglobin A_{1C} is a measure of the amount of glycosylation (presence of sugar) on the hemoglobin molecule. Since the life-cycle of the hemoglobin molecule is 3 months, this test is an excellent way to assess overall control of diabetes for the previous 3 months.
Identify the factors or components of the regimen that are the most difficult for the patient and consult with the diabetes nurse educator or teaching service, if available. The regimen may need to be modified to be more acceptable to the patient. The patient has to live with it every day, so it has to fit his or her life-style.	There are many different insulin regimens, meal patterns, and monitoring methods available. Consider all alternatives with the patient to find a realistic regimen that works for the patient.
Assess for financial difficulties, psychosocial problems, family/relationship problems, and psychiatric disorders and assist with obtaining resources. Consult social services, if available.	Diabetes is a very expensive disease to manage. Blood glucose test strips cost approximately 50–75 cents per strip. Other supplies such as insulin and syringes all add up to a large monthly sum.
Alert patient about support groups or group education programs that may be beneficial in coping with and managing diabetes.	

▼

DISCHARGE PLANNING/CONTINUITY OF CARE

- Assure understanding of self-management plan, especially if any modifications have been made.
- Refer to a home health agency if continued assistance with care or learning is required.
- Assist in obtaining prescriptions and supplies and establishing a plan for refilling prescriptions.
- Arrange follow-up with a physician, diabetes nurse educator, and dietitian to continue management and teaching after discharge.
- Provide information on local diabetes support groups and educational programs.
- Refer to the local chapter of the American Diabetes Association for further information.

REFERENCES

Dinsmoor, R. S. (1993). Hypoglycemia without warning. *Diabetes Self-Management*, March–April, pp. 6–8.

Gutherie, D. (1988). *Diabetes education: A core curriculum for health professionals.* Chicago, IL: American Association of Diabetes Educators.

Kreines, K. (1992). Diabetes management during same-day surgery and procedures. *Clinical Diabetes*, *10*(4), 52–54.

Lebovitz, H. (1991). *Therapy for diabetes mellitus and related disorders.* Alexandria, VA: American Diabetes Association.

Lorber, D., Curley, A., & Nazario, M. (1990). Discharge planning and diabetes. *Practical Diabetology*, *9*(4), 18–22.

▼

DIABETES MELLITUS: INITIATING INSULIN

Bonnie Allbaugh, RN, MS, CDE

Insulin is necessary for normal carbohydrate, protein, and fat metabolism. Exogenous insulin is required for people with insulin-dependent (Type I) diabetes since they do not produce enough of this hormone to sustain life. People with non-insulin-dependent (Type II) diabetes may need supplemental exogenous insulin when they have decreased insulin production or decreased insulin sensitivity, especially during times of illness, surgery, and stress. Insulin is often required for treatment of secondary diabetes, that is, occurring with other diseases and treatments such as pancreatic disease and high doses of steroid medications.

ETIOLOGIES

- New diagnosis of insulin-dependent (Type I) diabetes
- Treatment failure of oral hypoglycemics in non-insulin-dependent (Type II) diabetes
- Illness, surgery, or other stresses in Type II diabetes
- Secondary diabetes, that is, high-dose steroids and pancreatic disease

CLINICAL MANIFESTATIONS

- Consistent hyperglycemia
- Thirst, polyuria
- Ketonuria, ketonemia
- Marked weight loss

CLINICAL/DIAGNOSTIC FINDINGS

- Blood glucose > 200 mg/dL
- Elevated hemoglobin $A_{1}c$
- Presence of ketones in urine and/or blood

OTHER PLANS OF CARE TO REFERENCE

Effects of Hospitalization and Surgery on Diabetes Mellitus

▼

NURSING DIAGNOSIS: KNOWLEDGE DEFICIT—INSULIN USE

Related To
- Lack of exposure to information
- New diagnosis
- New treatment method

Defining Characteristics

Anger about diagnosis
Anxiety regarding injection
Fear of complications
Lack of questions
Many questions
Previous refusal to use insulin
Myths regarding need for insulin

Patient Outcomes

The patient will
- demonstrate correct preparation, administration, and site selection of insulin injection.
- state expected effect, action times, and side effects of insulin.
- describe own action plan for storage of insulin and disposal of syringes.
- demonstrate correct technique for blood glucose monitoring.
- demonstrate understanding of blood glucose values by defining blood glucose target ranges and action plan when out of ranges.
- list the common signs of hypoglycemia and own action plan for treatment and prevention.
- demonstrate urine testing for ketones.
- define when urine ketone testing is needed and the significance of ketones in the urine.
- define plan for on-going care and names of health care providers available for questions and concerns.

Nursing Interventions	Rationales
Assess for willingness to learn, cognitive and physical abilities (especially sight), and any concerns about or previous experience with injections.	Blurred vision lasting for several weeks is common when blood sugar is normalized and will return to normal. Building on previous experience, correcting misinformation, and encouraging participation in the learning experience are key adult learning principles.
Consult a diabetes teaching service for assistance, if available.	Certified diabetes educators are specialists in diabetes education.
Provide handouts and samples of equipment. Use audiovisual aids to supplement information.	Written materials are helpful for later reference.
Explain reason insulin is needed, its action, and expected effect.	Individualizing information enhances learning and acceptance.
Discuss species and types of insulin to be used, explaining differences in action and appearance (clear/cloudy).	Human insulin is preferred for those starting insulin therapy, especially if expected to be used intermittently. Fast-acting insulin onset, 30 min; peak, 3–4 hr; duration, 6–8 hr. Intermediate acting insulin onset, 1 hr; peak, 8–10 hr; duration, 18–24 hr.
Describe and demonstrate the sizes and types of syringes available. Recommend the syringe size appropriate for the expected dose of insulin.	Awareness of differences in syringe sizes can prevent incorrect doses using unfamiliar syringes.
Demonstrate drawing up insulin, including 1. cleaning hands and injection site 2. wiping top of bottle with alcohol 3. rolling intermediate insulin	
4. adding air equal to the dose	Equalizing air prevents formation of a vacuum in insulin bottle.
5. if mixing insulins, drawing fast insulin into syringe first	Inadvertent mixing of fast insulin into intermediate insulin bottle is less dangerous than vice versa

Nursing Interventions	Rationales
Demonstrate injection process, including	
1. 90° angle into subcutaneous tissue and 45° angle if thin	Intramuscular injection is not recommended due to faster absorption.
2. no aspiration and no rubbing of site after injection	Rubbing speeds absorption and action time.
Demonstrate recommended injection sites, including abdomen, arms, thighs, and buttocks. Explain reason for site rotation. Encourage rotation within one area for each injection rather than random rotation.	Prevents lipohypertrophy or lipoatrophy. Absorption is fastest in the abdomen, followed by the arms, thighs, and buttocks. Using one area per injection results in more predictable absorption and action time.
Observe performance of skills and give positive reinforcement.	Performing skill is essential to learning.
Describe syringe disposal:	
1. Place in a puncture-resistant disposal container.	Firm plastic bottles such as empty detergent bottles are acceptable.
2. Dispose of two-thirds full container meeting local regulations.	Many pharmacies, hospitals, and clinics will dispose of containers.
If the patient prefers to reuse syringes, explain recommendations: 1. Recap after use. 2. Do not wipe or soak in alcohol. 3. Stop use if syringe is dull, bent, or comes in contact with any surface other than skin.	While manufacturers do not recommend syringe reuse, studies have found no infections or other problems when patients reuse their own syringes. It is not recommended with poor hygiene, decreased resistance to infection, acute concurrent illness, or open wounds on hands.
Recommend storage of insulin at room temperature while in use and in the refrigerator prior to opening. Keep within a range of 36–86 °F. Avoid using bottle longer than 30 days.	Insulin at room temperature is more comfortable. Potency will decrease after 30 days if kept at room temperature. If stored in refrigerator, potency is good until expiration date.
Define normal blood sugar values and coordinate with physician to set blood sugar goals with patient.	

Nursing Interventions	Rationales
Discuss symptoms of hyperglycemia and hypoglycemia, significance, treatment, and prevention.	
Assist patient in establishing a plan to prevent and treat hypoglycemia with blood glucose monitoring (BGM), carrying 15 g of glucose and understanding the effect of food and activity on blood sugar.	Recommended treatment is 15 g of fast-acting carbohydrate repeated in 10 min if blood glucose is less than 80 or if symptoms remain.
Instruct family on the use of the glucagon emergency kit.	Glucagon should be given immediately if the patient is unconscious or unable or unwilling to swallow.
Demonstrate use and provide with equipment and supplies for BGM.	Blood glucose monitoring is recommended for anyone using insulin.
Observe BGM technique and assess for accuracy by comparing to a simultaneous laboratory value.	Capillary-meter results are usually higher than laboratory values and should be within 15% of laboratory value.
Demonstrate ketone testing for patients with Type I diabetes. Instruct on use when ill or when blood sugar is higher than 250 mg/dL.	Ketones normally will not form in Type II diabetes.

▼

DISCHARGE PLANNING/CONTINUITY OF CARE

- Assure understanding and ability to inject correct dose, test blood sugar, and recognize and treat hypoglycemia and hyperglycemia.
- Provide with needed supplies and prescriptions and discuss a plan for refills. Be aware of insurance/health maintenance organization requirements for obtaining supplies and equipment.
- Consult a home health agency if assistance or ongoing teaching is required.
- Arrange follow-up physician and/or diabetes nurse educator for questions and continued management.
- Provide with information on diabetes support groups in the area, American Diabetes Association affiliate office, and publications and other ongoing diabetes assistive services.

REFERENCES

American Diabetes Association Position Statement: Insulin Administration. (1990). *Diabetes Care, 13*(Suppl. 1), 28–31.

Bantle, J., Weber, M., Rao, S., Challapadhyay, M., & Robertson, R. (1990). Rotation of the anatomic regions used for insulin injections and day-to-day variability of plasma glucose in Type I diabetic subjects. *JAMA, 13*, 1802–1806.

Guthrie, D. (1988). *Diabetes education: Core curriculum for health professional.* Chicago, IL: American Association of Diabetes Educators.

Tattersall, R. B. & Gale, E. A. (1990). *Diabetes clinical management.* New York: Churchill Livingstone.

Zehrer, C., et al. (1990). Reducing blood glucose variability by use of abdominal insulin injection sites. *Diabetes Educator, 16*(6), 474–477.

▼

DIABETIC KETOACIDOSIS AND HYPEROSMOLAR NONKETOTIC SYNDROME

Bonnie Allbaugh, RN, MS, CDE

Diabetic ketoacidosis (DKA) and hyperosmolar nonketotic syndrome (HNKS) are acute, potentially life-threatening complications of diabetes mellitus. Hyperglycemia is the major presenting symptom in both situations due to lack of or ineffective insulin. When insulin is not available, glucose cannot migrate into the cells. Diabetic ketoacidosis, a complication of Type I, insulin-dependent, diabetes (IDDM), results from cellular metabolism of fat since glucose is not available. By-products of this metabolic process are ketone bodies (organic acids) that cause metabolic acidosis.

Commonly seen in the elderly, HNKS has a high mortality rate. It is usually seen in Type II, non-insulin-dependent, diabetes (NIDDM) and is characterized by severe hyperglycemia and dehydration.

In most cases of DKA and HNKS, the patient will require intensive care initially. However, in less severe cases and following immediate therapy, care will be provided on general medical-surgical units.

ETIOLOGIES

- DKA
  - illness/infection
  - inadequate insulin dosage
  - newly diagnosed IDDM
- HNKS
  - new onset of NIDDM
  - diabetes insipidus
  - illness/infection
  - Central nervous system (CNS) damage
  - gastrointestinal hemorrhage
  - protracted diarrhea
  - protracted vomiting

  - nutrition support-tube feedings of high-protein mixtures and total parenteral nutrition

CLINICAL MANIFESTATIONS

- DKA
  - hyperglycemia
  - polyuria, polydipsia, polyphagia
  - Kussmaul respirations
  - tachypnea
  - tachycardia, hypotension
  - abdominal pain
  - nausea, vomiting
  - decreased alertness, coma
- HNKS
  - severe hyperglycemia
  - severe dehydration (thirst, dry skin and mucous membranes, poor skin turgor)
  - focal neurological changes (hemiparesis, aphasia, seizures)
  - confusion, decreased alertness
  - coma

CLINICAL/DIAGNOSTIC FINDINGS

- DKA
  - serum glucose > 250 mg/dL
  - serum pH < 7.35
  - low serum bicarbonate
  - elevated ketones in urine and blood
  - serum electrolyte disturbances
- HNKS
  - serum glucose > 600 mg/dL
  - elevated serum osmolality to 350 mOsm/kg or higher
  - serum electrolyte disturbances
  - no or rare ketones

OTHER PLANS OF CARE OF REFERENCE

- Effects of Hospitalization and Surgery on Diabetes Mellitus
- Diabetes Mellitus: Starting Insulin

▼

NURSING DIAGNOSIS: FLUID VOLUME DEFICIT

Related To

- Osmotic diuresis from hyperglycemia
- Vomiting and diarrhea

Defining Characteristics

Thirst (may not be apparent in elderly with HNKS)
Hypotension, tachycardia
Decreased urine concentration
Dry skin and mucous membranes
Weight loss
Output greater than input
Oliguria if severe dehydration

Patient Outcomes

The patient will

- not experience thirst.
- demonstrate normal skin turgor.
- have a stable weight.
- have a balanced intake and output.
- have normalized blood glucose values.

Nursing Interventions	Rationales
Infuse prescribed intravenous (IV) solutions.	Initially isotonic saline is administered at very fast rates (250–500 mL/hr) to increase volume quickly and maintain sodium balance.
Assess for response to fluid replacement by monitoring 1. vital signs frequently 2. hourly urine output until stable at 30 mL/hr 3. breath sounds for adventitious sounds, dyspnea, and shortness of breath 4. central venous pressure (CVP), if placed 5. jugular vein distention 6. level of alertness Alert physician to any signs of fluid volume overload and adjust the prescribed IV rate accordingly.	Elderly patients and those with severe dehydration of HNKS may not be able to tolerate the rapid reperfusion usually tolerated by younger patients with DKA.

Nursing Interventions	Rationales
Monitor and record intake and output and urine specific gravity.	Urine specific gravity is an early indicator of changes in dehydration.
Frequently monitor laboratory values: hemoglobin, hematocrit, white blood cell (WBC) count and differential, blood urea nitrogen (BUN), creatinine, glucose, and electrolytes, especially potassium.	Initially laboratory values will be increased because of hemoconcentration. As dehydration is corrected, the true value is apparent. If hemoglobin and hematocrit are abnormally low, bleeding may be suspected. If the WBC count is elevated, an infection may be present. Potassium may be normal or high initially but will drop with rehydration.
Monitor glucose serum and/or capillary values. Alert physician when glucose is 250–300 mg/dL and anticipate changing to an IV infusion containing dextrose.	Blood glucose will also drop with fluid replacement. Use of solutions containing dextrose will allow a more gradual decrease in the blood sugar, which protects the brain from cerebral edema. Cerebral edema can occur if blood glucose drops suddenly, because glucose in the cerebral spinal fluid changes more slowly.
When potassium drops and adequate renal function has been established, alert physician and anticipate adding potassium to the IV infusions.	Potassium moves out of the serum and into the cells when insulin becomes available.
Monitor fluid status and infuse IV fluids until blood glucose is stabilizing and the patient is able to eat and drink adequately.	

▼

NURSING DIAGNOSIS: ALTERED NUTRITION—LESS THAN BODY REQUIREMENTS

Related To

- Lack of glucose metabolism caused by absence of insulin
- Use of fat/protein for energy needs
- Protein loss with diuresis

Defining Characteristics

Weight loss
Ketoacidosis (if DKA)
Hyperglycemia
Abdominal pain, nausea, and vomiting
Diuresis

Patient Outcomes

The patient will

- have a stable weight.
- eat an adequate diet.
- have decreasing ketonuria.
- have stable and near normal blood glucose range.

Nursing Interventions	Rationales
Administer insulin intravenously by bolus and/or continuous infusion or other routes as prescribed.	Initially in DKA and HNKS insulin is usually given as a continuous IV infusion after an IV bolus loading dose of 5–10 units. Use only regular insulin, intravenously, and human insulin is recommended to prevent antibody formation.
Adjust prescribed insulin drip rate to allow for a slow blood glucose decline to normal.	An insulin infusion of 1–8 U/hr results in a 50–100 mg/dL decrease when the patient is adequately hydrated.
Monitor blood glucose by meter using capillary or venous whole blood at least hourly until stable. Regularly compare meter results to laboratory values to assure accuracy.	Blood glucose monitoring by meter has greater potential for inaccuracy due to blood drop size, human error, hematocrit changes, and meter error. Whole blood glucose values compared simultaneously with serum are expected to be higher by up to 15%.
Assess for signs and symptoms of hypoglycemia.	Hypoglycemia can occur if blood sugar decreases too rapidly.

Nursing Interventions	Rationales
In DKA, monitor serum ketone values and test urine for ketones with each void or every 2–4 hr if an indwelling catheter is present.	Urine test for ketones use nitroprusside, which changes color in the presence of acetoacetate. The other ketone bodies, acetone and β-hydroxybutyrate, are only detected in serum tests. Urine tests will remain positive longer than blood because ketones clear more slowly from the urine.
Provide oral intake when tolerated, advancing diet from liquids to solid food as soon as possible.	

▼

NURSING DIAGNOSIS: HIGH RISK FOR DECREASED CARDIAC OUTPUT

Risk Factors

- Cardiac arrhythmias
- Hyperkalemia/hypokalemia
- Fluid and electrolyte imbalance
- History of congestive heart failure (CHF) and coronary artery disease
- Renal insufficiency
- Elderly

Patient Outcomes

The patient will

- not experience cardiac arrythmias.
- have a pulse at regular or normal rate.
- have a electrolytes in normal range.

Nursing Interventions	Rationales
Assess for changes in blood pressure and pulses.	
If cardiac monitored, observe for arrhythmias and waveform changes.	Hyperkalemia may show a peaked T wave, flat P wave, prolonged PR interval and QRS, atrial arrest, and ventricular arrhythmias. Hypokalemia may show ST depression, inverted T waves, large U wave, and ectopic beats.

Nursing Interventions	Rationales
Assess serum potassium, other electrolytes, and bicarbonate regularly.	In DKA, metabolic acidosis is usually corrected by fluid and insulin replacement. Only in cases of life-threatening acidosis is sodium bicarbonate administered. Acidosis that is corrected too quickly can result in cerebral edema.
Administer prescribed IV or oral potassium and alkaline phosphorous supplement.	

NURSING DIAGNOSIS: HIGH RISK FOR ALTERED CEREBRAL TISSUE PERFUSION

Risk Factors

- Hypoglycemia
- Cerebral edema
- Acid-base imbalance

Patient Outcomes

The patient will
- be alert and oriented.
- recognize and prevent hypoglycemia.

Nursing Interventions	Rationales
Carefully titrate the insulin and glucose infusions to maintain a blood glucose above 120–150 mg/dL while IV insulin is used. Review signs and symptoms of hypoglycemia with the patient and assess regularly (shaky, sweaty, rapid pulse, confusion, slurred speech). If hypoglycemia occurs, treat immediately by 1. decreasing the insulin infusion and increasing the rate of the glucose infusion 2. if no IV, and patient alert, giving 15–20 g of fast-acting carbohydrate (3–4 glucose tablets, 4 oz of juice or nondiet soda) 3. giving glucagon intramuscularly or dextrose 50% intravenously until alert, following protocol or as prescribed. (See Table 32.1).	
Throughout management for DKA and HNKS, assess and report any changes in alertness, level of consciousness, speech ability, and sensation and motion of all extremities.	In DKA, cerebral edema can occur with rapid changes in glucose level. In HNKS, lethargy and slowed thought processes are common and may continue for several weeks after recovery.

▼

NURSING DIAGNOSIS: HIGH RISK FOR KNOWLEDGE DEFICIT/ INEFFECTIVE MANAGEMENT OF THERAPEUTIC REGIMEN

Risk Factors

- Complex treatment regimen
- Chronic illness requiring constant management
- Difficult life changes
- Economic difficulties
- Personal/family conflicts
- Knowledge deficit
- Denial
- Psychosocial issues

Table 32.1 • Standard for Treating Hypoglycemia

1. If glucose is under 70 mg/dL and patient is alert:
   - Give 4–6 oz of juice or 1 fruit exchange.
   - If NPO, give 10 mL of dextrose 50% (D_{50}) if IV access is available.
   - If NPO and no IV access available, give 1 mL glucagon intramuscularly or subcutaneously.
   - If at night or longer than 1 hr to next meal, give an additional 1 bread and 1 protein exchange. If predialysis on a protein restrictive diet, give 2 breads instead of 1 bread and 1 protein.
   - If occurs in early a.m., do not use breakfast as the treatment source. The patient needs an additional fruit source. You may order breakfast early, but you must still treat the hypoglycemia with juice or 1 fruit exchange.
2. If glucose is under 70 mg/dL and patient is not alert:
   - Give 10 mL of D_{50} IV.
   - Give 20 mL of D_{50} IV if glucose is under 40 mg/dL.
   - If no IV access, give 1 mL glucagon intramuscularly or subcutaneously and establish access.
3. Recheck glucose in 15 min.
4. Recheck glucose in 15 and 30 min if IV glucose or parenteral glucagon was given.

Note: Consider Na^+, K^+, protein, or fluid restriction when determining treatment. See guidelines in the text or talk with a dietitian to help determine treatment.

▼

Patient Outcomes

The patient will

- identify components of the regimen which are most difficult.
- agree to follow a modified treatment regimen.
- describe signs and symptoms, prevention, and correction of hypoglycemia and hyperglycemia.
- obtain regular follow-up.
- perform skills required for new regimen.

Nursing Interventions	Rationales
Assess understanding and usual practices in self-management of diabetes, recognizing and respecting the current knowledge and efforts the patient has used. Focus on sick-day care and what the patient did in this incident.	Patients with a long history of diabetes may have developed unique and successful ways to manage their diabetes. However, they may not have had an opportunity to receive recent information on diabetes. Hospitalization provides an opportunity for an update. Do not assume the patient with DKA is not knowledgeable and in control of his or her diabetes. An illness with a rapid onset (e.g., flu, vomiting) can cause DKA to occur in 4–6 hr in a person with well-controlled diabetes.
Discuss any ways the patient could have responded differently to prevent or decrease the onset of DKA and HNKS. Review a plan for sick-day care, including 1. taking insulin even if vomiting 2. checking blood sugars every 4 hr when vomiting or ill 3. contacting physician or nurse for guidance and/or supplement usual dose of insulin with additional regular insulin as prescribed by physician 4. checking urine ketones if blood sugar is over 250 mg/dL or when vomiting or with diarrhea 5. drinking large amounts of fluids (if unable to eat solid food, drinking juices or nondiet soda to prevent hypoglycemia, see Table 32.2) 6. If unable to eat regular diet, using foods that settle the stomach (e.g., dry toast, crackers, warm soda)	

Nursing Interventions	Rationales
If the patient with HNKS is starting insulin, see Initiation of Insulin. Carefully assess patient's ability to learn this detailed new skill and break the learning into small accomplishable steps. If the patient is unable to learn it effectively, include family and consider a referral to a home health agency.	Patients with HNKS may have difficulty learning because of temporary altered though processes. Usually normal abilities will return several weeks after successful treatment.
Observe the level of glycosylated hemoglobin (hemoglobin A_{1c}) to indicate level of blood sugar control over the previous 3 months. Discuss the A_{1c} result and possible factors affecting it with the patient.	The hemoglobin A_{1c} is a measure of the amount of glycosylation (presence of sugar) on the hemoglobin molecule. Since the life cycle of the hemoglobin molecule is 3 months, this test is an excellent way to assess overall control of diabetes.
Identify the factors or components of the regimen that are the most difficult for the patient and consult with a diabetes nurse educator or teaching service, if available, to modify the regimen to be more acceptable to the patient. The patient has to live with it every day, so it has to fit his or her life-style.	There are many different insulin regimens, meal patterns, and monitoring methods available. Consider all alternatives to find a regimen that works for the patient.
Assess for financial difficulties, psychosocial problems, family/relationship problems, and psychiatric disorders and assist with obtaining resources. Consult social services, if available.	Diabetes is a very expensive disease to manage. Blood glucose test strips cost approximately 50 cents per strip. Other supplies such as insulin and syringes all add up to a large monthly sum.
Alert patient about support groups or group education programs that may be beneficial in coping with and managing diabetes.	

▼

DISCHARGE PLANNING/CONTINUITY OF CARE

- Assure understanding of self-management plan, especially illness care and any new skills or change in the regimen.

- Refer to a home health agency if continued assistance with care or learning is required.
- Assist in obtaining prescriptions and supplies and establishing a plan for refilling prescriptions.
- Arrange follow-up with a physician and diabetes nurse to continue management after discharge.
- Provide with information on support groups and educational programs in the area on diabetes.
- Refer to the local chapter of the American Diabetes Association for further information.

Table 32.2 • Suggested Foods For Treating Hypoglycemia

1 fruit =	120 mL orange juice (1)
	80 mL cranberry juice
	80 mL grape juice
	180 mL regular Sprite
1 bread =	3 graham crackers
	6 saltine crackers (2)
	1 slice bread
1 meat =	¼ cup cottage cheese (2,3)
	1 oz (slice) cheese (2,3)
	1 tbsp peanut butter (1,2,3)
1 fruit and 1 meat =	240 mL 2% milk (1,3)

Note: (1) = high in K^+; (2) = high in Na^+; (3) = high in protein.

REFERENCES

Fleckman, A. (1991). Diabetes ketoacidosis. *Practical Diabetology, 10*(3), 1–8.

Gutherie, D. (1988). *Diabetes education: A core curriculum for health professionals.* Chicago, IL: American Association of Diabetes Educators.

Lebovitz, H. (1991). *Therapy for diabetes mellitus and related disorders.* Alexandria, VA: American Diabetes Association.

Matz, R. (1988). Hyperosmolar non-acidotic uncontrolled diabetes: Not a rare event. *Clinical Diabetes,* 6(2), 29–37.

Sabo, C. & Michael, S. (1989). Diabetic ketoacidosis: Pathophysiology, nursing diagnosis, and nursing interventions. *Focus on Critical Care, 16*(1), 21–28.

Common Neurological Conditions and Procedures

▼

ALTERED CONSCIOUSNESS

Andrea Strayer, RN, MS, CNRN

Consciousness consists of arousal (alertness) and content (awareness). The reticular activating system is a physiological entity which enables a person to be aroused. The cerebral cortex enables thought, expression, and higher cortical functions. Altered consciousness indicates brain dysfunction or failure. Consciousness is the most sensitive indicator of neurological change. A change in the level of consciousness can occur rapidly or very slowly; it can be subtle or severe.

ETIOLOGIES

- Mass lesions
  - traumatic brain injury
  - destructive lesions of the thalamus
  - hemorrhage
  - infarction
  - tumor
  - abscess
- Metabolic, diffuse, or multifocal causes
  - encephalitis
  - uremia
  - hypoglycemia
  - hypoxia
  - ischemia
  - sedative drugs; barbiturates, ethanol, opiates, tranquilizers
  - electrolyte imbalance

CLINICAL MANIFESTATIONS

- Confused: requires repetition of instruction, disoriented
- Lethargy: oriented but slow to respond, slowed mental processes

- Obtundation: readily arousable with stimulation, very drowsy, can follow simple commands
- Stupor: requires vigorous stimuli to respond, requires continued stimuli to keep awake
- Coma: appears to be in sleeplike state, does not respond appropriately to stimuli
- Persistent vegetative state: has sleep-wake cycles, but at no time is aware of self or environment

CLINICAL/DIAGNOSTIC FINDINGS

- Head computerized tomography (CT) or head magnetic resonance imaging (MRI): will show a mass lesion
- Laboratory data: will delineate metabolic disorders
  - hyper/hypoglycemia
  - complete blood count: elevated white blood cell (WBC) count
  - electrolytes: hypo/hypernatremia, hypercalcemia, hypomagnesia
  - arterial blood gases: respiratory or metabolic alkalosis or acidosis, hypoxemia
  - elevated liver enzymes
  - elevated blood urea nitrogen (BUN) and creatinine
  - elevated thyroid function tests
  - toxicology screen

OTHER PLANS OF CARE TO REFERENCE

- Nutrition Support: Enteral Nutrition

▼

NURSING DIAGNOSIS: DECREASED INTRACRANIAL ADAPTIVE CAPACITY

Related To compromised intracranial fluid compensatory mechanisms

Defining Characteristics

Increased intracranial pressure
Increased lethargy, somnolence
Decreased mental status
Pupil changes
Vital sign changes: widening pulse pressure

Patient Outcomes

The patient will
- demonstrate a decrease in intracranial pressure.
- demonstrate orientation to person, place, and time.

- demonstrate normal pupillary reaction and accommodation.
- demonstrate vital signs within their normal limits.

Nursing Interventions	Rationales
Elevate the head of bed at least 30°.	Elevating the head of the bed and maintaining the patient's head and neck in an upright position promotes venous drainage, decreasing intracranial pressure. Additionally, it will promote oxygenation and help prevent aspiration.
Maintain the patient's head in neutral alignment.	
Provide the patient with rest periods between cares; do not cluster patient care activities.	By not clustering stimulation to patients, it helps keep their intracranial pressure low.
Perform a neurological exam as often as is warranted. This may be hourly when the patient is unstable. Assessment of level of consciousness, mental status, cranial nerves, pupils, motor strength, reflexes, sensation, and vital signs should be included in a comprehensive exam. Routine checks should be tailored to fit the patient's needs.	
Notify physician immediately of any changes in the neurological exam.	
Maintain a quiet environment; visitors may need to be limited while the patient is unstable.	Less stimulation will help keep the intracranial pressure down. This is only necessary when the patient is unstable. For instance, a patient in a chronic vegetative state requires stimulation.

▼

NURSING DIAGNOSIS: INEFFECTIVE AIRWAY CLEARANCE

Related To

- Increased lethargy
- Impaired airway protection
- Decreased or absent spontaneous cough

Defining Characteristics
Abnormal breath sounds
Change in rate and/or depth of respirations
Tachypnea

Patient Outcomes
The patient will maintain a patent airway, as evidenced by
- normal breath sounds
- normal rate and depth of respirations

Nursing Interventions	Rationales
Assess respiratory status, including observing rate and rhythm; auscultate breath sounds at least every 4 hr.	Provides objective data on which to base interventions.
Provide pulmonary care, including cough and deep breath, oral or nasotracheal suctioning, as warranted, at least every 4 hr.	Promotes oxygenation.
Turn the patient from side to side; do not lie flat on back.	Prevents airway occlusion and promotes drainage of secretions.

▼

NURSING DIAGNOSIS: HIGH RISK FOR INJURY

Risk Factors
- confusion
- lethargy

Patient Outcomes
The patient will be free of injury.

Nursing Interventions	Rationales
Keep all side rails up, bed in low position.	
Reorient the patient frequently.	
Place the patient in a room close to the nurses' station.	
Ask the family to bring familiar objects to put in the room.	
Keep a light on in the patient's room and the door open.	
Make sure the call light and essential items are always within reach.	
Observe the patient frequently.	
Utilize a bed monitor that will alert you when the patient is getting out of bed.	
Consider all of the above before using soft restraints or a posey vest.	

▼

DISCHARGE PLANNING/CONTINUITY OF CARE

- Coordinate with the discharge planning nurse or social worker, if available, to plan discharge arrangements for caregiver, home health agency, or nursing home.
- Assure care provider understands and can perform ongoing care needed.
- Assure arrangements are made to obtain supplies, equipment, and medication prescriptions.
- Arrange follow-up with physician or nurse practitioner for continued management and postdischarge care. Assure telephone numbers are provided if questions or problems develop.

ACKNOWLEDGMENT

This work was supported by the Department of Veteran Affairs.

REFERENCES

Barker, E. & Moore, K. (1992). Neurological assessment. *RN, 55*(4), 28–34.

Cammermeyer, M. & Appledorn, C. (Eds.). (1990). *Core curriculum for neuroscience nursing* (3rd ed). Chicago, IL: American Association of Neuroscience Nurses.

Hickey, J. (1992). *The clinical practice of neurological and neurosurgical nursing* (3rd ed). Philadelphia, PA: Lippincott.

Lower, J. (1992). Rapid neuroassessment. *American Journal of Nursing, 92*(6), 38–45.

Plum, F. & Posner, J. (1980). *The diagnosis of stupor and coma* (3rd ed). Philadelphia, PA: Davis.

Sullivan, J. (1990). Neurological assessment. *Nursing Clinics of North America, 25*(4), 795–806.

▼

AMYOTROPHIC LATERAL SCLEROSIS

Andrea Strayer, RN, MS, CNRN

Also known as Lou Gehrig's disease, amyotrophic lateral sclerosis (ALS) is an incurable, progressive degenerative disease of the nervous system. The degenerative changes occur in the anterior horn cells of the spinal cord, corticospinal tracts, motor nuclei of the brain stem, the Betz cells, and precentral cells of the frontal cortex. The initial symptoms are usually weakness and wasting of the upper extremities. As the disease progresses, speech and swallowing muscles also become involved, making communication, eating, and managing oral secretions difficult. In the final stages, the patient is immobile and has severe respiratory depression. Death occurs approximately 3 years after onset, usually from aspiration, infection, or respiratory failure. Sensation and intellect are not impaired.

ETIOLOGIES

- Unknown

CLINICAL MANIFESTATIONS

- Muscle weakness, wasting, and atrophy
- Muscle spasticity and hyperreflexia
- Muscle fasciculations
- Dysarthria and dysphagia
- Dyspnea

CLINICAL/DIAGNOSTIC FINDINGS

- History and neurological exam
- Electromyogram: fibrillations
- Rule out other disease processes

OTHER PLANS OF CARE TO REFERENCE

- Prevention and Care of Pressure Ulcers
- Nutrition Support: Enteral Nutrition

▼

NURSING DIAGNOSIS: IMPAIRED PHYSICAL MOBILITY

Related To muscle weakness

Defining Characteristics

Decreased muscle strength and mass
Impaired coordination

Patient Outcomes

The patient will
- maintain proper body alignment.
- use assistive devices and compensatory techniques.

Nursing Interventions	Rationales
Assess for active and passive range of motion in all extremities, strength, ability to turn in bed, sitting tolerance, muscle tone, current transfer technique, use of assistive devices, and use of orthotic devices.	
Coordinate with physical therapy and occupational therapy for in-depth evaluation, assistive devices, splints, and mobility.	Physical and occupational therapists are experts in evaluating and treating mobility problems as well as in choosing the best assistive devices.
Encourage to perform active range-of-motion exercises twice daily. Perform passive range-of-motion exercises twice daily when patient is not able to move in full range.	Assists in maintenance of muscle tone and strength.
Position in proper body alignment.	Most patients wish to be able to stay in their home and be independent as long as possible.

Nursing Interventions	Rationales
Assess living situation. Make recommendations to enhance the patient's safety. Ramps, grab bars, and so on, may be helpful.	

NURSING DIAGNOSIS: IMPAIRED SWALLOWING

Related To neuromuscular impairment

Defining Characteristics

Evidence of difficulty in swallowing
Evidence of aspiration

Patient Outcomes

The patient will

- experience no aspiration.
- maintain an acceptable nutritional status.
- follow swallowing guidelines to ensure safe eating.

Nursing Interventions	Rationales
Assess appetite, weight loss, head alignment, ability to handle own secretions, coughing after food or fluid intake, voice quality, and amount of time to eat a meal. Ask what foods, if any, the patient experiences difficulty with and how the foods are prepared at home.	A comprehensive assessment is necessary to determine the degree of swallowing impairment. It is important to ask the patient how they are managing their diet at home; they most likely have compensated for swallowing difficulties by food selection and preparation.
Assess for fever, breath sounds, cough, and congestion.	Assessment for signs and symptoms of an aspiration pneumonia will allow for quick and effective intervention. This may mean diet modification and/or antibiotic therapy.
Examine cranial nerves V (sensory discrimination and ability to chew), VII (muscles of face for symmetry, lip closure, drooling), IX and X (soft palate, position of uvula, gag reflex, hoarseness), and XII (tongue).	All are involved in coordinating a normal swallow.

Nursing Interventions	Rationales
Consult speech therapist, dietitian, and occupational therapist (if available) for evaluation and recommendations for dysphagia. Including texture, consistency, and temperature of food.	A team approach provides comprehensive and consistent treatment.
Promote safe swallowing: 1. Provide oral hygiene and dentures. 2. Position with head upright, chin tucked forward. Patient should remain upright 30 min after meals, if possible. 3. Ensure presence of suction if needed. 4. Allow adequate time to eat.	

▼

NURSING DIAGNOSIS: INEFFECTIVE BREATHING PATTERN

Related To
- Respiratory muscle weakness
- Fatigue

Defining Characteristics
Dyspnea
Tachypnea
Shallow respirations
Use of accessory muscles

Patient Outcomes
The patient will
- demonstrate normal rate, rhythm, and depth of respirations.
- exhibit adequate oxygenation.

Nursing Interventions	Rationales
Assist in obtaining adequate amount of rest.	Helps decrease fatigue.
Suction as needed to keep airway clear.	
Administer prescribed oxygen.	

Nursing Interventions	Rationales
Encourage head of bed to be elevated.	Assists with ventilation and oxygenation.
Provide for an adequate nutritional status.	Helps decrease muscle fatigue.

▼

NURSING DIAGNOSIS: IMPAIRED VERBAL COMMUNICATION

Related To neuromuscular degeneration

Defining Characteristics

Dysarthria/anarthria
Dyspnea

Patient Outcomes

The patient will

- exhibit an effective communication mechanism.
- demonstrate the ability to communicate needs.

Nursing Interventions	Rationales
Coordinate with the speech therapist to devise an appropriate and effective means of communication.	
Establish a calm, unhurried environment for communication.	

▼

NURSING DIAGNOSIS: TERMINAL ILLNESS RESPONSE

Related To diagnosis of amyotrophic lateral sclerosis

Defining Characteristics

Asking many questions
Asking few questions
Exaggerated behavior
Fear of disease and dying

Patient Outcomes

The patient will

- demonstrate adequate coping mechanisms.
- verbalize his or her diagnosis and its implications.

Nursing Interventions	Rationales
Establish trust and rapport by arranging for consistent care providers.	
Assess patient's perception of the illness and treatment plan. Clarify any misunderstandings.	Baseline of current knowledge.
Encourage to ask questions and raise concerns.	Allows the patient to be in control, gives permission to express dissatisfaction, and builds trust and communication outlets.
Encourage to keep a notebook of information received and questions they wish to ask.	A system to keep track of information.
Involve in care planning as much as possible. Encourage independence as possible.	Allows some control over environment and life.
Assess family support systems and their ability to cope.	
Involve family and significant others as patient desires. Encourage them to allow the patient to do as much independently as possible. Provide support and realistic outcomes.	
Answer questions honestly.	
Explore the treatment options and their role in decision making: 1. Provide information and support on advanced directives. 2. Assist in devising appropriate questions to discuss with the physician.	With the progression of the disease process discussions may center on long-term mortality and decisions regarding the dying process. With information and support introduced slowly, patients and families can together explore these difficult issues while the patient is still able.
If acceptable to the patient, consult a counselor or clergy.	
Discuss imminent respiratory failure, and assist with advance directive and decisions for life support.	It is most helpful to discuss what, if any, life support they wish to have in the initial stages of the disease.

DISCHARGE PLANNING/CONTINUITY OF CARE

- Assure patient and care providers understand and can carry out self-management plan at home.
- Assure arrangements are made to obtain supplies, equipment, and prescribed medications.
- Arrange follow-up with physician or nurse practitioner for continued management and postdischarge care. Assure telephone numbers are provided if questions or problems arise.
- Coordinate with the discharge planning nurse or social worker, if available, to plan discharge arrangements for care given, home health agency, or long-term care facility.
- Provide with addresses of ALS support groups:
  The ALS Association
  21021 Ventura Blvd. #321
  Woodland Hills, CA 91364
  Muscular Dystrophy Association
  National Headquarters
  3561 East Sunrise Drive
  Tucson, AZ 85718

REFERENCES

Cammermeyer, M. & Appeldon, C. (Eds.). (1990). *Core curriculum for neuroscience nursing* (3rd ed). Chicago, IL: American Association of Neuroscience Nurses.

Hickey, J. (1992). *The clinical practice of neurological and neurosurgical nursing* (3rd ed). Philadelphia, PA: Lippincott.

Kim, T. (1989). Hope as a mode of coping in amyotrophic lateral sclerosis. *Journal of Neuroscience Nursing, 21*(6), 342–347.

BRAIN TUMORS

Andrea Strayer, RN, MS, CNRN

Brain tumors affect the brain by compressing and infiltrating normal brain tissue. This results in cerebral edema, neurological deficits, and seizures. There is no known cure for brain tumors. Brain tumors can be classified by malignancy, histological origin, primary or metastatic, location, and neuroembryonic origin. See Table 35.1 for a summary of common adult brain tumors.

ETIOLOGIES

- Unknown

CLINICAL MANIFESTATIONS

- Headache
- Seizures
- Vomiting
- Papilledema
- Mental status changes
- Visual changes
- Motor deficits
- Personality changes

CLINICAL/DIAGNOSTIC FINDINGS

Head computerized tomography (CT) scan or head magnetic resonance imaging (MRI): Visualize the mass.

OTHER PLANS OF CARE TO REFERENCE

- Craniotomy
- Alterations in Consciousness
- Basic Standard for Preoperative and Postoperative Care

Table 35.1 • Common Adult Brain Tumors

Astrocytoma (grades I and II)
- Complete surgical removal rare, but may prolong life
- Irradiation for some; possibly chemotherapy
- 6–7 years prognosis, more possible

Glioblastoma Multiforme (also known as astrocytoma grades III and IV)
- Surgery and debulking to decrease intracranial pressure and relieve cerebral compression
- Irradiation for some; possibly chemotherapy also
- 1–2 years prognosis

Ependymoma (grades I–IV)
- Arises from lining of ventricles
- Causes rapid increase in intracranial pressure from cerebrospinal fluid obstruction
- Tumor of children and young adults
- Surgery, if accessible, irradiation or chemotherapy for some
- 1 month prognosis for malignant; 7–8 years for benign

Oligodendroglioma (grades I–IV)
- Surgery and irradiation treatment of choice
- 5 or more years prognosis

Meningioma
- Complete removal surgically, if possible; irradiation if complete resection not possible
- Many years prognosis, especially with complete resection

Metastatic brain tumor
- Surgery, if resectable; irradiation may be an option
- Poor prognosis

Primary cerebral lymphoma
- Irradiation
- 2 years prognosis

Pituitary adenoma
- Surgery and/or irradiation
- Will see visual problems and endocrine disorders
- Prognosis very good

▼

▼

NURSING DIAGNOSIS: KNOWLEDGE DEFICIT—DIAGNOSIS

Related To

- New diagnosis
- Fear
- Lack of exposure to information

Defining Characteristics

Many questions
Few questions
Exaggerated behaviors

Patient Outcomes

The patient will

- verbalize his or her diagnosis and its implications.
- describe available treatment options.

Nursing Interventions	Rationales
Ask patients to describe what they have been told about the diagnosis.	This gives you a baseline of their current knowledge.
Clarify the patient's understanding of the diagnosis and treatment options.	This gives you the opportunity to clarify misconceptions and repeat things they were not sure about.
Clarify the patient's understanding of the pros and cons of the treatment options.	This gives the patient the freedom to be in control.
Encourage to ask questions and raise concerns.	It is important with the vast amounts of information that they have a system for keeping track of it all.
Encourage to keep a notebook of information received and questions they wish to ask.	

NURSING DIAGNOSIS: HIGH RISK FOR INEFFECTIVE INDIVIDUAL COPING

Risk Factors

- New diagnosis of possible terminal illness
- Potential poor prognosis
- Lack of support people

Patient Outcomes

The patient will

- develop effective coping mechanisms.
- vent fears, frustrations, questions, or concerns.

Nursing Interventions	Rationales
Allow time to vent fears and ask questions. Be reassuring.	The patient needs time to adjust to the diagnosis.
Provide emotional support.	
Consult counselor or clergy.	
Assess family support systems and their ability to cope.	At this time, the family may also need additional resources to help cope.
Provide with addresses of a national support group: American Brain Tumor Association; 3725 Talman Avenue; Chicago, IL 60618. National Brain Tumor Foundation; 323 Geary Street, Suite, 510; San Francisco, CA 94102	

DISCHARGE PLANNING/CONTINUITY OF CARE

- Coordinate follow-up with radiation oncology as indicated.
- Arrange for referral to a home health agency if continued care, monitoring, or teaching is needed.
- Provide with information on the American Cancer Society, support groups, hospice care, and I Can Cope.
- Assure follow-up appointments with physician or nurse practitioner for continued care.

REFERENCES

Adams, B., Clancey, J., & Eddy, M. (1991). Malignant glioma: Current treatment perspectives. *Journal of Neuroscience Nursing*, *23*(1), 15–19.

Amato, C. (1991). Malignant glioma: Coping with a devastating illness. *Journal of Neuroscience Nursing*, *23*(1), 20–22.

Cammermeyer, M. & Appeldorn, C. (Eds). (1990). *Core curriculum for neuroscience nursing* (3rd ed). Chicago, IL: American Association of Neuroscience Nurses.

Hickey, J. (1992). *The clinical practice of neurological and neurosurgical nursing* (3rd ed). Philadelphia, PA: Lippincott.

Willis, D. (1991). Intracranial astrocytoma: Pathology, diagnosis and clinical presentation. *Journal of Neuroscience Nursing*, *23*(1), 7–14.

▼

CENTRAL NERVOUS SYSTEM INFECTIONS: MENINGITIS AND ENCEPHALITIS

Andrea Strayer, RN, MS, CNRN

Meningitis and encephalitis are the primary central nervous system (CNS) infections encountered. Bacterial meningitis (septic meningitis) is very serious and can be life threatening. The invading organisms create an inflammatory reaction in the meninges and ventricles. Viral meningitis (aseptic meningitis), caused by any number of viruses, tends to be a mild infection. However, viral encephalitis, which is an inflammation of the brain, has a high mortality rate. A brain abscess is a localized collection of pus which acts as a mass lesion causing edema in surrounding tissue. *Staphylococcus aureus* is the most common posttrauma and postsurgical infection. Other bacteria are associated with infection from primary sites such as congenital heart disease. Yeast, fungi, and protozoa are being seen more in the immunocompromised host. Due to the rarity of brain abscesses, this section will focus on meningitis and encephalitis.

ETIOLOGIES

- Spread via the bloodstream from a primary foci such as a middle-ear infection or sinusitis or inoculation from an insect bite
- Compound cranial fractures
- Laceration of the dura mater
- Contamination of a head or spinal incision
- Enteroviruses (viral infections)
- Toxic substances (viral encephalitis)

CLINICAL MANIFESTATIONS

- Bacterial
  - fever
  - severe headache

  - decreased level of consciousness
  - stiff neck
  - possible seizures
- Viral
  - fever
  - headache
  - drowsiness and occasionally confusion
  - signs of meningeal irritation, neck stiffness, photophobia
  - possible nausea and vomiting, weakness, muscle soreness

CLINICAL/DIAGNOSTIC FINDINGS

Cerebrospinal fluid

- Increased white blood cells (WBCs) (only slightly with viral)
- Increased protein (bacterial)
- Decreased glucose (bacterial)
- Culture bacteria present (bacterial)
- Pressure on lumbar puncture may be elevated

OTHER PLANS OF CARE TO REFERENCE

- Alterated Consciousness
- Lumbar Puncture

▼

NURSING DIAGNOSIS: ALTERED CEREBRAL TISSUE PERFUSION

Related To

- Inflammatory process
- Cerebral edema
- Hydrocephalus

Defining Characteristics

Increased intracranial pressure
Alteration in consciousness

Patient Outcomes

The patient will demonstrate alertness and orientation to time, place, and person.

Nursing Interventions	Rationales
Elevate head of bed to at least 30°.	Increase venous drainage, helping to decrease intracranial pressure.
Position the patient's head in a neutral position.	

Nursing Interventions	Rationales
Monitor the neurological status very closely. The neurological exam includes assessment of level of consciousness, mental status, pupils, cranial nerves, motor strength, reflexes, and sensation.	
Notify the physician of any deterioration in neurological status.	If there is a decline, the physician may order diagnostic studies or additional medications.
Administer intravenous antimicrobials as prescribed.	

▼

NURSING DIAGNOSIS: PAIN

Related To meningeal irritation

Defining Characteristics

Headache
Neck and back pain
Photophobia

Patient Outcomes

The patient will verbalize
- decreased photophobia
- neck and back pain
- headache.

Nursing Interventions	Rationales
Assess pain and restlessness on a regular basis.	Effective pain control will help decrease intracranial pressure and increase the patient's comfort.
Administer analgesics as indicated. Nonsteroidals may be scheduled. Acetaminophen with codeine may be used for severe headaches. Stronger narcotics are contraindicated due to clouding of consciousness.	The medications administered should not interfere with the neurological exam.

Nursing Interventions	Rationales
Provide the patient with comfort measures, such as dark, quiet room and positioning. Approach the patient in a calm, quiet manner.	
Assess effectiveness of interventions regularly.	

DISCHARGE PLANNING/CONTINUITY OF CARE

- Arrange follow-up with physician or nurse practitioner for continued management and postdischarge care. Provide telephone numbers of whom they should contact with questions or problems.
- Assist the patient in obtaining prescriptions, especially if analgesics are still required.
- Refer the patient to a home health care agency if continued nursing care, teaching, or assistance is needed after discharge.

ACKNOWLEDGMENT

This work was supported by the Department of Veteran Affairs.

REFERENCES

Cammermeyer, M. & Appeldorn, C. (Eds.). (1990). *Core curriculum for neuroscience nursing* (3rd ed). Chicago, IL: American Association of Neuroscience Nurses.

Hickey, J. (1992). *The clinical practice of neurological and neurosurgical nursing* (3rd ed). Philadelphia, PA: Lippincott.

Mocsny, N. (1992). Toxoplasmic encephalitis in the AIDS patient. *Journal of neuroscience nursing*, 24(1), 30–33.

Mocsny, N. (1992). Cryptococcal meningitis in patients with AIDS. *Journal of neuroscience nursing*, 24(5), 265–268.

Twomey, C. (1992). Brain abscess: An update. *Journal of Neuroscience Nursing*, 24(1), 34–39.

GUILLAIN-BARRÉ SYNDROME

Andrea Strayer, RN, MS, CNRN

The Guillain-Barré syndrome (GBS) is a progressive disorder that affects primarily the motor component of the peripheral nerves. The patient will present with complaints of bilateral and symmetrical symptoms, usually weakness and numbness. The most common presentation starts in the extremities and progresses proximally. It can occur in either an ascending or descending pattern. Intravenous gamma-globulin and plasmaphoresis are treatments used to decrease the autoimmune response to the peripheral nerves. For either to be effective, the treatment must be started within 2 weeks of the first symptom. Approximately 75% of patients afflicted with GBS will recover with no residual impairment.

ETIOLOGIES

- Unknown
- Thought to be an autoimmune disorder
- 60–70% report a mild respiratory or gastrointestinal (GI) infection 1–3 weeks before onset
- Vaccinations (antirabies and swine flu) have also been implicated

CLINICAL MANIFESTATIONS

- Bilateral and symmetrical weakness and numbness
- Degree of severity varies
- Initial progressive phase
  - onset of first symptom to the point where there is no further deterioration (1–3 weeks)
- Plateau phase
  - period during which maximum symptoms exist (days to 2 weeks)
- Recovery phase
  - period of remyelination and axonal regeneration
  - return to maximal function (6 months to 2 years)

CLINICAL/DIAGNOSTIC FINDINGS

- Increased protein in cerebrospinal fluid
- Nerve conduction
  - slowed or blocked in 80%
  - velocity 60% of normal

OTHER PLANS OF CARE TO REFERENCE

Prevention and Care of Pressure Ulcers

▼

NURSING DIAGNOSIS: KNOWLEDGE DEFICIT—DISEASE PROCESS AND RECOVERY COURSE

Related To
- Lack of exposure
- Unfamiliarity with resources

Defining Characteristics
Fear
Many questions
Few questions
Exaggerated behavior

Patient Outcomes
The patient will
- verbalize knowledge of the disease process.
- describe medical and nursing plan of care.

Nursing Interventions	Rationales
Discuss the usual disease course, frequency of nursing assessment, procedures such as an electromyelogram (EMG), and supportive care, especially during the progressive and plateau phases.	The patient and family will be less anxious if they know what to expect.

Nursing Interventions	Rationales
Discuss expected length of hospitalization before they are ready for rehabilitation (can be up to 6–8 weeks.	Patients will need to stay in the acute care setting until they are completely stabilized and have begun early rehabilitation participation. If they begin their rehabilitation program too soon, they may relapse.

▼

NURSING DIAGNOSIS: HIGH RISK FOR INEFFECTIVE BREATHING PATTERN

Risk Factors

- Muscle demyelination
- Increased fatigue
- Anxiety

Patient Outcomes

The patient will

- maintain adequate ventilation.
- demonstrate freedom from respiratory distress.

Nursing Interventions	Rationales
Assess rate and rhythm of respirations; auscultate breath sounds; and monitor vital capacity, negative inspiratory force, and pulse oximetry at least every 4 hr.	Adequate ventilation is of primary importance. If the vital capacity, negative inspiratory force, and/or PaO_2 fall, the patient may first have oxygen ordered. If oxygenation continues to deteriorate, the patient will need the support of a ventilator.
Monitor arterial blood gases.	The thought of being on a ventilator can be very frightening, and the patient will need support and guidance.
Notify a physician immediately of respiratory distress and/or marked changes in respiratory assessment.	

Nursing Interventions	Rationales
Discuss intubation and ventilation if this is a necessary procedure for the patient. Include methods of communication used while on a ventilator and what it will feel like (suctioning, coughing). Instruct that muscle strength will need to return before being able to come off the ventilator.	

▼

NURSING DIAGNOSIS: HIGH RISK FOR PAIN IN EXTREMITIES

Risk Factors

- Acute muscle degeneration

Patient Outcomes

The patient will demonstrate adequate pain control.

Nursing Interventions	Rationales
Assess pain regularly using a scale from 0 to 10.	A scale is helpful for pain assessment continuity.
Perform range-of-motion exercises every 4 hr.	Range-of-motion exercises may not only help with the pain and discomfort the patient feels, but also keeps joints loose and prevents deformities during the immobilized period.
Turn from side to side at least every 2 hr, utilizing proper body alignment.	Proper body alignment is necessary to prevent contractures. In the immobilized patient, turning at least every 2 hr is a must.
Massage muscles to help alleviate pain.	
Medicate for pain, as needed, preferably using nonsteroidal analgesics. Acetaminophen with codeine can be used with discretion.	Constipation and GI upset are side effects of codeine. Narcotics may interfere with respiratory status.

▼

DISCHARGE PLANNING/CONTINUITY OF CARE

- Assure understanding of self-management plan.
- Describe the rehabilitation process.
- Coordinate with the rehabilitation clinical nurse specialist, social worker, or discharge planner for discharge to a rehabilitation center or a home health agency for continued rehabilitation.
- Arrange for follow-up with physician or nurse practitioner.

ACKNOWLEDGMENT

This work was supported by the Department of Veteran Affairs.

REFERENCES

Anderson, S. (1992). Guillain-Barré syndrome: Giving the patient control. *Journal of Neuroscience Nursing*, *24*(3), 158–162.

Cammermeyer, M. & Appeldorn, C. (Eds.). (1990). *Core curriculum for neuroscience nursing* (3rd ed). Chicago, IL: American Association of Neuroscience Nurses.

Hickey, J. (1992). *The clinical practice of neurological and neurosurgical nursing* (3rd ed). Philadelphia, PA: Lippincott.

Ropper, A. (1992). The Guillain-Barré syndrome. *New England Journal of Medicine*, *326*(17), 1130–1136.

Van Der Meche, F., Schmitz, P., & the Dutch Guillian-Barré Group. (1992). A randomized trial comparing intravenous immune globulin and plasma exchange in Guillain-Barré syndrome. *New England Journal of Medicine*, *326*(17), 1123–1129.

▼

LUMBAR PUNCTURE

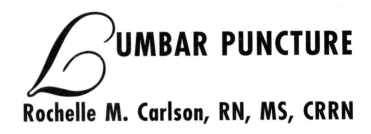

Rochelle M. Carlson, RN, MS, CRRN

A lumbar puncture (LP) is the introduction of a sterile needle into the subarachnoid space at either level L_3–L_4 or L_4–L_5 using strict aseptic technique. The procedure is more commonly performed for diagnostic purposes but may also be used as a therapeutic measure.

ETIOLOGIES

- Diagnostic indications
  - examination of the characteristics of the cerebrospinal fluid (CSF)
  - measurement of the pressure of CSF
  - visualization of the parts of the nervous system radiographically by injection of contrast medium
- Therapeutic indications
  - intrathecal administration of anesthetic, antibiotics, steroids, or other medications

CONTRAINDICATIONS

- Infection at the site of lumbar puncture
- Greatly increased intracranial pressure

CLINICAL MANIFESTATIONS

- Fever
- Nuchal rigidity
- Change in level of consciousness
- Muscle weakness
- Other abnormal findings on neurological examination
- Pain

Table 38.1 • Normal and Abnormal Characteristics of Cerebrospinal Fluid

Characteristic	Normal	Abnormal
Color	Clear, colorless	Cloudy: may be due to presence of bacteria or white blood cells (WBCs). Yellow: xanthochronic, most often due to red blood cell (RBC) breakdown.
RBC	None	Presence could be due to a traumatic tap or subarachnoid hemorrhage.
WBC	0–5/mm^3, agranulocytes	Increased WBC count associated with meningitis, tumor, multiple sclerosis, infarct, abscess, or subarachnoid hemorrhage.
Glucose	50–80 mg/100 mL	Decreased level may be suggestive of bacteria in CSF Increased level: no significance.
Protein	15–45 mg/100 mL	Increased level associated with tumor, infection, hemorrhage, and demyelinating disease. Decreased level: no significance.
Chloride	120–130 mEq/L	Low concentration associated with meningitis
Pressure	70–180 mmH_2O	More than 200 mmH_2O often seen with tumor, cerebral edema, hydrocephalus, cerebral hemorrhage, abscess, or cyst. Less than 50 mmH_2O seen in spinal block.
Culture and sensitivity	No bacteria	Presence of bacteria or fungus seen in meningitis or abscess. Sensitivity used to help determine appropriate antimicrobial therapy.

▼

CLINICAL/DIAGNOSTIC FINDINGS

See Table 38.1

▼

NURSING DIAGNOSIS: KNOWLEDGE DEFICIT—LUMBAR PUNCTURE PROCEDURE

Related To lack of exposure to procedure

Defining Characteristics

Many questions
Lack of questions
Fear of complications
Anxiety about possible diagnostic findings

Patient Outcomes

The patient will

- explain why the procedure is necessary.
- describe preprocedure preparation.
- demonstrate correct positioning during the procedure.
- describe postprocedure plan of care.
- identify health care providers to contact if questions arise following the procedure.

Nursing Interventions	Rationales
Assess the patient's understanding and fears regarding the procedure.	
Provide written as well as oral instruction when possible.	Written materials are helpful for later reference.
Explain why the procedure is indicated for this patient.	Clear explanations can prevent misunderstandings and decrease anxiety.
Describe desired outcome: diagnostic findings or therapeutic response.	
Discuss possible complications of the procedure.	Information about complications is necessary for informed consent for procedures.
Instruct the patient to be well hydrated before the procedure.	Dehydration may contribute to a postprocedure spinal headache.

Nursing Interventions	Rationales
Describe the procedure and the position that the patient will assume for the procedure (fetal position with the back at the edge of the bed or sitting on the edge of the exam table leaning forward).	These positions allow for greatest access to the subarachnoid space by separating the vertebral bodies.
Explain postprocedure care (flat position, drinking plenty of fluids, vital signs, and neurological checks).	Postprocedure care is aimed at recognizing and minimizing complications.
Inform the patient of who to call if questions arise pre- or postprocedure.	

▼

NURSING DIAGNOSIS: HIGH RISK FOR PAIN

Risk Factors

- Positioning
- Introduction of the spinal needle
- Leakage of CSF

Patient Outcomes

The patient will

- experience no pain or mild pain.
- notify a health care professional if experiencing postprocedure pain.

Nursing Interventions	Rationales
Assess pain level and location (headache when assuming an upright position, low back pain, pain radiating into the legs) pre- and postprocedure.	
Position flat for 4–24 hr following the procedure.	Post-LP headaches are thought to be caused by leakage of CSF from the LP site. A flat position is believed to decrease the chances of CSF leakage. The length of time a patient should lay flat is decided by patient history and physician preference.

Nursing Interventions	Rationales
Encourage a large intake of fluids postprocedure	Extra fluids will potentiate the body making more CSF to replace the fluid that was withdrawn in the procedure.
Administer analgesics as prescribed when pain does occur.	Acetaminophen is used for mild pain while narcotics may be used for severe pain.
Reassure the patient that back pain and extremity pain are usually transitory.	

▼

NURSING DIAGNOSIS: HIGH RISK FOR INFECTION/ INCREASED INTRACRANIAL PRESSURE

Risk Factors

- Break in aseptic technique during LP procedure
- Elevated CSF pressure prior to LP procedure

Patient Outcomes

The patient will

- be free from infection postprocedure.
- not have a rise in intracranial pressure postprocedure

Nursing Interventions	Rationales
Assess for vital signs, neurological status (level of consciousness, orientation, sensation, movement, and strength), respiratory pattern, and presence of nuchal rigidity preprocedure.	
Assist the physician as needed during the procedure to maintain aseptic technique.	The physician will be performing the following steps: sterile draping, cleansing the site, administering local anesthesia, measuring pressure and gathering fluid into sterile containers or instilling medication.
If necessary, assist in holding the patient in position.	The patient needs to remain still during the procedure to maintain asepsis and to prevent trauma.

Nursing Interventions	Rationales
Apply a Band-Aid after removal of the needle to protect the puncture site from pathogens.	
Assess for fever, nuchal rigidity, and redness or warmth at the site of needle insertion following the procedure. 1. Notify physician if these symptoms of infection are present. 2. Teach outpatients to notify nurse or physician if these symptoms occur.	
Assess vital signs, neurological status, and respiratory patterns at least every 30 min for the first 2 hr and then every hour for the next 2 hr following the procedure or as prescribed by the physician. 1. Notify physician if symptoms of increased intracranial pressure are present 2. Teach outpatients to notify nurse or physician if change in level of consciousness or disturbances in sensation or motor function occur.	

▼

DISCHARGE PLANNING/CONTINUITY OF CARE

- Assure that the patient understands symptoms (e.g., persistent headache, fever, and redness or warmth at site of insertion) to report to nurse or physician.
- Report assessment data and care given to next shift of nurses.
- Ensure that a driver is available for patients going home following the procedure. A LP commonly performed in outpatient as well as inpatient settings.
- Provide written information, including phone number of nurse or physician to call, if patient is going home after procedure.
- Arrange follow-up with physician for continued management and postdischarge care.

REFERENCES

Cammermeyer, M. & Appeldorn, C. (Eds.). (1990). *Core curriculum for neuroscience nursing*. Chicago, IL: American Association of Neuroscience Nurses.

Hickey, J. V. (1992). *The clinical practice of neurological and neurosurgical nursing* (3rd ed). Philadelphia: Lippincott.

Snyder, M. (Ed.). (1991). *A guide to neurological and neurosurgical nursing* (2nd ed). Albany, NY: Delmar.

▼

MULTIPLE SCLEROSIS

Elizabeth A. Bruckbauer, RN, MS

Multiple sclerosis (MS), an inflammatory disease of the central nervous system (CNS), is a progressive, sometimes disabling disorder of young people (average onset in early thirties) characterized by exacerbations and remissions. Inflammation of the myelin sheath surrounding the axon and nerve fibers of the brain and spinal cord results in decreased thickness of the sheath, reducing efficiency of impulse transmission. Although the function of the sheath may be regained by natural recovery, continued exacerbations, with destruction of the myelin sheath and formation of hard scar (or plaque), can result in eventual impairment in cognitive or physical function.

ETIOLOGIES

Unknown. Research theories include
- immune or autoimmune response
- postviral infection syndrome
- genetic predisposition

CLINICAL MANIFESTATIONS

- Multiple and varied sensory, motor, cerebellar, cognitive, and psychological symptoms
- Disturbances of sensation, gait, and monocular loss of vision most common early symptoms
- Pattern of exacerbations and remissions
- Progressive cognitive and physical disability with eventual impairment in or loss of independence

CLINICAL/DIAGNOSTIC FINDINGS

- History of attacks of neurological symptom(s) lasting at least 24 hr, separated by at least 1 month, affecting differing parts of the CNS
- Abnormal neurological signs
- Localization of lesions by computerized tomography (CT) scan or magnetic resonance imaging (MRI)
- Delays in visual-, auditory-, and somatosensory-evoked response potentials
- Oligoclonal bands in cerebrospinal fluid that are not concurrently present in serum

▼

NURSING DIAGNOSIS: HIGH RISK FOR IMPAIRED PHYSICAL MOBILITY AND SELF-CARE DEFICITS

Risk Factors

- Exacerbations producing increased muscle weakness, incoordination, altered balance, and/or cognitive impairments
- Bedrest as part of hospital or home treatment
- Family or professional caregivers providing more than necessary physical care to patient; imposing dependency

Patient Outcomes

The patient will

- function at optimal physical ability within the limitations of his or her disability.
- identify and utilize appropriate therapy services to improve and maintain physical abilities.
- identify and utilize appropriate adaptive equipment or utensils to improve and maintain physical abilities.
- be able to direct caregivers to provide assistance which promotes independence.

Nursing Interventions	Rationales
Assess physical function at each admission/discharge utilizing standardized rating scales whenever possible.	Changes in level of function signal exacerbations and remissions. Detection of declining function and early intervention can preserve independence. Areas of impairment vary widely with individuals; assessment of specific needs is essential.

Nursing Interventions	Rationales
Utilize turning, positioning, and range-of-motion exercises.	Prevent complications of immobility.
Assist and encourage the patient to care for self to fullest potential.	Avoid contributing to "learned helplessness."
Mobilize appropriate rehabilitation services to increase independence and prevent loss of function.	
Teach patient and family members to allow patient to function to maximum ability, providing assistance only when patient is clearly unable to perform a task.	

▼

NURSING DIAGNOSIS: HIGH RISK FOR ALTERED THOUGHT PROCESSES AND SENSORY/PERCEPTUAL DEFICITS

Risk Factors

Potential for progressive destruction of neurosensory pathways in the central and/or peripheral nervous system.

Patient Outcomes

The patient will

- identify altered thought processes and utilize appropriate interventions to improve function.
- identify impaired sensory/perceptual function and utilize appropriate interventions to improve function.

Nursing Interventions	Rationales
Assess communication, problem-solving, memory, and judgment skills in the context of ability to express needs and thoughts coherently, follow directions, sequence self-care tasks, recognize and utilize familiar objects, and learn new material.	
Refer to neuropsychology, speech pathology, and/or occupational therapy, as available, for formal cognitive testing when impairment is suspected.	
Assess for visual, auditory, kinesthetic, gustatory, tactile, and/or olfactory impairments that may contribute to changes in functional abilities.	
Refer for formal sensory/perceptual testing when impairment is suspected.	
Increase awareness of patient and family members about the potential for these deficits and possible impact on function.	

▼

NURSING DIAGNOSIS: ALTERED URINARY AND/OR BOWEL ELIMINATION

Related To

- Neuromotor and neurosensory impairments
- Impaired mobility
- Declining cognitive abilities

Defining Characteristics

Urinary retention or incontinence
Bowel retention or incontinence
Lack of awareness of incontinence
Incontinence or retention due to inability to manage clothing or transfers involved in toileting

Patient Outcomes

The patient will

- eliminate stool and urine on a regular and predictable basis.
- maintain urinary and bowel continence.
- utilize assistive devices as needed to maintain independence in toileting.
- recognize the need to eliminate urine and stool.

Nursing Interventions	Rationales
Assess bowel function for incontinence or constipation.	A regulatory program of QD or QOD biscodyl suppository may prevent incontinence or treat chronic constipation
Assess dietary habits that may contribute to constipation.	Increasing dietary intake of high-fiber foods (fruits, vegetables, and whole grains) and increasing fluid intake may relieve constipation.
Evaluate need for stool softeners and/or bulk-forming products as part of a regulatory bowel program.	
Develop and implement a teaching plan with the patient to understand the need for a regulatory bowel program and to utilize diet, suppositories, and medications appropriately.	
Teach proper insertion of suppository, need for consistency in daily regimen, dietary sources of fiber, and medication usage and side effects.	

Nursing Interventions	**Rationales**
Assess urinary symptoms, including hesitancy, frequency, loss of sensation, incontinence, and retention. Also inquire about history of urinary tract infection or urolithiasis. Record frequency and amount of fluid intake and urinary output.	Incontinence in MS may result from urinary retention with overflow (flaccid bladder) or involuntary detrusor contractions (spastic bladder). Determining the type of bladder dysfunction is imperative in determining interventions. A spastic bladder (characterized by small-volume, frequent voiding pattern) may be treated with anticholinergic drugs (oxybutynin, imipramine, or propantheline) to reduce smooth-muscle contractions and a toileting regimen emptying of the bladder before involuntary contractions occur.
If urinary retention is suspected, measure postvoiding urine volumes over a 48-hr period.	Residual urine volumes above 100 mL is indicative of a flaccid bladder and may be treated by the crede method (manual pressure applied to the abdomen over the bladder to express urine), digital stimulation of the anus, and cholinergic drugs such as Bethanechol chloride to improve bladder contractions.
Institute an intermittent catheterization regimen for patients with high residual urine volumes (>150 mL consistently) or urinary retention that does not respond to measures given in the previous intervention. Catheterize every 4–6 hr to prevent overdistension of the bladder and reduce incidence of infection.	Detrusor/external sphincter dyssynergia (incoordination between bladder contraction and sphincter relaxation) results in retention.
Teach clean intermittent self-catheterization to patients who are physically and cognitively able to manage the routine.	Outside of the hospital environment, washing hands and catheterization supplies with soap and water is sufficient to prevent infection. Impairments in fine motor coordination, balance, and cognition may necessitate teaching to a caregiver instead of the patient.

Nursing Interventions	Rationales
Evaluate physical ability to manage clothing, toilet transfers, and hygiene and assist patient to adapt clothing and equipment to his or her level of function. Involve occupational and physical therapies as needed.	
Evaluate declining cognitive function as a contributor to incontinence. Devise a toileting schedule for patients who are unable to respond to normal body signals to eliminate. Involve caregivers in carrying through the schedule for profoundly impaired patients.	
Utilize indwelling catheters only when absolutely necessary.	Indwelling catheters promote urinary infection and can result in erosion of the urethra with long-term use.
Adult diapers and external incontinence devices may be necessary for some patients. Inspection of the skin for signs of irritation and breakdown and thorough, regular cleansing are essential to maintain skin integrity.	

▼

NURSING DIAGNOSIS: SEXUAL DYSFUNCTION

Related To

- Progressive neurological impairment
- Impaired physical mobility
- Caregiver role impairment of relationship with partner
- Poor body image related to disability

Defining Characteristics

Verbalization of problem
Inhibited sexual desire
Impaired relationship with partner as caregiver

Patient Outcomes

The patient will

- identify factors contributing to altered sexual activity.
- express thoughts and feelings about altered sexual function.
- express thoughts and feelings about altered relationship with partner.
- express feelings of loss related to disability that may interfere with sexual identity.
- explore alternative means of sexual expression within the limitations of disability.

Nursing Interventions	Rationales
Include assessment of sexual function in initial assessment of overall physical function.	
Promote an atmosphere of openness to communication of sexual concerns through active listening and nonjudgmental responses.	
Assure privacy for discussion of sexual matters.	
Include partner in discussions, with patient's consent.	
Assist patient and partner to identify causes of sexual dysfunction (emotional, psychological, and physical).	
Assist patient to express thoughts and feelings about altered body image that may impact sexual identity.	
Assist patient and partner to identify and grieve losses in relationship resulting from changes in roles and assumption of caregiver role by partner.	
Encourage patient and partner to identify and explore mutually agreeable alternative means of sexual expression, within the limitations of patient's disability.	
Refer for professional sexual counseling when patient and partner are in need of extensive assistance in identifying and expressing thoughts and feelings.	

▼

NURSING DIAGNOSIS: FATIGUE

Related To

- Combination of upper motor neuron weakness
- Spasticity
- Malfunctioning nerve fibers
- Increased core temperature
- Depression (sometimes)

Defining Characteristics

Feeling of tiredness after activity
Increased weakness with exposure to heat
Spontaneous, overwhelming exhaustion

Patient Outcomes

Patient will be able to

- describe a plan for structuring his or her day to incorporate energy conservation techniques, paced activities, and rest to avoid fatigue.
- identify potential causes of overheating and define a plan for avoiding and treating overheating.

Nursing Interventions	Rationales
Assess for symptoms of fatigue that interfere with or follow activity.	
Monitor patients involved in intensive therapy programs for increasing fatigue.	Therapies may need to be scheduled to allow for rest periods between sessions if patient fatigues easily.
Assist patient to modify daily schedule to create balance between activity and rest.	
Assess for underlying depression that may contribute to fatigue.	
Teach patient to avoid hot baths/showers and saunas and to treat overheating with ice packs, cool bath/shower, or air conditioning.	Increased core temperature results in muscle weakness, sometimes compromising physical function.

Nursing Interventions	Rationales
Refer to occupational therapy for teaching energy conservation techniques.	

▼

NURSING DIAGNOSIS: INEFFECTIVE DENIAL

Related To uncertain nature of progressive illness.

Defining Characteristics

Refusal to participate in self-care and/or rehabilitative activities during exacerbations; prefers to wait for remission
Views permanent progression as an exacerbation, unrealistically expecting remission
Anger toward professional/family caregivers who present adaptive rather than curative approaches

Patient Outcomes

The patient will

- express feelings of loss for altered physical function.
- participate in rehabilitative therapy and self-care activities to the maximum of remaining ability.
- identify and utilize appropriate coping mechanisms for dealing with loss.

Nursing Interventions	Rationales
Assist the patient to identify feelings of fear and anxiety over uncertain nature of disease.	
Allow patient to make choices in care whenever possible to increase feelings of control.	
Provide clear interpretation of symptoms whenever possible.	
Provide straightforward prognostic information when recovery of function is not the expectation.	
Refer for psychological assessment when necessary.	

▼

NURSING DIAGNOSIS: HIGH RISK FOR CAREGIVER ROLE STRAIN

Risk Factors

- Family member with significantly increased care needs on discharge
- Severity of disability requiring significant, long-term physical care
- Unpredictability of disease progression
- Cognitive and/or psychological impairments that reduce the patient's ability to cooperate with care
- Past history of dysfunctional family relationship between caregiver and care receiver
- Lack of respite for caregiver
- Caregiver's competing role commitments

Caregiver Outcomes

The caregiver will

- define the limitations of own involvement in caring for the patient.
- identify and mobilize family and community resources for caring for the patient and/or for respite care.
- identify available support system for self.

Nursing Interventions	Rationales
Assess patient and caregiver interactions for signs of verbal and/or physical abuse.	
Allow patient and caregiver to express feelings about their relationship privately.	
Encourage and support expression of feelings of loss of aspects of relationship and burden of increased responsibility of caregiver.	
Assist caregiver to define reasonable limitations to his or her involvement in caring for family member.	
Develop and implement a teaching plan with the patient and caregiver to address areas of care unfamiliar to caregiver.	
Assist caregiver to define additional family and/or community services needed.	
Arrange for necessary community support services or refer to social services and/or discharge planner to facilitate arrangements.	

▼

DISCHARGE PLANNING/CONTINUITY OF CARE

- Refer patient and family to local chapter of the National Multiple Sclerosis Society for further information and support.
- Refer to a home health care agency for continued nursing, attendant, and therapy care.
- Assist patient to identify community agencies for provision of adaptive equipment and home modifications.
- Arrange for follow-up appointments with physician postdischarge.

REFERENCES

Bartels DesRosier, M., Catanzaro, M., & Piller, J. (1992). Living with chronic illness: Social support and the well spouse perspective. *Rehabilitation Nursing*, *17*(2), 87–91.

Clark, C. (1991). Nursing care for multiple sclerosis. *Orthopaedic Nursing, 10*(1), 21–32.

Erickson, R. P., Lie, M. R., & Wineinger, M. A. (1989). Rehabilitation in multiple sclerosis. *Mayo Clinic Proceedings, 64*, 818–828.

Swanson, J. W. (1989). Multiple sclerosis: Update in diagnosis and review of prognostic factors. *Mayo Clinic Proceedings, 64*, 577–586.

▼

PARKINSON'S DISEASE

Maureen R. Anderson RN, BSN, CRRN

Parkinson's disease is a neurological disorder which is chronic and progressive. It affects 1% of the population over the age of 50. It is characterized by the lack of dopamine in the extrapyramidal area of the brain, which is responsible for controlling movement.

ETIOLOGIES

- Idiopathic-degeneration of dopaminergic neurons in the substania nigra secondary to an undetermined biological process
- Secondary (parkinsonism): can usually be contributed to a cause
  - drug induced
  - neurotoxins
  - strokes
  - tumors
  - metabolic

CLINICAL MANIFESTATIONS

- Primary
  - tremor
  - rigidity
  - bradykinesia
  - postural instability
- Secondary
  - micrographia
  - stooped posture
  - swallowing and speeech difficulties
  - constipation
  - cognitive changes
  - depression

CLINICAL/DIAGNOSTIC FINDINGS

Exclusion of other diagnosis by

- magnetic resonance imaging (MRI) and computerized tomography (CT) scan: to rule out tumor, bleeding, hydrocephalus, or other positive findings
- Serum blood tests: to rule out toxic conditions or endocrine or metabolic dysfunction
- Positron emission tomography (PET) scan: can show decreased dopamine intake in the brain

▼

NURSING DIAGNOSIS: IMPAIRED PHYSICAL MOBILITY

Related To neurological impairment

Defining Characteristics

Inability to purposefully move within the physical environment, including bed mobility, transfer, and ambulation
Reluctance to attempt movement
Limited range of motion
Impaired coordination

Patient Outcomes

The patient will

- demonstrate the appropriate use of adaptive equipment to enhance mobility.
- maintain optimal level of mobility, as evidenced by increasing or maintaining activity level.
- avoid complications of immobility.

Nursing Interventions	Rationales
Assess for current level of activity, functional abilities, active and passive range of motion in all joints, and the effect of Parkinson symptoms such as tremor, rigidity, and balance on mobility	Assessment provides a baseline of patient's functional abilities.
Encourage patient to perform active range of motion (ROM) of joints twice a day; assist as needed.	Range of motion prevents contractures, increases flexibility, and strengthens muscles.

Nursing Interventions	Rationales
Provide a safe and obstruction-free environment by providing a call light and maintaining side rails up when in bed and providing a clear pathway from bathroom to bed and into hallway.	A safe environment will prevent accidents and aid in increasing mobility.
Assist in use of adaptive equipment if needed, such as a walker, cane, or wheelchair.	Adaptive devices can assist in safe and improved mobility.
Encourage ambulation several times a day and assist if needed.	Ambulation increases flexibility and can aid in preventing complications of immobility.
Encourage independence in activities of daily living (ADLs) by providing sufficient time and assist as needed.	Bradykinesia, rigidity, and tremor can increase the time needed to perform ADLs.
Encourage correct posture and taking large steps while picking up feet with ambulation.	Correct posture and large steps will prevent a shuffling gait and stooped posture.
Place colored tape on floor one step width apart in tight areas such as bathrooms if "freezing" occurs frequently or encourage side-to-side rocking and taking steps forward by placing heels down first.	Freezing occurs when a Parkinson patient wishes to move but cannot initiate the movement. Colored tape will give visual cues to help reinitiate ambulation along with rocking side to side.
Provide a hard straight-back chair with arm rests in room.	A hard straight chair will assist in independence rising from a chair.
Consult occupational and/or physical therapy as needed.	Occupational and physical therapy can evaluate and treat mobility problems, including teaching of exercise programs and use of assistive devices such as canes or walkers.

▼

NURSING DIAGNOSIS: SELF-CARE DEFICIT—BATHING/HYGIENE, DRESSING/GROOMING, TOILETING, FEEDING

Related To

- Neuromuscular impairment
- Impaired mobility status

Defining Characteristics

Bathing/hygiene
Inability to wash body or body parts
Inability to obtain or get to water source
Inability to regulate temperature flow

Dressing/grooming
Impaired ability to put on or take off necessary items of clothing
Impaired ability to obtain or replace articles of clothing
Impaired ability to fasten clothing

Toileting
Inability to get to toilet or commode
Inability to sit on or rise from toilet or commode
Inability to manipulate clothing for toileting
Inability to carry out proper toilet hygiene

Feeding
Inability to bring food from a receptacle to the mouth

Patient Outcomes

Patient will

- perform activity at expected optimal level as evidenced by defining and working toward functional goals.
- demonstrate increased ability to perform activity.
- demonstrate ability to cope with the necessity of needing assistance.
- demonstrate appropriate use of adaptive equipment.

Nursing Interventions	Rationales
Assess current level of functioning, including assistive equipment and effect of Parkinson symptoms.	Assessment assists in providing a baseline of current function.
Provide ample time for activities and assist as needed.	Bradykinesia and other Parkinson symptoms can cause need for increased times to perform activities.
Encourage family and significant others to promote independence in ADLs as much as possible.	Encouraging independence enhances a patient's self-esteem and decreases his or her sense of disability.
Provide all needed equipment within close reach or as directed by the patient.	Providing needed items close to patients prevents falls or accidents and decreases time needed to perform activities.

Nursing Interventions	Rationales
Provide assistive equipment as needed, that is, button hooker, long-handle sponge, zipper pull, built-up eating utensils.	Assistive devices can help increase independence.
Bathing/grooming	
1. Provide grab rails within easy access in shower or bath. 2. Provide nonslip surfaces at bottom of tub or shower stall.	Grab bars and nonslip surface can prevent loss of balance and falls.
Dressing	
1. Encourage use of loose-fitting clothes, such as pullover tops, clothes that close in the front, easy zippers, and velcro items.	Loose clothing provides ease of dressing and can increase independence.
Toileting	
1. Maintain adequate intake and output.	Adequate intake and output helps maintain appropriate bowel and bladder function.
2. Instruct in use of elevated toilet seat, bedside commode, or external collecting devices.	A bedside commode is helpful for those who freeze in bathrooms and more convenient at night. Elevated toilet seat makes getting up easier. External collecting devices are useful for males who have difficulties with incontinence.
Feeding	
1. Encourage patient use of dentures and glasses.	Dentures and glasses will aid the patient in eating.
2. Set up tray and assist with opening of packages and cutting up of food as needed.	Assisting in setting up meals can increase independence in eating.
3. Assist in providing optimal position for eating.	Appropriate positioning is necessary when eating to prevent aspiration or choking.

NURSING DIAGNOSIS: CONSTIPATION

Related To immobility and drug therapy

Defining Characteristics

Frequency less than usual pattern
Hard-formed stools
Reported feeling of rectal fullness
Straining at stool

Patient Outcomes

Patient will be able to pass a soft-formed stool on a regular basis.

Nursing Interventions	Rationales
Assess regular bowel pattern, including last bowel movement, consistency, bowel sounds, use of medications, and diet.	Assessment assists in providing baseline data on bowel status.
Encourage sufficient fluid intake of at least 2 L/day unless contraindicated.	Appropriate fluid intake maintains bowel patterns and promotes proper stool consistency.
Provide a diet high in fiber and bulk, including such foods as bran, raw fruits, and vegetables. Consult Dietary if needed.	A high-fiber diet increases bulk of stool and stimulates peristalsis to promote regularity.
Assist in promoting a regular time for bowel movements.	A regular time for bowel movements helps establish a regular bowel program.
Encourage use of toilet or commode instead of a bedpan.	Using a commode or a toilet is more effecient in emptying bowels because of gravity.
Administer medications as prescribed: 1. Metamucil 2. Docusate or Docusate with Casanthranol oil	Mild laxatives can soften stool and promote regular bowel movements.

▼

NURSING DIAGNOSIS: IMPAIRED VERBAL COMMUNICATION

Related To inability to articulate words

Defining Characteristics

Phonation and pronunciation difficulties
Soft, whispered speech
Slurred, slow speech

Patient Outcomes

Patient will

- demonstrate increased ability to express self as evidenced by using other forms of communication.
- verbalize decreased frustration with communication.

Nursing Interventions	Rationales
Assess current method of communication, including use of communication devices.	
Encourage patient to read from newspaper or books, exaggerating the enunciation of every syllable.	Exaggerating syllables can promote better verbalization.
Encourage use of short sentences or single words.	Exhaling and forcing out words can make a voice appear stronger.
Encourage patient to speak slowly and to forcefully blow out each syllable.	
Allow patient adequate time for verbalization.	
Encourage use of picture board or other communication devices as needed.	
Provide an appropriate response to attempts to speak. 1. Do not pretend to understand. 2. Ask "are you saying . . ." to clarify verbalization.	

Nursing Interventions	Rationales
Suggest discussing with physician a speech referral if problem is severe or there is a need for communication devices.	Communication devices can greatly enhance communication.

▼

NURSING DIAGNOSIS: SELF-ESTEEM DISTURBANCE

Related To

- Effects of Parkinson's disease
- Changes in social roles
- Changes in relationships with others

Defining Characteristics

Self-negating verbalization
Evaluates self as unable to deal with events
Denial of problems obvious to others
Hesitant to try new things or situations

Patient Outcomes

Patient will

- express feelings regarding self and disability.
- participate in ADLs and therapies.
- communicate with family members.
- participate in education and support groups.

Nursing Interventions	Rationales
Assess current level of self-esteem, perception of self, level of participation in care, and past coping methods.	Assessment provides a baseline of patient's current status. Past successful coping strategies can be utilized.
Encourage expression of thoughts and concerns regarding diagnosis and life-style changes.	Listening effectively helps establish a trusting relationship.
Encourage support and visits of friends and family.	
Encourage participation in ADLs.	Promoting independence in ADLs can reassure the patient of the ability to be independent even with a disability.

Nursing Interventions	Rationales
Keep patient and family current regarding diagnosis, treatment, and progress.	Treating the patient and family as an important part of the team will help them cope better.
Encourage participation in support groups.	
Encourage recreational activities.	

▼

NURSING DIAGNOSIS: KNOWLEDGE DEFICIT—SELF-CARE AND MEDICATION THERAPY

Related To
- New diagnosis
- Treatment
- Lack of previous exposure to information

Defining Characteristics
Anger about diagnosis
Lack of or many questions
Fear of complications

Patient Outcomes
Patient/family will
- demonstrate understanding about Parkinson's disease, causes, symptoms, and treatment.
- state appropriate interventions regarding symptoms of Parkinson's disease
- state prescribed medications, dosages, side effects, schedules, and reason for use.

Nursing Interventions	Rationales
Assess patient/family willingness to learn, current knowledge level concerning disease causes, symptoms, treatment, and outcomes.	Assessment provides a baseline of current knowledge and helps to initiate teaching plan
Reemphasize explanation of disease, causes, symptoms, and treatment.	Reinforcement helps patient/family learning.
Discuss how symptoms of disease impact on current life-style.	Discussion of situation helps patient and family communicate about the disease.

Nursing Interventions	Rationales
Provide written information about Parkinson's disease as available.	Protein can interfere with the absorption of levodopa. 1. Fatigue can exacerbate symptoms. 2. Hard candy increases saliva and frequent hygiene prevents oral complications. 3. Anticholinergics or tricyclic antidepressants can help decrease drooling.
Teach patient or family necessary information on how to manage symptoms of Parkinson, including self-care deficit, physical issues, speech difficulties, bowel and bladder programs, and the following additional items: 1. Use of a blender is needed if swallowing is a problem. 2. Avoid high-protein meals during the day. 3. Encourage regular rest periods between activities. 4. Encourage use of gum or hard candy and frequent oral hygiene if dry mouth is a problem. 5. Encourage use of tissues, frequent oral hygiene, or discussion with physician regarding medications if drooling is a problem.	
Assess baseline knowledge of medications.	

Nursing Interventions	**Rationales**
Provide the following information regarding medications, as needed: *Preventive medications* 1. Selegiline (eldepryl deprenyl), monoamine oxidase (MAO) inhibitor type B • usual dosage 5 mg twice daily, usually taken at 8:00 a.m. and 12 noon because it can have a slight amphetamine effect. • side effects include insomnia and nervousness. • found to be helpful, slowing the progression of the disease and enhancing the effect of Sinemet. *Levodopa replacements* 1. Sinemet (carbidopa/levodopa) • carbidopa decreases nausea and vomiting (also inhibits conversion of levodopa to dopamine until reaching the brain) • levadopa is the dopamine replacement. • usual dosage is 25/100 three times daily to maximum of eight tablets a day (Sinemet also comes in 25/250, 10/100, and the controlled-release form, Sinemet CR; combination of different types of Sinemet may also be used). • Side effects include nausea and vomiting, orthostatic hypotension, difficulty sleeping or vivid dreams, dyskinesias (abnormal movements), and wearing-off effect. The wearing-off effect is when the medication peaks and then quickly wears off, requiring shorter dose intervals. Sinemet CR helped this side effect.	

Nursing Interventions	**Rationales**
Dopamine agonists 1. bromocriptine (Parlodel) • imitates the action of dopamine, often used with Sinemet • usual dosage is 2.5–5 mg three times a day but can go up to 20 mg three times a day. • side effects similar to levodopa but can also cause mental disturbances, anxiety, and confusion 2. pergolide (Permex) • effect longer than bromocriptine; also stronger (has more effect on speech-related difficulties) • usual dosage 1–2 mg three times daily • side effects similar to bromocriptine *Anticholinergics* 1. trihexyphenidyl (Artane) • useful in treating tremors, rigidity, and drooling • enhances levodopa by blocking cholinergic receptors in brain • side effects include dry mouth, constipation, and mental confusion • usual dosage 1–5 mg twice daily. *Other medications* 1. amantadine hydrochloride (Symmetrel) • antiviral agent thought to increase release of dopamine in brain • side effects include leg edema • usual dosage 100 mg two to three times a day.	

▼

DISCHARGE PLANNING/CONTINUITY OF CARE

- Assure ability to perform safe self-care at home.
- Provide patient with needed prescription and supplies and a plan for refills when needed.
- Refer to a home health agency if continued nursing care or therapy is needed.
- Arrange for home equipment from a vendor if necessary, for example, a wheelchair, cane, or walker.
- Arrange follow-up with physician for questions and evaluation after discharge.
- Provide phone number and name of person for patient to call with questions after discharge.
- Provide list of Parkinson support groups in the area and Parkinson foundations and organizations.

REFERENCES

Hanak, M. (1992). *Rehabilitation nursing for the neurological patient.* New York: Springer.

Hickey, J. (1992). *The clinical practice of neurological and neurosurgical nursing* (3rd ed). Philadelphia, PA: Lippincott.

Marr, J. (1991) The experience of living with Parkinson's disease. *Journal of Neuroscience Nursing*, 23(8), 325–329.

Mumma, C. (Ed.). (1987). *Rehabilitation nursing: Concepts and practice, a core curriculum* (2nd ed). Skokie, IL: Rehabilitation Nursing Foundation.

▼

SEIZURE DISORDERS

Andrea Strayer, RN, MS, CNRN

Seizures are an excessive, synchronous, uncontrolled discharge of neurons in the brain which interferes with normal functioning. Clinical manifestations occur when a sufficient number of neurons have been recruited. Seizures are not a disease; they are a symptom of a problem within the brain. The mechanism which initiates a seizure is unclear. Epilepsy is a chronic seizure disorder. Eighty percent of persons with epilepsy have been diagnosed before the age of 20. Approximately 80% of patients who have epilepsy are well controlled on medications.

ETIOLOGIES

- Genetic predisposition
- Cerebral trauma
  - traumatic brain injury
  - birth injury
- Cerebrovascular
  - stroke
  - hemorrhage
- Infection
  - meningitis
  - encephalitis
- Lesions
  - tumors
  - arteriovenous malformations
- Biochemical
  - drug induced
  - electrolyte imbalance
  - vitamin deficiency
  - metabolic disorders
  - endocrine disorders
- Idiopathic

CLINICAL MANIFESTATIONS

Simple partial seizure
- Consciousness is not impaired; restricted to one part of one hemisphere
- May involve: involuntary movements of one part of the body, strange smell or taste, fearful feeling
- Best described as an experience by the patient
- Lasts a moment to minutes

Complex partial seizure
- Almost always involves an alteration in consciousness: restricted to one hemisphere
- Most common manifestation of epilepsy
- May involve automatisms such as lip smacking, fumbling with clothing, mumbling, repetitive speech, or pacing
- May have an aura (simple partial seizure) before a complex partial seizure
- After the seizure, may be confused, sleepy, and/or combative

Secondarily generalized seizure
- Begin as simple or complex partial and progresses to generalized seizure

Generalized seizure
- Involves both hemispheres of the brain:
- tonic-clonic seizure
  - most frequently encountered of generalized seizures
  - tonic phase is extension of trunk and extremities; may include stridor, cry, moan, or cyanosis
  - clonic phase is rhythmic muscular contractions
- absence: simple seizure
  - may have mild tonic, clonic, atonic, autonomic components or just impairment of consciousness alone
  - usually less than 30 s of unresponsiveness
  - may be associated with eyelid fluttering, decreased tone, increased tone, automatisms, or a combination of above; almost always begins before puberty
- absence: complex seizure
  - more prolonged and involved than simple
- myoclonic seizure
  - shortest of generalized seizures; single myoclonic jerk during which consciousness is not lost
- clonic seizure
  - muscle contraction and relaxation usually lasting several minutes
- tonic seizure
  - abrupt increase in muscle tone, loss of consciousness, and autonomic signs
  - lasts 30 s to several minutes

- atonic seizure
  - abrupt loss of muscle tone followed by postictal confusion; injury likely to occur if seizures go on uncontrolled

Status epilepticus

- Seizures that occur at a frequency that prevents the patient from fully recovering from one seizure before having another
- Medical emergency

CLINICAL/DIAGNOSTIC FINDINGS

- Patient history: descriptive of seizures; thorough history the best diagnostic tool
- Electroencephalogram (EEG): may be abnormal
- Head computerized tomography (CT) or head magnetic resonance imaging (MRI): may be abnormal

▼

NURSING DIAGNOSIS: HIGH RISK FOR INJURY

Risk Factors

- Generalized seizure
- Postictal confusion

Patient Outcomes

The patient will be without injury.

Nursing Interventions	Rationales
Institute seizure precautions, following hospital policy. Protect the patient from harm during a seizure: 1. Do not try to restrain or put anything in the mouth. 2. If a generalized seizure, protect head and limbs from hitting objects. 3. Turn to side to keep airway open and allow saliva to drain. 4. Provide privacy. 5. Be reassuring.	

Nursing Interventions	Rationales
Protect the patient from harm during the postictal period by gently guiding away from danger. Never approach in an aggressive manner.	After a seizure, patients are often confused. The length of time a patient remains confused varies, usually lasting only a few minutes.
Observe the length of time the seizure lasts, where (body area) it begins, where it progressed to, what extremities are involved, and if patient is able to answer orientation question. Report all observations during the event.	

▼

NURSING DIAGNOSIS: KNOWLEDGE DEFICIT—DIAGNOSIS AND TREATMENT

Related To

- Fear and anger of diagnosis
- Anxiety of unpredictability of seizures
- New medications
- Social stigma associated with seizures

Defining Characteristics

Many questions
Few questions
Exaggerated behavior

Patient Outcomes

Patient will

- explain the etiology for the seizures.
- describe what to do to prevent the recurrence of seizures.
- verbalize how to maintain a seizure calendar.
- state antiepileptic medications, dosing, potential side effects, and who to call if problems develop.

Nursing Interventions	Rationales
Discuss the specific seizure type diagnosed and its implications.	

Nursing Interventions	Rationales
Advise patient to tell family, friends, and at least one co-worker as to what to expect when a seizure occurs.	
Discuss any life-style changes the patient will need to adjust to.	Each state has its own driving laws; refer to your Department of Transportation. Patients may need to change or adjust their occupation.
Discuss antiepileptic medication(s), why they are indicated, and side effects: 1. phenytoin (Dilantin); side effects: drowsiness, ataxia, hystagmus, gingival hyperplasia 2. phenobarbital; side effects: drowsiness 3. carbamazepine (Tegretol); side effects: diplopia, gastrointestinal (GI) upset, hyponatremia, ataxia, nystagmus 4. primidone (Mysoline); side affects: drowsiness, ataxia 5. valproic acid (Depakene); side effects: GI upset, weight gain, hand tremor, hair loss, decreased platelets (dose related)	Antiepileptic medications raise the threshold for seizures.
Encourage patients to carry a list of the name and dose of their medication on their person.	
Discuss safety precautions, including avoiding bathing in a bath tub and wearing medical alert identification.	
Demonstrate how to use a seizure calendar, including the date and time of their seizures, what they were doing, and precipitation event.	An accurate seizure history will help discover seizure trends.

Nursing Interventions	Rationales
Discuss with family members what to observe for during the seizure and seizure first aid.	Family/friends are the best historians. They will also be less anxious if they are taught appropriate first aid.

▼

NURSING DIAGNOSIS: INEFFECTIVE INDIVIDUAL COPING

Related To

- New onset of seizures
- New diagnosis of epilepsy
- Poorly controlled seizures

Defining Characteristics

Verbalization of inability to cope
Inability to problem solve
Alteration in societal participation
Inappropriate use of defense mechanisms

Patient Outcomes

The patient will

- develop effective coping mechanisms.
- vent fears, frustration, questions, or concerns.

Nursing Interventions	Rationales
Allow time to vent and ask questions. Be reassuring.	The patient needs time and assistance to develop effective coping mechanisms.
Provide emotional support.	
Consult a counselor.	
Assess family support systems and their ability to cope.	

▼

DISCHARGE PLANNING/CONTINUITY OF CARE

- Discuss when and how to reach the appropriate health care providers.
- Provide with information on community resources and support groups

which are affiliates of the Epilepsy Foundation of America. They are prepared to help newly diagnosed patients.

- Assure patient has a follow-up appointment with a physician or nurse practitioner.
- Establish a plan for taking and refilling prescribed medications.

ACKNOWLEDGMENT

This work was supported by the Department of Veteran Affairs.

REFERENCES

Cammermeyer, M. & Appeldorn, C. (Eds). (1990). *Core curriculum for neuroscience nursing* (3rd ed). Chicago, IL: American Association of Neuroscience Nurses.

Dilorio, C. Faherty, B., & Manteuffel, B. (1993). Learning needs of persons with epilepsy: A comparison of perceptions of persons, with epilepsy, nurses, and physicians. *Journal of Neuroscience Nursing, 25*(1), 22–29.

Engel, J. (1989). *Seizures and epilepsy.* Philadelphia, PA: Davis.

Hartshorn, J. & Byers, V. (1992). Impact of epilepsy on quality of life. *Journal of Neuroscience Nursing, 24*(1), 24–29.

Hickey, J. (1992). *The clinical practice of neurological and neurosurgical nursing* (3rd ed). Philadelphia, PA: Lippincott.

▼

SPINAL CORD INJURY

Maureen R. Anderson, RN, BSN, CRRN
Rochelle M. Carlson, MS, RN, CRRN

A spinal cord injury occurs as a result of excessive forces exerted on the spinal column and its supporting structures (vertebrae and soft tissues). Hyperflexion, hyperextension, compression, and excessive rotation are types of forces that may cause fracture and/or dislocation of the vertebrae or disruption of the ligaments supporting the vertebral bodies. The body responds with hemorrhage, edema, and metabolic by-products causing ischemia and necrosis of the spinal neurons and ultimately damage to the spinal cord.

ETIOLOGIES

In order of decreasing incidence:
- motor vehicle accidents
- falls
- gunshot wounds
- sports injuries (including diving accidents)

CLINICAL MANIFESTATIONS

- Quadriplegia: injury to the cervical segments of the spinal cord resulting in at least some paralysis or paresis to the arms and legs and impairment to the bowel and bladder
- Paraplegia: injury to the thoracic, lumbar, or sacral segments of the spinal cord resulting in at least some paralysis or paresis to the legs and impairment to the bowel and/or bladder
- Complete lesion: total loss of sensation and motor function below the level of injury
- Incomplete lesion: some preservation of sensory function or motor function or both functions seen below the level of injury
- Spinal shock: loss of reflexes and vasomotor tone below the level of

injury; occurs immediately following the injury and usually lasts 1–6 weeks, may last days to months

CLINICAL/DIAGNOSTIC FINDINGS

Evidence of vertebral fracture, dislocation, or spinal cord abnormality on x-ray, computerized tomography (CT) scan, or magnetic resonance imaging (MRI)

OTHER PLANS OF CARE TO REFERENCE

- Prevention and Care of Pressure Ulcers
- Thrombophlebitis/Deep-Vein Thrombosis

▼

NURSING DIAGNOSIS: HIGH RISK FOR INEFFECTIVE AIRWAY CLEARANCE

Risk Factors
- Neurological impairment, spinal cord injury thoracic 12 and above
- Ineffective cough
- Immobility

Patient Outcomes
The patient will
- demonstrate effective coughing and an increased air exchange.
- maintain clear lungs.

Nursing Interventions	Rationales
Assess current lung status, respiratory rate, breath sounds, secretions, and cough.	Assessment assists in providing baseline data.
Provide cough assist method of enhancing cough or instruct patient in method:	Cervical injured persons have impaired respirations due to weakness or paralysis of chest and abdominal muscles, along with a decreased ability to cough.

Nursing Interventions	Rationales
1. staff • Place cupped hands over stomach or abdomen. • Ask patient to take a deep breath; when the patient exhales, push upward and inward on abdomen. 2. patient • Use pillow or other supportive object over abdomen. • Inhale deeply; while exhaling push upward and in.	A cough is more efficient with a good cough assist.
Encourage deep-breathing exercises or if needed resistance breathing exercises through respiratory therapy.	Deep breathing keeps the lungs well expanded and prevents pulmonary complications. Resistance exercises improve the strength and functioning of respiratory muscles.
Encourage use of abdominal binder when up in chair.	Abdominal binders make the diaphragm more dome shaped, helping it to work more effectively.
Maintain adequate hydration, 2–3 L if not medically contraindicated.	Hydration helps keep secretions thin, thus making them easier to mobilize.
Assist in changing positions every 2–3 hr if in bed.	Turning or position changes help mobilize secretions.
Monitor for symptoms of upper airway infections, that is, shortness of breath, fever, difficulty bringing up sputum, or chest pain with breathing.	A decreased ability to cough and clear secretions cause increased risk of possible influenza complications.
Encourage influenza vaccines every fall.	

▼

NURSING DIAGNOSIS: DYSREFLEXIA

Related To

- Bladder distention
- Bowel distention

- Skin irritation
- Lack of patient and caregiver knowledge

Defining Characteristics

Spinal cord injury thoracic 7 and above
Paroxysmal hypertension (sudden increase in blood pressure >140/90)
Bradycardia, heart rate < 60
Tachycardia, heart rate > 120
Diaphoresis above level of injury
Red splotches on skin above level of injury
Pallor below level of injury
Chilling
Others: goose pimples, blurred vision, chest pain, nasal congestion

Patient Outcomes

Patient will

- demonstrate knowledge of signs and symptoms and treatment of dysreflexia.
- prevent episodes of dysreflexia.
- manage episodes of dysreflexia appropriately if they occur.

Nursing Interventions	Rationales
Assess current level of knowledge about dysreflexia, including signs, symptoms, and treatment.	Assessment provides a baseline of knowledge and provides a starting point for patient education.
Maintain and promote bowel, bladder, and skin programs.	Appropriate management of bowel, bladder, and skin can prevent dysreflexia.
Discuss causes of dysreflexia along with signs and symptoms.	Information about causes and symptoms can help prevent dysreflexia.
Discuss treatment of dysreflexia:	
1. When a dysreflexic episode occurs, set patient up at 90°.	Elevating the head of bed or sitting at a 90° angle will cause blood pressure to decrease.
2. Check blood pressure and pulse; if systolic blood pressure exceeds 160 or diastolic blood pressure is greater than 110, give medication as prescribed by physician for dysreflexia.	Monitoring blood pressure helps to assess whether episode is resolving or medication is needed. If blood pressure is uncontrolled, a stroke can occur.

Nursing Interventions	Rationales
3. Check urinary system. Empty bladder using anesthetic lubricant, that is, lidocaine jelly. Check Foley/condom catheter for kinks and plugs. If catheter is plugged, insert new Foley.	A distended bladder is the usual cause of dysreflexia in 90% of cases. An anesthetic lubricant decreases sensory input to the urinary system.
4. Check rectum for stool using anesthetic lubricant. Do not digitally stimulate.	Distended bowel is the second most frequent cause of dysreflexia. An anesthetic lubricant decreases sensory input to the rectal area.
5. Check skin for open areas. Check positioning of body in chair or bed. Look for injury to other areas of the body.	Decubitus ulcers, tight clothing, injuries, or improper positioning can cause dysreflexia.
6. Notify physician if source of dysreflexia cannot be found and pressure remains elevated.	Sustained high blood pressure can be a life-threatening situation resulting in a stroke.

▼

NURSING DIAGNOSIS: BOWEL INCONTINENCE

Related To neurogenic (reflexic or areflexic) bowel

Defining Characteristics

Involuntary passage of stool
Sensory loss of urge to defecate

Patient Outcomes

The patient will

- easily pass a soft-formed stool on a regular basis.
- not pass stool at an unpredictable time.

Nursing Interventions	Rationales
Obtain previous and current history of bowel elimination pattern (frequency, time of day, facilitating factors, color, consistency, laxative, or enema usage).	Data will assist in establishing bowel program consistent with previous patterns.
Assess nutritional habits (fluid and fiber intake, food preferences).	

Nursing Interventions	**Rationales**
Assess and treat for diarrhea or constipation before initiating a bowel program.	Diarrhea causes urgency resulting in incontinence, and a fecal impaction allows liquid stool to seep out.
Perform physical exam of abdomen for distention and bowel sounds and of rectum for presence of stool, hemorrhoids, sphincter tone, and sensation.	Intact sphincter tone indicates that the patient has a reflexic bowel and is coming out of spinal shock.
Encourage fluid intake of 2000–2400 mL every 24 hr if otherwise not contraindicated.	Adequate fluid intake will help prevent constipation.
Provide for a high-fiber diet (fruits, vegetables, whole grains, and cereals). Consult a dietitian as needed.	High-fiber diet will help prevent constipation.
Administer medications as prescribed: 1. psyllium mucilloid 2. docusate 3. docusate with casanthranol	Maintain stool consistency when possible without medications. Often a bulk former such as psyllium mucoloid and a stool softener such as docusate are necessary when initiating a bowel program. Docusate with casanthranol adds a mild stimulant which is sometimes effective for an areflexic bowel
Choose an appropriate bowel program (reflexic or areflexic bowel).	Reflexic bowel program should be used for spinal cord injury (SCI) levels above T12. Areflexic bowel program should be used for SCI levels L1 and below. An SCI level at T12 is a "mixed" bowel and may require components from both bowel programs.
Initiate *reflexic* bowel program if indicated: 1. Provide for privacy. 2. Position on left lateral side.	A reflexic bowel is also referred to as an upper motor neuron (UMN) or spastic bowel. The sacral reflex arc is intact.

Nursing Interventions	Rationales
3. Administer a bisacodyl suppository every day or every other day at the same time of the day.	It is most effective to begin a bowel program using a suppository to stimulate a movement. After spinal shock has resolved and the bowel program is established, stimulating the reflexic bowel by just digital stimulation should be attempted.
4. Position on a commode within 20 min.	Do not use a bedpan. The patient does not have adequate sensation to prevent skin breakdown.
5. Perform digital stimulation.	Stimulation of the reflex arc will assist in moving stool out of the rectum.
6. Repeat digital stimulation every 5 min for up to four times if the patient has not evacuated stool.	
7. Apply incontinence pads to patient and repeat the bowel program at the same time the following day if there was no movement.	The bowel program should begin with a daily program until there is no incontinence. An every other day program can be initiated if this is most consistent with previous patterns or the amount of stool is less on the alternative day. The time of day should coincide with the previous pattern and, if possible, within 30 min of a meal to take advantage of the gastrocolic reflex to stimulate peristalsis. It may take a few days to a week to establish an effective bowel program.
Initiate an *areflexic* bowel program if indicated:	An areflexic bowel is also called a lower motor neuron (LMN) or flaccid bowel. Sacral reflex arc is not intact. The bowl program is usually more difficult to establish because reflex emptying is not possible.
1. Provide for privacy. 2. Position on a commode or toilet.	

Nursing Interventions	Rationales
3. Instruct to perform the Valsalva maneuver (take a deep breath, tighten abdominal muscles, and bear down during exhalation).	The Valsalva maneuver is contraindicated for patients with a cardiac history.
4. Manual removal of stool may be necessary if the patient is not able to evacuate stool by him or herself.	
5. Apply incontinence pads and repeat the program at the same time the following day if there was no bowel movement.	

NURSING DIAGNOSIS: URINARY RETENTION

Related To

- Spinal cord injury of the sacral segments (cauda equina injury)
- Spinal shock
- Medications that paralyze the bladder

Defining Characteristics

No sensation of bladder filling
No motor reflex of bladder emptying
Increased bladder capacity
Bladder distention
Difficulty or inability to initiate urination
Negative bulbocavernosus reflex
Residual urine

Patient Outcomes

The patient will

- empty his or her bladder on a routine basis without incontinence or renal impairment.
- be free from urinary tract infections.

Nursing Interventions	Rationales
Assess previous and current voiding patterns (frequency, nocturia, incontinence, force and quality of stream, sensation of bladder fullness).	

Nursing Interventions	Rationales
Monitor intake and output.	
Perform physical exam to check for bladder distention and bulbocavernosus reflex.	Presence of a bulbocavernosus reflex would indicate that the spinal reflex arc is intact and that spinal shock is resolving.
Prepare the patient for possible diagnostic tests (cystometrogram/electromyogram, cystoscopy, ultrasound, urinalysis and culture, intravenous pyelogram).	A cystometrogram describes how well the detrusor muscle responds to bladder filling. An electromyogram can define detrusor sphincter dyssynergia. A cystoscopy looks for anatomical obstruction. An ultrasound may be used to measure postvoid residual. A urinalysis and culture will rule out a urinary tract infection. An intravenous pyelogram is a baseline study of the upper urinary system. A patient may have all or only some of these tests ordered.
Assess daily for signs and symptoms of a urinary tract infection (fever, cloudy urine, odorous urine, increased spasticity, increased incontinent episodes, flank pain, hematuria).	Urine stasis promotes bacterial growth. Both ICPs and indwelling Foley catheters provide a method for bacteria to be introduced into the bladder.
Provide for clear, noncarbonated, decaffeinated fluids. Encourage cranberry and apple juice; discourage a large intake of juices with pulp.	Caffeine, carbonation, and pulp increase the alkalinity of the urine. Alkaline urine contributes to infection and the formation of renal calculi. Cranberry and apple juice promote acid urine.

Nursing Interventions	Rationales
Establish a fluid schedule of 2000–2400 mL/day. Eighty percent of the fluids should be taken between the hours of 7 a.m. and 7 p.m. according to a fluid schedule.	An adequate fluid intake will flush the urinary system and help prevent infection and calculi formation. Taking in a greater percentage of fluids during the day will decrease the volume of urine made at night and will decrease night time voiding and catheterizations. A schedule of fluid intake will allow a schedule of voids/catheterizations in order to predictably keep urine volumes below 500 mL.
Administer prescribed medications:	
1. cholinergics	A cholinergic, such as Urecholine, may be prescribed to help stimulate the detrusor muscle to contract.
2. Ditropan	A bladder antispasmodic agent, such as Ditropan, may be used to decrease the number of bladder contractions and may cause urinary retention. It is sometimes used for female patients who have uncontrolled reflex incontinence.
3. ascorbic acid 4. methenamine hippurate	Ascorbic acid and methenamine hippurate are used to help acidify the urine
Initiate a bladder program. Instruct on methods to empty the bladder:	These methods exert abdominal pressure on the bladder, forcing the urine to be expelled.
1. Valsalva maneuver	The patient should perform the Valsalva maneuver and attempt to void. The procedure should be repeated until the bladder is empty.

Nursing Interventions	Rationales
2. Credé maneuver	The Credé maneuver is performed by placing one hand on top of the other just below the level of the umbilicus. The patient should then press down and firmly toward the pelvic arch. This should be repeated until no more urine is expelled.
3. anal stretch maneuver	The anal stretch is performed by sitting on the toilet or commode and inserting one to two gloved, lubricated fingers into the anal sphincter. The fingers should then be spread apart and hold the sphincter distended.
Obtain postvoid residuals.	
Initiate intermittent catheterization program (ICP) if patient is unable to void or if residual volumes are greater than or equal to 100–150 mL.	The ICP in the hospital should be sterile because of the many virulent organisms with which the patient may come in contact. A clean technique may be used at home. An ICP maintains bladder muscle tone and provides for complete evacuation of the bladder.
Adjust catheterization times to keep bladder volumes below 500 mL.	Volumes greater than 500 mL promote bacterial growth. Usually catheterizing every 3–6 hr will maintain an acceptable bladder volume. If the patient has a Foley catheter in prior to initiating the ICP, the Foley should be emptied at 3–4 hr intervals and the times recorded to give a baseline for an ICP schedule.
Instruct to attempt to void prior to each catheterization.	
Discontinue intermittent catheterization when patient is able to empty bladder with 50 mL or less residual urine.	

Nursing Interventions	Rationales
Insert an indwelling Foley catheter for drainage only when other options have failed or are inappropriate.	An indwelling catheter places the patient at higher risk for infection, limits independence, and is a greater hindrance to normal sexual relations.

▼

NURSING DIAGNOSIS: REFLEX INCONTINENCE

Related To spinal cord injury above the level of reflex arc

Defining Characteristics

No sensation of bladder filling
Inhibited bladder contractions or spasms at regular intervals
Decreased bladder capacity
Positive bulbocavernosus reflex

Patient Outcomes

The patient will

- be able to empty his or her bladder on a routine basis without incontinence or renal impairment.
- be free from urinary tract infections.

Nursing Interventions	Rationales
Please refer to the interventions and rationale for urinary retention *except* follow the interventions below for methods of emptying the baldder.) Instruct on methods to empty the bladder:	In a reflex bladder, the spinal reflex arc is intact. Voluntary control over voiding is not possible. Voiding is possible by manually triggering the reflex arc by cutaneous stimulation.
1. suprapubic tapping	Suprapubic tapping is performed by lightly tapping over the bladder with one hand. Tapping should continue until a good stream starts or for 3–5 min.
2. light pulling of pubic hairs	
3. digital rectal stimulation	
4. stroking inner thigh	

Nursing Interventions	Rationales
Use external condom catheters and bed/leg bags for males to facilitate maintaining continence.	Use of external condom catheters allows male SCI patients to spontaneously void without embarrassment of incontinence. Often the number of intermittent catheterizations is decreased, thereby decreasing the risk of infection.
Use incontinence pads or adult briefs for females only if unable to attain continence by other methods.	Use of incontinence pads or adult briefs places the patient at high risk for impaired skin integrity. It also decreases self-esteem.

▼

NURSING DIAGNOSIS: HIGH RISK FOR IMPAIRED SKIN INTEGRITY

Risk Factors
- Physical immobility
- Incontinence
- Altered sensation

Patient Outcomes
Patient will maintain intact skin integrity.

Nursing Interventions	Rationales
Assess current skin status, including bony prominences, temperature, dryness, sensation level, spasticity, and nutritional status.	Assessment provides a baseline of current skin status.
Reposition the patient initially every 2 hr: 1. If skin shows redness after 2 hr in one position and does not fade after 1 hr after repositioning, increase frequency of turns. 2. If patient has developed skin tolerance, repositioning may occur every 3–4 hr.	Skin tolerance needs to occur gradually in order to prevent skin breakdown.
Encourage weight shifts when up in wheelchair every 30 min to 2 hr; assist as needed.	Weight shifts relieve pressure on skin.

Nursing Interventions	Rationales
Provide for skin protection: pressure-reducing mattress on bed, elbow, and heel protectors and pressure-reducing cushion in wheelchair.	Protective skin mechanisms aid in preventing skin breakdown.
Provide adequate nutrition and hydration. Calorie intake of 2000–3000 a day and fluid intake of 2000–2500.	Adequate nutrition and hydration help prevent skin breakdown.
Establish appropriate bowel and bladder programs. (Refer to alterations in elimination.)	Excrement can irritate skin, causing an increased risk for breakdown.
Provide mirror for self-inspection of skin.	
Inspect skin after position changes or every 2 hr when in bed.	Early detection of skin redness can prevent further injury to skin.

▼

NURSING DIAGNOSIS: HIGH RISK FOR ALTERED PERIPHERAL TISSUE PERFUSION

Risk Factors
Decrease or interruption of venous blood flow.

Patient Outcomes
Patient will not develop a deep-vein thrombosis (DVT).

Nursing Interventions	Rationales
Assess circulation and bilateral lower extremities, including temperature warmth, redness, pedal pulses, capillary refill, movement, and sensation.	
Perform leg measurements every morning before getting up. Mark each leg at largest circumference of thigh and calf.	Consistent leg measurements done at the same time every day can help detect a DVT.

Nursing Interventions	Rationales
Report to physician any changes in leg measurements greater than 2 cm or an increase in edema, warmth, coolness, redness, absent, or decreased pedal pulses.	
Encourage use of antiembolism thigh-high stockings.	Antiembolism stockings improve venous blood flow.
Place prescribed intermittent pneumatic compression devices on at night while hospitalized.	Intermittent pneumatic compression devices move superficial venous blood deep where the veins return blood to the heart.
Maintain adequate fluid intake of 2–3 L/day if not contraindicated.	Adequate fluid intake prevents dehydration.
Maintain high activity level if possible.	Activity and movement will enhance venous circulation.

▼

NURSING DIAGNOSIS: IMPAIRED PHYSICAL MOBILITY

Related To neurological impairment

Defining Characteristics

Inability to purposefully move within the physical environment, including bed mobility, transfers, and ambulation
Limited range of motion
Decreased muscle strength, control, and/or mass
Impaired coordination
Increased tone and hyperreflexia

Patient Outcomes

The patient will

- maintain proper body alignment.
- maintain or improve passive range of motion in all extremities.
- uses assistive devices and compensatory techniques to facilitate movement in a safe manner.
- manage spasticity to allow for optimal function.

Nursing Interventions	Rationales
Assess for active and passive range of motion in all extremities, strength in extremities, ability to turn in bed, sitting tolerance, muscle tone, current transfer technique, use of assistive devices, and use of orthotic devices.	
Consult physical therapy and occupational therapy for in-depth evaluation, stretching and strengthening, assistive devices, and patient instruction in mobility.	Physical therapists and occupational therapists are experts in evaluating and treating mobility problems as well as in choosing the best assistive device.
Position in a functional alignment when in bed or when up in a wheelchair (knees slightly flexed, abduct arms with elbows in slight flexion, wrist in neutral position, elevate arms and hands when possible, one pillow under head when possible, prevent external leg rotation, ankles should be in a 90° position, and avoid pillows under the knee).	Functional alignment will help prevent contractures.
Position prone periodically if tolerated and not contraindicated.	Prone position will help prevent contractures of the hips.
Reposition in bed or wheelchair as frequently as necessary to prevent skin breakdown, contractures, and discomfort.	Some patients may need to change position initially as frequently as every 15 min. The average is about every 2 hr at first and tolerance may progress to every 4 hr.
Encourage patient to perform active range of motion twice daily as able.	Active range of motion helps to strengthen muscles and joints, prevent contractures, and decrease spasticity.
Perform passive range of motion twice daily when patient is not able to move in full range.	Passive range of motion helps to prevent contractures and decrease spasticity.

Nursing Interventions	Rationales
Progress mobility as tolerated:	Patients with SCI often become very hypotensive when assuming an upright position because of decreased vasomotor tone from spinal shock and prolonged bedrest.
1. Apply abdominal binder and antiembolism stockings.	Abdominal binder and antiembolism stockings will prevent pooling of blood in lower extremities and abdomen.
2. Cardiac chair will be necessary for first times up in a chair. 3. Begin at 30° angle. 4. Monitor blood pressure and pulse rate. 5. Limit time up in chair to 15 min three times a day initially. 6. Increase increments by 15 min as tolerated. 7. Increase angle of cardiac chair when blood pressure and pulse rate are stable and when patient has no complaints of dizziness.	
8. Provide patient with a wheelchair after patient has been able to sit at 90° in cardiac chair. Lock wheelchair prior to transfers.	Wheelchair provides greater accessibility and independence.
Transfer quadripllegic patient by "airplaning" the patient (nurse should face the patient, lock patient's knees between own knees, bend knees, keep back straight, and put arms around patient's rib cage. Patient should tuck hands inside close to body or put arms around nurses rib cage.)	Position of airplane transfer uses good body mechanics for nurse (weight is close to center of gravity) and safety for patient. A second person may assist by standing behind the patient and boosting the buttocks during the lift.
Elevate quadriplegic's hands and arms on a lap board when in wheelchair.	Elevation helps prevent edema.

Nursing Interventions	Rationales
Transfer paraplegic patient using a sliding board for assistance.	Allows greater independence for patient and less strain for nurse. Requires upper body strength of patient.
Encourage patient to propel self in wheelchair or to independently control motorized wheelchair when able.	Allows greater independence for patient. A physical therapist should recommend the proper chair.
Provide methods for controlling spasticity:	Uncontrolled spasticity interferes with function.
1. range of motion	
2. preventing contributing factors (e.g., urinary tract infection, skin breakdown, improper positioning, impaction, ingrown toenails, fractures)	Contributing factors are noxious stimuli which stimulate the nociceptive flexion reflex.
3. employing methods to decrease continuous spasms • clonus: press on knee, lift toe • extensor spasm: curl toes or hands • flexor spasm: gradual range and stretching	Continuous spasms interfere with proper movement.
Administer spasticity medications as prescribed:	
1. baclofen (Lioresal)	Baclofen acts centrally on the central nervous system (CNS) to decrease spasticity. It reduces transmission of impulses from the spinal cord to skeletal muscle by promoting pre- and postsynaptic inhibition. Side effects include transient fatigue, confusion, and drowsiness. Baclofen must be tapered: abrupt withdrawal can cause hallucinations.

Nursing Interventions	Rationales
2. dantrolene sodium (Dantrium)	Dantrolene sodium acts locally on the muscle by decreasing intracellular calcium, thereby weakening the muscle contraction. Side effects include drowsiness, fatigue, dizziness, transient hepatitis, and chronic anorexia. Liver function tests should be monitored.
3. diazepam (Valium)	Diazepam acts as a CNS depressant by enhancing presynaptic inhibition throughout the CNS. It releases the inhibitory neurotransmitter γ-aminobutyric acid (GABA). Side effects include depression and lethargy. It should be tapered as seizures can occur with abrupt withdrawal. Depression can occur with discontinuation following long-term use.

▼

NURSING DIAGNOSIS: SELF-CARE DEFICIT—BATHING/HYGIENE, DRESSING/GROOMING, TOILETING, FEEDING

Related To

- Neuromuscular impairment
- Impaired mobility status

Defining Characteristics

Bathing/hygiene

Inability to wash body or body parts
Inability to obtain or get to water source
Inability to regulate temperature flow

Dressing/grooming

Impaired ability to put on or take off necessary items of clothing
Impaired ability to obtain or replace articles of clothing
Impaired ability to fasten clothing

Toileting

Unable to sit on or rise from toilet or commode
Unable to manipulate clothing for toilet
Unable to carry out proper toilet hygiene

Feeding
Inability to bring food from a receptacle to the mouth

Patient Outcomes

Patient will
- perform activity at expected optimal level.
- demonstrate increased accuracy and speed in performing activity.
- demonstrate ability to cope with the necessity of needed assistance.
- demonstrate appropriate use of adaptive equipment.

Nursing Interventions	Rationales
Assess current level of functioning, including assistive equipment and level of spinal cord injury.	Assessment provides a baseline of current functional status.
Consult occupational therapy for patient evaluation, assistive device selection, patient instruction in use of assistive devices, and home environment evaluation to determine need for adaptations.	Occupational therapists are experts in choosing adaptive devices for self-care and in home environment assessments.
Provide ample time for activities and assist as needed.	Time constraints can cause frustration.
Provide all needed equipment within close reach or position items as directed by patient.	Laying out appropriate clothing items decreases the amount of time needed to dress.
Provide assistive equipment as needed, that is, tendon splint, built-up eating utensils, bath sponge, universal cuff, zipper puller, and so on.	Assistive devices can help increase independence.
Encourage independence in appropriate activities.	Independence in activities promotes self-esteem.
Offer frequent encouragement.	Encouragement reinforces progress.
Bathing/hygiene 1. Assist in transferring to and from commode and bed as needed.	
Dressing/grooming 1. Encourage use of sweat suits and loose clothing.	Loose clothing is easier to put on independently.

Nursing Interventions	Rationales
2. Encourage use of high-top tennis shoes several sizes larger than normal.	High-top tennis shoes prevents foot drop. Shoes several sizes larger are needed to prevent skin breakdown.
3. Dress lower extremities in bed and upper extremities when up in chair.	Finding the most efficient method of dressing increases independence.
Toileting 1. Assist in transfers to and from commode as needed.	
Feeding: 1. Set up tray; assist in opening of packages and cutting up of food as needed. 2. Assist in providing optimal position for eating.	Appropriate positioning is important when eating to prevent aspiration and choking.

▼

NURSING DIAGNOSIS: SELF-ESTEEM DISTURBANCE

Related To

- Spinal cord injury
- Change in social roles
- Changes in relationships with others

Defining Characteristics

Self-negation verbalization
Evaluates self as unable to deal with events
Denial of problems obvious to others
Hesitant to try new things or situations

Patient Outcomes

The patient will

- express feelings regarding self and disability.
- participate in activities of daily living (ADLs) and therapies.
- communicate with family members.
- participate in education and support groups.

Nursing Interventions	Rationales
Assess current level of self-esteem, perception of self, level of participation in care, and past coping methods.	Assessment provides a baseline of patient's current status. Past successful coping strategies can be identified and utilized.
Encourage expression of thoughts and concerns regarding diagnosis and life-style changes.	Listening effectively helps establish a trusting relationship.
Encourage support and visits of friends and family.	
Encourage participation in ADLs.	Promoting independence in ADLs can reassure the patient of the ability to be independent even with a disability.
Keep patient and family current regarding diagnosis, treatment, and progress.	Treating the patient and family as an important part of the team will help them cope better.
Encourage participation in support groups.	
Encourage participation in recreational activities.	

▼

NURSING DIAGNOSIS: KNOWLEDGE DEFICIT—SELF-CARE

Related To
- New diagnosis/treatment
- Lack of previous exposure to information about SCI

Defining Characteristics
Anger about diagnosis
Lack of questions
Many questions
Inappropriate or exaggerated behaviors
Anxiety

Patient Outcomes
The patient will
- verbalize understanding of SCI, causes, functional outcome, and treatment.
- direct others or become independent in all aspects of SCI management.

Nursing Interventions	Rationales
Assess current level of knowledge of SCI, patient's and family members' willingness to learn, causes, treatments, and functional outcomes.	Allows for identifying and addressing misconceptions that may have already occurred.
Discuss how injury impacts on current life-style. Schedule periodic patient/family conferences with the health care team caring for the patient to allow time for asking questions and for giving consistent messages.	Enables fuller participation in the recovery process by the patient and family.
Teach the patient necessary information to direct attendants or to become independent in managing SCI (e.g., bowel program, bladder program, spasticity management, positioning and transferring techniques, dysreflexia, skin protection, DVT prevention, respiratory maintenance): 1. Prioritize teaching by beginning with critical skill and skills that the patient wants to learn. 2. Allow for the caregivers to demonstrate the skills. 3. Discuss common problems and ways to solve them.	
Provide written information and audiovisual aids if available.	
Plan day or weekend passes for the patient to go home before discharge	Allows for integration of learning in the home setting before discharge.

▼

DISCHARGE PLANNING/CONTINUITY OF CARE

- Assure patient's ability to perform or direct safe self-care at home.
- Refer to a home health agency if continued nursing care, occupational therapy, physical therapy, or home health aide assistance is needed.

- Arrange for home equipment from a vendor if necessary (e.g., wheelchair, cushion, commode, sliding board, hoyer lift).
- Assist patient in obtaining prescriptions and medical supplies and in establishing a plan for refilling prescriptions and supplies when needed.
- Arrange follow-up with physician for questions and evaluation after discharge.
- Provide phone number and name of person for patient to call with questions after discharge.
- Provide patient with information on spinal cord injury groups in the area.
- Refer to the local chapter of the National Spinal Cord Injury Association for further information.

REFERENCES

Cammermeyer, M. & Appeldorn, C. (Eds.). (1990). *Core curriculum for neuroscience nursing* (3rd ed). Chicago, IL: American Association of Neuroscience Nurses.

Hanak, M. (1992). *Rehabilitation nursing for the neurological patient.* New York: Springer.

Hickey, J. V. (1992). *The clinical practice of neurological and neurosurgical nursing* (3rd ed). Philadelphia, PA: Lippincott.

Mumma, C. M. (Ed.). (1987). *Rehabilitation nursing: Concepts and practice: A core curriculum* (2nd ed). Skokie, IL: Rehabilitation Nursing Foundation.

▼

STROKE/CEREBRAL VASCULAR ACCIDENT

Rochelle M. Carlson, RN, MS, CRRN

A stroke is a syndrome in which blood flow to the brain is disrupted because of cerebral vascular abnormalities. The result is a gradual or sudden onset of neurological impairment that lasts for more than 24 hr. The severity and permanence of neurological deficits may vary greatly and depend on the rapidity of onset, size of the lesion, etiology, and presence of collateral circulation. This plan focuses on the postacute and rehabilitation phases of stroke. (See Altered Consciousness, p. 373, for assessment and interventions during the acute phase of stroke.)

ETIOLOGIES

- Thrombus
- Embolus
- Hemorrhage

RISK FACTORS

- Hypertension
- Smoking
- Heart disease
  - myocardial infarction
  - congestive heart failure
  - left ventricular hypertrophy
  - atrial fibrillation
  - valvular heart disease/prosthesis
  - endocarditis
- Hyperlipidemia
- Diabetes
- Drug and alcohol abuse
- Over the age of 65
- Male gender

- Black race
- Past history of other strokes or transient ischemic attacks (TIAs)
- Oral contraceptives
- Obesity
- Polycythemia

CLINICAL MANIFESTATIONS

- Middle cerebral artery syndromes
  - hemiplegia and sensory impairment on the contralateral side
  - upper extremity affected more than lower extremity
  - aphasia
  - homonymous hemianopsia
  - change in level of consciousness
  - spatial perceptual problems
- Anterior cerebral artery syndromes
  - sensorimotor deficit of contralateral foot and leg
  - minor upper extremity involvement
  - urinary incontinence
  - perseveration and cognitive impairment
  - lack of spontaneity, flat affect, slowness
  - distractibility
- Posterior cerebral artery syndromes
  - homonymous hemianopsia
  - visual perceptual problems
  - perseveration
  - possible sensory loss
  - mild hemiparesis
- Vertebrobasilar artery syndromes
  - dysphagia and dysarthria
  - ipsilateral numbness of the face and Horner's syndrome
  - impaired pain and temperature sensation
  - nystagmus, diplopia
  - ataxia, vertigo
- Carotid artery syndromes
  - fleeting blindness
  - bruit (from stenosis)
  - contralateral hemiplegia and sensory loss
- Hemorrhage
  - elevated blood pressure (initially very high)
  - headache
  - nausea
  - vomiting
  - change in level of consciousness

CLINICAL/DIAGNOSTIC FINDINGS

- Hemorrhage or occluded vessel on head computerized tomography (CT) scan or magnetic resonance imaging (MRI)
- Narrowing of vessel, thrombosis formation, aneurysm, or arterial venous malformation on cerebral arteriogram or by digital subtraction angiography
- Slowing of brain waves on electroencephalogram (EEG)
- Elevated serum cholesterol and triglycerides in thrombotic stroke
- Narrowing or occlusion of carotid arteries by Doppler study

OTHER PLANS OF CARE TO REFERENCE

- Altered Consciousness
- Seizure Disorder
- Nutritional Support: Enteral Nutrition
- Prevention and Care of Pressure Ulcers
- Thrombophlebitis/Deep-vein Thrombosis

▼

NURSING DIAGNOSIS: ALTERED CEREBRAL TISSUE PERFUSION

Related To interruption of flow: arterial (progression or recurrence of stroke)

Defining Characteristics

Change in level of consciousness and/or orientation
Increased intracranial pressure
Progressive motor and/or sensory impairments
Cushing's triad (hypertension, bradycardia, respiratory irregularities)
Pupillary changes (sluggish response, dilated)
(See Clinical Manifestations for specific characteristics.)

Patient Outcomes

The patient will

- have level of consciousness and orientation that improves or remains unchanged.
- demonstrate a normal intracranial pressure.
- demonstrate a normal or unchanged pupillary response.
- demonstrate normal vital signs.
- maintain an intact airway and adequate oxygenation.

Nursing Interventions	Rationales
Assess neurological, cardiac, and respiratory status (vital signs, level of consciousness, orientation, motor function, sensation, cranial nerve assessment, pupillary reactions, breath sounds, oxygen saturation, and arterial blood gases and telemetry if prescribed). Assess every 2–4 hr until patient is stable or as prescribed by physician. Notify physician immediately of any change in status.	
Position with head of bed at 30° if there is increased intracranial pressure.	Gravity promotes drainage from the head and decreases intracranial pressure.
Maintain blood glucose levels in normal range. Administer prescribed insulin if necessary.	Hyperglycemia can extend the stroke and worsen the motor outcome.
Maintain blood pressures in prescribed range. Avoid rapid blood pressure drops.	If the patient has had an embolic or thrombotic stroke, blood pressures should range about 150–170 systolic and 90–100 diastolic to ensure adequate perfusion. Patients with a hemorrhagic stroke will need lower blood pressures; the physician should write specific orders. Rapid blood pressure drops lower cerebral perfusion.
Administer supplemental oxygen as ordered. Provide suctioning if necessary.	Hypercapnia and hypoxemia increase intracranial pressure.
Administer intravenous (IV) fluids as prescribed (usual is two thirds normal maintenance dose of isotonic fluids; no dextrose).	A lower than usual dose of IV fluids prevents fluid overload, which would contribute to cerebral edema. Dextrose in the IV solution will add to hyperglycemia.
Minimize temperature elevations through the use of prescribed cooling blankets, antipyretics, and fans.	Increased temperature increases metabolic rate and need for oxygen.

Nursing Interventions	Rationales
See Altered Consciousness for care of the stroke patient during the neurologically unstable period.	

▼

NURSING DIAGNOSIS: IMPAIRED VERBAL COMMUNICATION

Related To neurological deficits following stroke

Defining Characteristics

Difficulty expressing thoughts verbally
Speaks or verbalizes with difficulty
Stuttering
Slurring
Difficulty forming words or sentences

Patient Outcomes

The patient will

- communicate needs using alternate verbal and nonverbal method of communication.
- express decreased frustration with communicating.

Nursing Interventions	Rationales
Assess spontaneous speech for fluency, word use, grammatical errors, rhythm, melody, word content, and articulation. Assess comprehension through simple and complex, yes-no, auditory as well as written commands. Assess ability to repeat, name, self-correct, read aloud, and write. Assess handedness, native language spoken, level of education, and current and previous methods of communication.	Dysphasia/aphasia is the expressive loss of comprehension and/or production of verbal and/or written language. There are several types of aphasia that range from mild to severe impairment. With Wernicke's aphasia the patient predominantly has fluent (sometimes nonsensical) speech but impaired comprehension; damage has been to the dominant temporal and parietal lobe. Broca's aphasia is characterized by impaired expression with mild comprehension impairment; damage has been to the left frontal lobe. Accurate assessment is necessary because nursing interventions are directed at the specific type of communication disorder.

Nursing Interventions	Rationales
Physically examine movement of the pharynx, tongue, face, lips, muscle tone, presence of drooling, and cranial nerves VII (facial), X (vagus), and XII (hypoglossal).	A patient's communication problem may be due to dysarthria, which is an impairment caused by disturbed muscular control.
Consult a speech therapist for comprehensive evaluation and treatment.	Speech therapists are experts in providing therapy for communication disorders. The entire health care team should work together to provide a consistent communication approach to the patient.
Establish a calm, unhurried environment: 1. Recognize frustration; allow to ventilate. 2. Ensure respect and dignity (do not "talk down" to the patient). 3. Anticipate and validate needs. 4. Reinforce efforts and maintain a positive outlook. 5. Provide glasses, hearing aids, and dentures for communication. 6. Decrease distractions. 7. Do not pretend to understand. 8. Establish eye contact if culturally appropriate. 9. Use humor when appropriate.	A relaxed environment enhances communication and promotes self-esteem.
Promote communication for patients who *do not* have a comprehension deficit: 1. Help the patient to speak when frustrated but do not be overly helpful.	 Acknowledges frustration without decreasing self-confidence.
2. Stimulate communication during routine activities. 3. Offer opportunities to hear speech. 4. Encourage participation in group activities.	Decreases isolation and normalizes speech in every-day routines.

Nursing Interventions	Rationales
5. Do not interrupt. 6. Allow mistakes. 7. Allow a longer response time; listen.	Self-confidence is increased when patient is allowed to speak.
8. Provide paper and pen if able to write.	Writing may be a more effective communication method for dysarthric patients. Written communication will be impaired for dysphasic patients.
Promote communication for patients *with* a comprehension deficit:	
1. Stimulate speech in few, brief periods. 2. Limit the frequency and duration of group activities.	Enhances comprehension by limiting fatigue. Patient may be able to understand first three or so words and then fatigue and lose comprehension.
3. Use touch, patience, and calm tone if severely impaired. 4. Get attention before speaking (say name or touch).	Decreases anxiety and fear. Patients often feel very isolated and lost if severely impaired.
5. Speak in slow, distinct, simple, direct speech that requests yes-no responses.	Limits the amount of words on which to concentrate; communicates the most important messages.
6. Use gestures, pantomime, and other body language.	Nonverbal communication is more easily understood.
7. Provide pictures and drawings.	Pictures and drawings are especially helpful for those who are more severely impaired.

▼

NURSING DIAGNOSIS: IMPAIRED SWALLOWING

Related To neuromuscular impairment

Defining Characteristics

Evidence of difficulty in swallowing, for example, stasis of food in oral cavity, coughing, choking
Evidence of aspiration

Patient Outcomes

The patient will
- experience no aspiration
- maintain serum albumin within normal limits and appropriate weight for height.
- follow swallowing guidelines to ensure safe eating.

Nursing Interventions	Rationales
Assess appetite, weight loss, head alignment, ability to handle own secretions, drooling, nasal burning, tickling at the back of the throat, taste, coughing after food or fluid intake, holding food in the mouth, pocketing food on the affected side, voice quality, and amount of time to eat a meal.	A comprehensive assessment is necessary to determine the type of swallowing impairment.
Examine cranial nerve V (sensory discrimination and ability to chew food), cranial nerve VII (muscles of face for symmetry, lip closure, drooling), cranial nerves IX and X (soft palate for symmety or deviation, position of uvula, gag reflex, hoarseness), and cranial nerve XII (tongue for symmetry, deviation, atrophy).	Cranial nerves V (trigeminal), VII (facial), IX (glossopharyngeal), X (vagus), and XII (hypoglossal) are all involved in coordinating a normal swallow.
Assess for fever, breath sounds, cough, and congestion at least daily until patient is no longer at risk for aspirating.	Assessment for signs and symptoms of an aspiration pneumonia is necessary to determine if the dysphagia management program is effective and to intervene quickly if an infection does occur.
Consult speech pathologist, dietitian, and occupational therapist for evaluation and recommendations for dysphagia program, including texture and temperature of food.	A team approach provides comprehensive and consistent treatment of the complex problem of impaired swallowing.

Nursing Interventions	Rationales
Prepare patient for barium swallow study if recommended.	A barium swallow study is a video fluroscopic view of a patient's swallow. It helps in pinpointing the exact problem in swallowing. The patient will be asked to swallow foods of different consistencies (liquid, pudding, cookie) that have a little barium mixed in. No preparation is necessary. The patient may be given a mild laxative afterward to prevent constipation from the barium if necessary.
Promote safe swallowing:	
1. Provide oral hygiene and dentures; check denture fit.	
2. Position patient with head upright, chin tucked forward. Patient should remain upright for 30 min after eating if possible.	Correct positioning promotes a safe swallow. Remaining upright after a meal will decrease possible aspiration from reflux.
3. Ensure presence of suction machine if needed.	Suction patient if apparent aspiration occurs.
4. Start with therapeutic feedings (small amounts) and progress to full amounts to maintain nutrition.	Small feedings will enable swallow retraining without fatiguing the patient. Supplemental enteral nutrition may be needed during this time period.
5. Provide verbal cueing for dysphagia management if cognitively impaired.	Verbal cueing will help the patient stay on task.
6. Allow adequate time to eat but do not allow patient to eat for longer than 30 min.	Prevent fatigue from eating too long. Patient is at greater risk for aspirating when fatigued.
Follow specific guidelines for individualized dysphagia program as directed by speech pathologist, dietitian, and occupational therapist:	
1. Provide thickened liquids (nectars, milk shakes, slushes, commercial thickeners, or gelatin added to thin liquids).	Thickened liquids slow the time the bolus is in the oral cavity and allow the patient who has a delayed or absent swallow reflex more time to safely swallow.

Nursing Interventions	Rationales
2. Avoid acidic and carbonated foods and liquids.	These foods are irritants to the nasal mucosa for patient who has reflux of food or liquid into the nasal cavity.
3. Turn head toward affected side as much as possible when taking medications. 4. Place pills in applesauce, ice cream, or hot cereal.	These techniques help patients who have pooling of food and medication in vallecular sinus to swallow a more cohesive bolus along the side of the throat where musculature and sensation are intact.
5. Double swallow; drink frequently; intentional coughs.	Methods to help clear residue in the pharynx enable swallowing.
6. Avoid straws.	Straws speed up the transit time of liquids in the oral cavity.
7. Practice modified supraglottic swallow with patient: Take bolus, flex chin and tuck to neck, swallow bolus without breathing, double swallow, raise chin, and cough or clear throat.	The modified supraglottic swallow helps avoid aspiration for those who have delayed or absent swallow reflex.
8. Place food on unaffected side of mouth. 9. Instruct to move tongue to affected side to check for food.	Uses areas of intact musculature and sensation to prevent aspiration and pocketing of food.
10. Avoid sticky foods (syrup, peanut butter, pudding).	Sticky foods contribute to residue buildup on the pharyngeal wall.
11. Provide thermal stimulation (icing): Tap base of anterior facial arches with cold mirror or cold water.	Thermal stimulation helps to trigger a swallow reflex for patients who have difficulty initiating a swallow.
Consult with physician about nutritional support options (enteral or parenteral) if patient is unable to safely swallow to meet nutritional demands.	Aspiration is a life-threatening occurrence.

NURSING DIAGNOSIS: BOWEL INCONTINENCE

Related To neurological impairment

Defining Characteristics

Involuntary passage of stool

Patient Outcomes

The patient will

- easily pass a soft-formed stool on a regular basis.
- not pass stool at an unpredictable time.

Nursing Interventions	Rationales
Obtain previous and current history of bowel elimination pattern (frequency, time of day, facilitating factors, color, consistency, laxative or enema usage).	Data will assist in establishing bowel program consistent with patient's previous pattern.
Assess nutritional habits (fluid and fiber intake, food preferences).	Assess and treat for diarrhea and constipation.
Diarrhea causes urgency resulting in incontinence and a fecal impaction allows liquid stool to seep out.	Perform physical exam of abdomen for distention and bowel sounds and of rectum for presence of stool, hemorrhoids, and sensation.
Encourage fluid intake of 2000–2400 mL every 24 hr if otherwise not contraindicated.	Adequate fluid intake will help prevent constipation.
Provide for a high-fiber diet (fruits, vegetables, whole grains, and cereals). Consult dietitian as needed.	High-fiber diet will help prevent constipation.
Administer prescribed medications: 1. psyllium mucilloid 2. docusate 3. docusate with casanthranol	Maintain stool consistency when possible without medications. Often a bulk former such as psyllium mucilloid and a stool softener such as docusate are necessary when initiating a bowel program. Docusate with casanthranol adds a mild stimulant.

Nursing Interventions	Rationales
Initiate a bowel program: 1. Provide for privacy. 2. Position patient on left lateral side. 3. Remove stool if present in rectum.	
4. Administer a bisacodyl suppository at the time of the day that is consistent with previous bowel habits.	It is most effective to begin a bowel program using a suppository to stimulate a movement. A bowel program should begin with a daily program until there is no incontinence. An every other day or every third day program can be initiated if this is most consistent with previous patterns or the amount of stool is less on the alternate day. Timing within 30 min of a meal will take advantage of the gastrocolic reflex to stimulate peristalsis. Timing should also coincide with previous bowel habits for maximum effectiveness.
5. Assist the patient to the commode or toilet when sensation to defecate occurs (usually within 20 min).	
6. Perform digital stimulation if patient is not able to defecate; may repeat suppository and digital stimulation one time if needed.	Stimulation of the reflex arc will assist in moving stool out of the rectum. If no bowel movement is produced after a second trial, further assessment is needed.
Encourage the patient to defecate without a suppository on the second day and following days after initiating the bowel program:	
1. Administer a bisacodyl suppository only if the patient was not able to defecate in 4 hr of the scheduled time period.	Allowing a small amount of flexibility for patients who may be able to have spontaneous bowel movements reduces costs of medication, increases patient satisfaction, and discourages dependence on external stimulation.

Nursing Interventions	Rationales
2. Substitute a glycerin suppository for the bisacodyl suppository if the patient has had soft-formed stools with no incontinence for 5 consecutive days.	Glycerin suppositories are less irritating to the bowel wall. Their use is a step in weaning the patient from the need for external stimulation to produce a bowel movement.
3. Return to a bisacodyl suppository if unsuccessful with the glycerin suppository.	
4. Discontinue use of glycerin suppository if the patient has a consistent pattern of soft-formed stools with no incontinence.	Patients with a strong, consistent premorbid pattern may be able to achieve spontaneous bowel movements. Other patients may need to continue with either a bisacodyl or glycerin suppository.

▼

NURSING DIAGNOSIS: ALTERED URINARY ELIMINATION

Related To sensory motor impairment

Defining Characteristics

Frequency, retention, incontinence, urgency

Patient Outcomes

The patient will

- empty bladder on a routine basis without incontinence or renal impairment.
- be free from urinary tract infections.

Nursing Interventions	Rationales
Assess previous and current voiding patterns (frequency, nocturia, incontinence, force and quality of stream, sensation of bladder fullness), ability to use the toilet, and cognition to indicate need to void.	
Monitor intake and output.	

Nursing Interventions	Rationales
Perform physical exam to check for bladder distention, atrophic vaginitis, and urethritis.	Atrophic vaginitis or urethritis may indicate an estrogen deficiency and could contribute to irritation of urinary tract.
Prepare the patient for possible diagnostic tests (cystometrogram/electromyogram, cystoscopy, ultrasound, urinalysis and culture, intravenous pyelogram).	A cystometrogram describes how well the detrusor muscle responds to bladder filling. An electromyogram can define detrusor sphincter dyssynergia. A cystoscopy looks for anatomical obstruction. An ultrasound may be used to measure postvoid residual. A urinalysis and culture will rule out a urinary tract infection. An IV pyelogram is a baseline study of the upper urinary system. A patient may have all or only some of these tests ordered.
Assess daily for signs and symptoms of a urinary tract infection (fever, cloudy urine, odorous urine, increased spasticity, increased incontinent episodes, flank pain, hematuria).	Urine stasis promotes bacterial growth. Both intermittent catheterization programs and indwelling Foley catheters provide a method for bacteria to be introduced into the bladder.
Provide for clear, noncarbonated, decaffeinated fluids. Encourage cranberry and apple juice; discourage a large volume of juices with pulp.	Caffeine, carbonation, and pulp increase the alkalinity of the urine. Alkaline urine contributes to infection and the formation of renal calculi. Cranberry and apple juice promote acid urine.
Establish a fluid schedule of 2000–2400 mL/day. Eighty percent of the fluids should be taken between the hours of 7 a.m. and 7 p.m. according to a fluid schedule.	An adequate fluid intake will flush the urinary system and help prevent infection and calculi formation. Taking in a greater percentage of fluids during the day will decrease the volume of urine made at night and decrease nighttime voidings and catheterizations. A schedule of fluid intake will allow a schedule of voids/catheterizations in order to predictably keep urine volumes below 500 mL.

Nursing Interventions	Rationales
Administer prescribed medications:	
1. cholinergics	A cholinergic such as Urecholine may be prescribed to help stimulate the detrusor muscle to contract.
2. Ditropan	A bladder antispasmodic agent, such as Ditropan, may be used to decrease the number of bladder contractions and may cause urinary retention.
3. ascorbic acid 4. methanamine hippurate	Ascorbic acid and Methenamine hippurate are sometimes used to help acidity the urine.
Obtain postvoid residuals.	
Initiate intermittent catheterization (ICP) program if patient is unable to void or if residual volumes are greater than or equal to 100–150 mL.	The ICP in the hospital should be sterile because of the many virulent organisms with which the patient may come in contact. A clean technique may be used at home. The ICP maintains bladder muscle tone and provides for complete evacuation of the bladder.
1. Adjust catheterization times to keep bladder volumes below 500 mL.	Volumes greater than 500 mL promote bacterial growth. Usually catheterizing every 3–6 hr will maintain an acceptable bladder volume. If the patient has a Foley catheter in prior to initiating ICP, the Foley should be emptied at 3–4 hr intervals and the time recorded to give a baseline for an ICP schedule.
2. Instruct patient to attempt to void prior to each catheterization.	
3. Discontinue intermittent catheterization when patient is able to empty bladder with 50 mL or less residual urine.	

Nursing Interventions	Rationales
4. Insert an indwelling Foley catheter for drainage only when other options have failed or are inappropriate.	An indwelling catheter places the patient at higher risk for infection, limits independence, and is a greater hindrance to normal sexual relations.
Initiate a timed voiding schedule for patients with uninhibited bladder contractions:	Timed voiding will help to retrain the bladder to hold a larger amount of urine and will provide for behavior modification for cognitively impaired patients who benefit from structure.
1. Carefully assess voiding/incontinence pattern.	Patient's previous pattern may have been to void around specific events: upon awakening, before or after meals, and before going to sleep. Include these natural patterns in the timed voiding schedule.
2. Ensure method to communicate urge to void. 3. Provide opportunity to void every half hour to begin with and progress to every 2–4 hr. 4. Reduce time between voids if incontinent episode occurs. 5. Encourage patient to hold urine until next scheduled voiding time.	
Use commodes and urinals as acceptable alternatives to voiding on the toilet.	Enables a patient with limited mobility to gain continence.

Nursing Interventions	Rationales
Use containment devices only if patient is unable to attain continence by other methods: 1. Males may use external condom catheters and leg bags or adult briefs. 2. Females may use incontinence pads or adult briefs. 3. Protect skin by washing with soap and water at least once a day and with use of moisture barrier ointment.	Containment devices potentially may impair skin integrity and may lower patient's self-esteem.

▼

NURSING DIAGNOSIS: HIGH RISK FOR IMPAIRED SKIN INTEGRITY

Risk Factors

- Physical immobility
- Incontinence
- Altered sensation

Patient Outcomes

The patient will maintain intact skin integrity.

Nursing Interventions	Rationales
Assess current factors influencing skin status, including bony prominences, skin temperature and dryness, edema, sensation, incontinence, spasticity, and nutritional status.	
Reposition patient initially every 2 hr: 1. If skin shows redness after 2 hr in one position and does not fade after 1 hr after repositioning, increase frequency of turns. 2. If patient has developed skin tolerance, repositioning may occur every 3–4 hr.	

Nursing Interventions	Rationales
Assist the patient in shifting weight every 30 min to every 2 hr when up in wheelchair.	Weight shifts relieve pressure on the skin.
Provide for skin protection: 1. Apply pressure-reducing mattress on bed. 2. Apply elbow and heel protectors. 3. Provide pressure-reducing cushion in wheelchair.	Protective skin products aid in preventing skin breakdown.
Provide adequate nutrition (2000–3000 calories a day) and hydration (2000 mL a day).	Adequate nutrition and hydration help prevent skin breakdown.
Establish a bowel and bladder program to prevent incontinent episodes.	Excrement can irritate the skin, causing skin breakdown.

▼

NURSING DIAGNOSIS: HIGH RISK FOR INJURY: HEMORRHAGE

Risk Factors

Altered clotting factors

Patient Outcome

The patient will be free from injury (hemorrhage).

Nursing Interventions	Rationales
Assess risk for hemorrhage: Medication responses higher than therapeutically desired for warfarin, heparin, and aspirin; history of falls and excessive alcohol consumption.	Warfarin elevates the prothrombin time (PT); heparin elevates the partial prothrombin time (PTT), and aspirin and excessive alcohol consumption decrease platelet counts. A fall could cause a hemorrhage if clotting factors are altered.

Nursing Interventions	Rationales
Administer prescribed medications: warfarin, heparin, and/or aspirin.	A therapeutic dosage of warfarin is most often indicated for stroke prevention when the cause of the initial stroke was a cardioembolus or when a minor stroke has occurred and the patient is awaiting surgery for a proven carotid stenosis. Dose may begin with 5 mg daily and then is adjusted based on PT or on international normalized ratio (INR) which is a standardized prothrombin ratio. A therapeutic dosage of heparin is indicated to be administered IV from a progressing stroke, acute large-vessel thrombosis, or cardioembolic stroke. Dose begins with a 5000–10,000 bolus IV and is adjusted based on PTT. Aspirin is indicated when the cause of stroke is due to intercerebral thrombus caused by atherosclerotic plaque buildup. Dosage is usually 325 mg daily.
Draw PT, PTT, platelets, complete blood count (CBC) as prescribed. Evaluate for therapeutic ranges.	Baseline PT, PTT, platelets, and CBC could be drawn before treatment begins. Draw PT level 2–3 days after first warfarin dose (warfarin has a long half-life). Prothrombin time should then be drawn daily until it is in a stable therapeutic range (one and a half to two times or control or INR intensity of 2–3.5). After PT and warfarin dose are stable, PT should be drawn monthly at the same time of day to evaluate study blood level. Partial prothrombin time should be drawn 4 hr after first heparin dose and then drawn every 4–8 hr until PTT is in a stable therapeutic range (one and a half to two times control). After PTT and heparin dose are stable, PTT should be drawn daily at the same time to evaluate steady blood level.

Nursing Interventions	Rationales
Monitor for bleeding: 1. frank blood in stool or urine or coffee ground gastric residual 2. black tarry stools (check stool guaiacs) 3. nosebleeds 4. bleeding gums 5. easy bruising	These are early signs that anticoagulant level is higher than desired.
Monitor for signs and symptoms of intracerebral or subdural hemorrhage if patient has fallen.	Patient on anticoagulant or antiplatelet therapy is at increased risk for brain hemorrhage.
Avoid intramuscular (IM) injections with warfarin and heparin.	Intramuscular injection may potentiate bleeding into the muscle.
Monitor blood pressure closely if patient has a history of hypertension.	Increased blood pressure with anticoagulant therapy could put patient at risk for a hemorrhagic stroke.
Evaluate medication profile for drug interactions that may increase bleeding time: 1. warfarin: heparin, sulfonylureas, phenytoin, steroids, cimetidine, metronidazole, salicylates, amiodarone, allopurinol, heparin 2. heparin: warfarin, salicylates, dextran, steroids, nonsteroidal anti-inflammatories 3. consult pharmacist if any questions	

Nursing Interventions	Rationales
Teach the patient taking warfarin the following: 1. It is important to do monthly blood tests, including partial thromboplastin (PT) T. 2. Avoid hazardous activities and report falls and accidents to nurse or physician. 3. Report signs of bleeding (gums, urine, stools, nosebleeds). 4. Report unusual headache or change in cognition. 5. Report change in medications (including over-the-counter medications). 6. Do not take aspirin or nonsteroidal anti-inflammatories unless specifically prescribed by physician. 7. Wear Medic-Alert bracelet. 8. Avoid excessive alcohol consumption.	Patient and family need to know how to manage anticoagulant therapy to avoid serious hemorrhage.
Teach the patient who is taking aspirin the following: 1. Take with food or milk. 2. Monitor stools and urine for blood. 3. Avoid taking nonsteroidal anti-inflammatories. 4. Report any change in cognition. 5. Avoid excessive alcohol consumption.	Aspirin can irritate gastric mucosa and cause bleeding. Patient needs to understand side effects and that aspirin is not a benign medication.

▼

NURSING DIAGNOSIS: HIGH RISK FOR ALTERED PERIPHERAL TISSUE PERFUSION

Risk Factors

- Decreased or interruption of venous blood flow

Patient Outcomes

The patient will

- not experience a deep-vein thrombosis (DVT).
- demonstrate methods to promote circulation.

Nursing Interventions	Rationales
Assess blood pressure, circulation, pedal pulses, color, skin temperature, capillary refill, movement, and sensation, pain, and presence of Homan's sign in legs. Assess current understanding of DVT.	
Measure legs at the largest part of calf and thigh bilaterally every morning before getting up.	Leg measurements are smallest and most consistent in the morning because dependent edema increases leg circumference when an upright position has been maintained.
Report any changes in leg measurement greater than 2 cm or an increase in warmth, coolness, redness, edema, absent or decreased pedal pulse, onset of pain, or a positive Homan's sign to physician.	These are signs and symptoms of a DVT.
Encourage use of thigh-high antiembolism stockings.	Thigh-high anti-embolism stockings improve venous blood flow. Knee-high stockings tend to constrict the calf and/or popliteal area and should be avoided if possible.
Place prescribed intermittent pneumatic compression devices on at night or during prolonged bed rest during the day. Intermittent pneumatic compression devices move superficial venous blood flow deep where the veins return blood to the heart.	
Maintain adequate fluid intake of 2000–3000 mL/day if not contraindicated.	Adequate fluid intake prevents dehydration.
Maintain high activity level if possible.	Movement will enhance venous return.

Nursing Interventions	Rationales
Teach patient not to cross feet or legs and to avoid wearing clothing or catheter bags that constrict the legs.	Constrictive clothing and crossed legs and feet interfere with venous return.

▼

NURSING DIAGNOSIS: IMPAIRED PHYSICAL MOBILITY

Related To neurological impairment

Defining Characteristics

Inability to purposefully move within the physical environment, including bed mobility, transfer, and ambulation
Limited range of motion
Decreased muscle strength, control, and/or mass
Impaired coordination

Patient Outcomes

The patient will

- maintain proper body alignment.
- maintain or improve passive range of motion in all extremities.
- use assistive devices and compensatory techniques to facilitate movement in a safe manner.
- manage spasticity with assistance to allow for optimal function.

Nursing Interventions	Rationales
Assess for active and passive range of motion in all extremities, strength in extremities, ability to turn in bed, sitting tolerance, muscle tone, current transfer technique, use of assistive devices, and use of orthotic devices.	
Consult physical therapy and occupational therapy for in-depth evaluation, stretching and strengthening, assistive devices, splints, slings, and patient instruction in mobility.	Physical therapists and occupational therapists are experts in evaluating and treating mobility problems as well as in choosing the best assistive devices.

Nursing Interventions	Rationales
Position in a functional alignment when in bed or when up in a wheelchair (knees slightly flexed, abduct arms with elbows in slight flexion, wrist in neutral position, elevate arms and hands when possible, one pillow under head when possible, prevent external leg rotation, ankles should be in a 90° position, and avoid pillows under the knee).	Functional alignment will help prevent contractures.
Position prone periodically if tolerated and not contraindicated.	Prone position will help prevent contractures of the hips.
Reposition in wheelchair as frequently as necessary to prevent skin breakdown, contractures, and discomfort.	Some patients may need to change position initially as frequently as every 15 min. The average is about every 2 hr initially, and tolerance may progress to every 4 hr.
Encourage patient to perform active range of motion twice daily as able.	Active range of motion helps to strengthen muscle and joints and prevents contractures. It also helps to decrease spasticity.
Perform passive range of motion twice daily when patient is not able to move in full range. Use a steady, gentle, slow, continuous motion.	Passive range of motion helps to prevent contractures and reduces spasticity.
Apply heat or cold to extremities before movement as directed by the physician and physical or occupational therapist.	Heat or cold application may temporarily reduce some types of spasticity to allow for functional or therapeutic activities during that time.
Apply splints to spastic extremities as recommended by physical or occupational therapist. Monitor skin for breakdown and muscle tone for increased spasticity.	Splints are a static method of stretching an extremity to reduce muscle tone and prevent contractures. Monitoring the effectiveness of splints is necessary because they may actually increase spasticity and create pressure ulcers.

Nursing Interventions	Rationales
Teach patient to use relaxation techniques such as imaging if able.	Relaxation exercises can decrease frustration and muscle tone.
Administer medication as prescribed: 1. baclofen (Lioresal) 2. dantrolene sodium (Dantrium) 3. diazepam (Valium)	These medications are used as a last resort to decrease spasticity because their central nervous system (CNS) side effects are often more damaging to function than the spasticity itself. Baclofen acts centrally on the CNS to decrease spasticity. It reduces transmission of impulses from the spinal cord to skeletal muscle by promoting pre- and postsynaptic inhibition. Side effects include transient fatigue, confusion, and drowsiness. Baclofen must be tapered; abrupt withdrawal can cause hallucinations. Dantrolene sodium acts locally on the muscle by decreasing intracellular calcium, thereby weakening the muscle contraction. Side effects include drowsiness, fatigue, dizziness, transient hepatitis, and chronic anorexia. Liver function tests should be monitored. Diazepam acts as a CNS depressant by enhancing presynaptic inhibition throughout the CNS. It release the inhibitory neurotransmitter γ-aminobutyric acid (GABA). Side effects include depression and lethargy. It should be tapered as seizures can occur with abrupt withdrawal. Depression can occur with discontinuation following long-term use.

Nursing Interventions	Rationales
Progress patient's mobility as tolerated: 1. Apply antiembolism stocking to affected leg. 2. Cardiac chair may be necessary for first times up in a chair. 3. Begin at a 30° angle. 4. Monitor blood pressure and pulse. 5. Limit time up in chair to 15 min three times a day at first. 6. Increase increment by 15 min as tolerated. 7. Increase angle of cardiac chair when blood pressure and pulse rate are stable and when patient has no complaints of dizziness.	Patient may become hypotensive when first sitting because bedrest can decrease vasomotor tone.
Provide patient with a wheelchair after patient has been able to sit at 90° in cardiac chair.	Wheelchair provides greater accessibility and independence.
Transfer a hemiplegic patient by asking the patient to bear weight on the unaffected leg and pivot toward the unafffected side. [Nurse should brace the patient's legs with own legs; patient should be wearing ankle-foot orthosis (AFO) if needed.]	A hemiplegic patient has greater strength, coordination, and perception on the unaffected side, making a transfer in this direction less likely to result in a fall. Bracing the legs and wearing an AFO will support the lower leg and foot from giving way. The Bobath method promotes transfers to the affected side but should only be used if personnel have training in this method.
Elevate affected hand and arms on a lap board when in wheelchair.	Elevation helps prevent edema.
Encourage patient to propel self in wheelchair.	Allows greater independence for patient. A physical therapist should recommend proper chair.

Nursing Interventions	Rationales
Place gait belt on patient and hold on to back of belt while walking slightly behind and to the side of the unaffected side if patient is able to walk with or without assistive devices.	Gait belt provides a method for nurse to hold on to unsteady patient to prevent a fall. Walking near unaffected side promotes safety by drawing patient to strong side for steadying if a stumble occurs. (Walking near affected side is appropriate for some therapeutic purposes.)

▼

NURSING DIAGNOSIS: SELF-CARE DEFICIT—BATHING/HYGIENE, DRESSING/GROOMING, TOILETING, FEEDING

Related To

- Neuromuscular impairment
- Impaired mobility status

Defining Characteristics

Bathing/hygiene

Inability to wash body or body parts
Inability to obtain or get to water source
Inability to regulate temperature flow

Dressing/grooming

Impaired ability to put on or take off necessary items of clothing
Impaired ability to obtain or replace articles of clothing
Impaired ability to fasten clothing

Toileting

Inability to rise from toilet or commode
Inability to manipulate clothing for toileting
Inability to carry out proper toilet hygiene

Feeding

Inability to bring food from a receptacle to the mouth

Patient Outcomes

The patient will be able to

- perform activity at expected optimal level.
- demonstrate increased accuracy and speed in performing activity.
- demonstrate ability to cope with the necessity of needed assistance.
- demonstrate appropriate use of adaptive equipment.

Nursing Interventions	Rationales
Assess current level of functioning including use of assistive equipment and sensory/perceptual impairment.	
Consult occupational therapy for patient evaluation, assistive device selection, patient instruction in use of assistive devices, and home environment evaluation to determine need for adaptations.	Occupational therapists are experts in choosing adaptive devices for self-care and in home environment assessments.
Provide privacy and ample time for activities; assist as needed.	Time constraints cause frustration.
Provide all needed equipment within close reach or position items as directed by patient.	Allows independence and decreases time needed to dress.
Provide assistive equipment as needed.	Assistive devices can help increase independence.
Encourage independence in appropriate activities.	Independence in activities promotes self-esteem.
Offer frequent encouragement.	
Bathing/hygiene 1. Assist in transferring as needed. 2. Provide safety items: rubber mats, grab bars, and bath bench. 3. Provide assistive devices: long-handled sponge, soap on a rope, washing mitts, adapted toothbrush and razor holder, hand-held shower spray.	
Dressing/grooming 1. Encourage use of loose clothing. 2. Dress lower extremities when in bed and upper extremities when up in chair. 3. Dress affected side first to promote ease in dressing. 4. Lay out clothes in order of dressing.	Loose clothing is easier to put on independently. Promotes structure and decreases amount of choices needed in dressing for cognitively impaired.

Nursing Interventions	Rationales
5. Provide assistive devices: button hook, zipper pull, long shoehorn, stocking aids, velcro closures, and elastic shoe laces.	
Toileting 1. Assist in transfers to and from commode or toilet as needed. 2. Provide assistive devices: raised toilet seat, grab bars, and stool to elevate legs.	
Feeding 1. Set up tray; assist in opening of packages and cutting up of food as needed. 2. Provide assistive devices: plate guard, padded handle on utensils, suction device under plate or bowl, and rocker knife for cutting.	

NURSING DIAGNOSIS: UNILATERAL NEGLECT

Related To neurological event

Defining Characteristics

Consistent inattention to stimuli on affected side
Inadequate self-care
Inadequate positioning and/or safety precautions in regard to the affected side
Does not look toward affected side
Leaves food on plate on affected side

Patient Outcomes

The patient will

- attend to affected side with cues as needed.
- scan visual field to compensate for loss on affected side.
- prevent injury to affected side.
- utilize intact senses to compensate for deficits.
- use both sides of the body in activities.

Nursing Interventions	Rationales
Assess sensation and awareness of body parts, ability to distinguish between right and left, visual acuity and field cuts, attention span, insight into disability, disorientation, ability to abstract, impulsivity, ability to sequence steps, and effect of neglect on activities of daily living.	Unilateral neglect is most commonly caused by injury to the right parietal lobe. Patients with right-lobe impairment also display problems with spatial relationships, sensory interpretation, relationship of body parts, judgment, and impulsivity. Homonymous hemianopsia (loss of vision on the contralateral side) may be present with injury to either the right or left hemisphere of the brain.
Promote environmental safety during the initial phase of treatment: 1. Approach from the unaffected side. 2. Position so that unaffected visual field is toward activity. 3. Place items in on unaffected side (call light, food on tray, furniture, etc.).	Initially the patient is unaware of the deficit and will miss important items or fall into items not in the visual field at this stage.
Assist to compensate for the perceptual deficit gradually: 1. Teach about neglect and call attention to affected side. 2. Approach from midline or affected side and announce yourself. 3. Change environment by moving items out of visual field. 4. Teach patient to scan environment during meals and during activity by turning to affected side and moving eyes horizontally and vertically.	Integrating information from both sides of the body is important to safely manage in the world. The patient will become more impaired if not taught how to compensate for the deficit.
Encourage touching and looking at affected body parts.	Promotes acceptance and integration of affected side and decreases fear. Patients with unilateral neglect often attribute affected body parts to another person.

Nursing Interventions	Rationales
Teach how to look for and position affected extremities by looking for them in the bed, in the wheelchair, and when ambulating; use sling for affected arm if necessary.	Protects affected extremities from injury (e.g., getting caught in wheelchairs, side rails).
Encourage activities that use both sides of the body.	Promotes integration of right and left.
Provide a simple, uncluttered environment.	A simple environment decreases the amount of information to process.
Give verbal and visual cues to patients during all activities as needed: 1. Highlight affected side by placing a dot on affected glass lens or by drawing a line on affected side of reading material. 2. Give short, step-by-step commands and assist as necessary.	Cues may be necessary to draw the patient's attention to the affected side. Simple commands enable processing of the information.
Reorient as needed.	Disorientation is common because sensory input is impaired.
Recognize judgment impairments and impulsivity; do not overestimate abilities or believe patient's self-assessment of abilities.	The patient is often unaware of deficits and may not be safe with some activities.

NURSING DIAGNOSIS: GRIEVING

Related To

- Actual or perceived object loss: parts and processes of the body
- Family roles and responsibilities
-

Defining Characteristics

Verbal expression of distress and loss
Anger
Sadness
Crying
Difficulty in expressing loss
Labile affect
Interference with life functioning
Alterations in eating habits, sleep patterns, activity level, libido

Patient Outcomes

The patient will
- verbalize feelings of loss.
- sleep without disturbance.
- maintain weight.
- increase socialization.
- carry out necessary daily functions.
- decrease crying episodes.
- use coping mechanisms to move through the grief process.

Nursing Interventions	Rationales
Assess the meaning of the stroke to the patient and the impact of the loss of family functioning, the patient's body image following the stroke, social withdrawal, irritability, hopelessness, change in daily functions, sleep pattern changes, appetite changes, past losses, past coping patterns, social supports, and formal depression screens (e.g., Geriatric Depression Screen or Beck Depression Inventory).	Twenty to 60% of stroke patients have significant depression that seems to be related to the meaning of the disease to the patient and social supports. Patients with anterior damage and infarcts in the left hemisphere are at highest risk. The greatest severity and prevalence of depression is seen 6 months to 2 years following the stroke.
Establish a therapeutic relationship.	A consistent relationship promotes trust and encourages verbalization.
Actively listen and convey empathy.	
Encourage ventilation of feelings.	Expression helps the patient work through the loss.
Allow the patient to cry.	
Use therapeutic touch to convey caring and acceptance.	
Acknowledge and validate the meaning of the loss and the changes in family roles.	Recognizing the loss gives the patient permission to grieve and work through the loss.
Explain the grief reaction and that the stages are fluid and not necessarily sequential: 1. denial 2. bargaining 3. anger 4. depression 5. acceptance/resolution	Understanding the grief reaction helps to normalize the experience so that the patient does not feel all alone. It also gives a frame of reference for their feelings.

Nursing Interventions	Rationales
Encourage continuing daily tasks and functions as able: 1. Set achievable short-term goals. 2. Provide structure and routine. 3. Encourage participation in social activities.	Daily tasks can be used to point out successes and progress. The structure will decrease the amount of energy needed to perform the tasks. Social activities allow acceptance by others.
Reflect on past coping strategies and identify strategies that may be helpful in this situation.	Build on successfully coping through past experiences or suggest ways to approach this experience differently.
Teach problem-solving skills.	Knowing how to deal with problems gives control and hope.
Identify and mobilize support systems such as family, friends, support groups, clergy, and church groups.	
Consult and collaborate with psychology and social work for evaluation and on-going counseling.	A team approach is helpful in assisting the patient and family with the many emotional aspects of a stroke.
Monitor for suicidal ideation: 1. Make a contract if patient has a plan. 2. Protect patient with constant supervision and safe environment if actively suicidal. 3. Consult psychiatry for evaluation and treatment.	The patient may become so depressed that suicide appears to be the only option.

Nursing Interventions	Rationales
Administer medications as prescribed for depression: 1. tricyclic antidepressants 2. prozac	Antidepressant medications may be necessary if the patient withdraws, loses weight, and cannot carry out daily functions. Side effects of tricyclic antidepressants (e.g., orthostatic hypotension, blurred vision, urinary retention, constipation, and dry mouth) should be monitored closely in this population. Tricyclic antidepressants are often contraindicated because of underlying disease. Side effects of Prozac include anorexia, weight loss, and insomnia. Prozac should be administered in the morning.

▼

NURSING DIAGNOSIS: KNOWLEDGE DEFICIT—DIAGNOSIS AND CARE

Related To lack of exposure to information

Defining Characteristics

Many questions
Few questions
Inappropriate or exaggerated behaviors
Verbalization of not understanding stroke management
Anxiety

Patient Outcomes

The patient and family will

- demonstrate skills necessary to function at home.
- verbalize an understanding of stroke prevention, treatment, and rehabilitation.

Nursing Interventions	Rationales
Assess patient and family members current knowledge about stroke and their reaction to the disability.	Allows for identifying and addressing misconceptions that may have already occurred.

Nursing Interventions	Rationales
Provide comprehensive stroke education to patients and family members: 1. definition or description 2. causes 3. risk factors 4. how to decrease risk factors 5. warning signs 6. medical-surgical management 7. rehabilitation and prevention of complications 8. how stroke affects behavior 9. depression following stroke 10. family changes following stroke.	
Schedule periodic patient/family conferences with the health care team caring for the patient to allow time for asking questions and for giving consistent messages.	Enables fuller participation in the recovery process by the patient and family.
Teach patient and caregivers the skills necessary to function at home (e.g., medication administration, bowel and bladder programs, skin care, swallowing and diet guidelines, communication system, positioning, transfers, dressing, safety measures). 1. Prioritize teaching by beginning with critical skills and skills that the patient and/or caregiver wants to learn. 2. Allow for return demonstration of the skills. 3. Discuss common problems and ways to solve them.	
Provide written and audiovisual materials when possible.	
Plan day or weekend passes for the patient to go home before discharge.	Allows for integration of learning in the home setting before discharge.

▼

DISCHARGE PLANNING/CONTINUITY OF CARE

- Refer patient to a rehabilitation facility if further inpatient rehabilitation is necessary.
- Assure understanding by patient and caregiver of patient home management plan.
- Arrange for home equipment from vendor if necessary (e.g., wheelchair, cushion, commode, bath bench, hoyer lift, walker).
- Refer to a home health care agency if continued nursing care, occupational therapy, speech therapy, physical therapy, or home health aide assistance is needed.
- Arrange follow-up with physicians for continued management postdischarge. Ensure that a prothrombin time will be drawn and interpreted by a nurse or physician within the specified time if the patient is on warfarin therapy.
- Provide telephone number of a nurse or physician to call if problems or questions arise.
- Assist patient in obtaining prescriptions and medical supplies and in establishing a plan for refilling prescriptions and obtaining supplies.
- Provide patient and family with information on community resources that might be helpful: handicapped sticker, transportation options, adult day care, chore service, grocery delivery, telephone assurance, delivered meals, and lifeline.
- Provide with information on stroke support groups or educational programs in the area.
- Refer to local chapter of the American Heart Association or National Stroke Association for further information.

REFERENCES

Emick-Herring, B. & Wood, P. (1990). A team approach to neurologically based swallowing disorders. *Rehabilitation Nursing, 15*(3), 126–132.

Hickey, J. V. (1992). *The clinical practice of neurological and neurosurgical nursing* (3rd ed). Philadelphia, PA: Lippincott.

Kelly-Hayes, M. & Phipps, M. A. (Eds.). (1991). Stroke. *Nursing Clinics of North America, 26*(4), 929–1048.

Leonard, A. D. & Newburg, S. (1992). Cardioembolic stroke. *Journal of Neuroscience Nursing, 24*(2), 69–76.

Mumma, C. M. (Ed.). (1987). *Rehabilitation nursing: Concepts and practice: A core curriculum* (2nd ed). Skokie, IL: Rehabilitation Nursing Foundation.

▼

TRAUMATIC BRAIN INJURY

Rochelle M. Carlson, RN, MS, CRRN

A traumatic brain injury (TBI) is caused by an external force to the head which results in neurological impairment or death. The neurological impairment may be either temporary or permanent and may range from minor to severe. Brain injuries are classified into primary and secondary injuries. A primary injury is caused by the impact of the trauma and is described as either focal or diffuse. In focal injuries, a contusion, laceration, or hematoma is seen at the site of impact (coup injury) or at the side of the brain opposite from the impact (coup-contrecoup injury). A diffuse injury is the result of rapid acceleration, deceleration, and rotational forces which shear and stretch the nerve fibers in the brain. While a primary injury cannot be altered by the health care team, a secondary injury can often be influenced by interventions. A secondary injury is caused by events in the brain, such as cerebral edema and increased intracranial pressure, that occur in response to the primary injury and act to extend the destruction of the initial blow. Although any person can be a victim of TBI, the typical victim is male, 15–24 years of old, with a history of risk-taking behavior who has been drinking and driving. Complications of brain injury include hydrocephalus, epilepsy, and diabetes insipidus. This care plan should be initiated after the patient's neurological status has stabilized, which usually occurs in an intensive care or intermediate care setting. (See Altered Consciousness, p. 373, for assessment and interventions during the acute phase following a TBI.)

ETIOLOGIES

- Motor vehicle accidents (account for 50% of all TBIs)
- Alcohol and/or drug use and multiple trauma
- Falls
- Sports-related injuries
- Violent acts/assaults
- Environmental/occupational injuries

CLINICAL MANIFESTATIONS

- Concussion (temporary neurological impairment)
  - may be mild or severe
  - loss of consciousness for seconds to hours
  - posttraumatic amnesia
  - loss of reflexes
  - headache
  - visual disturbance
  - dizziness
  - confusion
  - irritability, drowsiness
- Diffuse axonal injury (DAI)
  - may be mild, moderate, severe
  - immediate loss of consciousness for greater than 6 hr
  - increased intracranial pressure
  - hypertension
  - elevated temperature
- Brain stem injury
  - damage to cranial nerves III–XII possible
  - coma
  - pupils nonreactive
  - decerebration
- Missile injury (penetration of the brain)
  - memory impairment
  - dementia
  - psychosis
  - seizures
  - focal symptoms (aphasia, paresis)
- Epidural hematoma
  - blood formation between the skull and dura mater
  - momentary unconsciousness
  - lucid period for a few hours to 1–2 days followed by a rapid decrease in level of consciousness
  - headache increasing in severity
  - vomiting
  - seizure
  - hemiparesis
  - vital sign changes (decreased pulse, widening pulse pressure)
- Subdural hematoma
  - formation of blood between the dura and arachnoid layer
  - may be acute, subacute, chronic
  - headache
  - decreasing level of consciousness
  - drowsiness
  - agitation
  - slow thinking

- confusion
- ipsilateral pupil fixed and dilated, if severe

- Intracerebral hemorrhage
  - decrease in level of consciousness
  - headache
  - hemiplegia on contralateral side
  - dilated pupil on ipsilateral side

CLINICAL/DIAGNOSTIC FINDINGS

- Serum blood alcohol level elevated
- Toxicology screens of serum and urine: evidence of drug use
- X-rays: skull fractures and possible C-spine fracture (5–20% of brain injury also have C-spine fracture)
- Computerized tomography (CT) scan and/or magnetic resonance imaging (MRI) scan: contusion, hematoma, edema, midline shift
- Angiography: contusion, hematoma (when CT not available)
- Electroencephalogram (EEG): focal damage; may determine brain death
- Evoked potentials: show extent of injury and disruption of neuronal pathway
- Lumbar puncture: usually contraindicated because of increased intracranial pressure

OTHER PLANS OF CARE TO REFERENCE

- Altered Consciousness
- Seizure Disorders
- Stroke/Cerebral Vascular Accident
- Thrombophlebitis/Deep-Vein Thrombosis
- Prevention and Care of Pressure Ulcers

▼

NURSING DIAGNOSIS: HIGH RISK FOR VIOLENCE—SELF-DIRECTED OR DIRECTED AT OTHERS

Risk Factors

- Traumatic brain injury (especially a frontal or temporal injury)
- Hallucinations
- Overstimulating environment
- Altered perception of environmental cues

Patient Outcomes

The patient will

- not bring harm to self or others.

- demonstrate a sense of control over his or her external and/or internal environment with assistance from others.

Nursing Interventions	Rationales
Assess physiological and neurological status at least every 8 hr. Assessment may need to be more frequent if patient shows a deterioration in status. Assessment should include vital signs, level of consciousness and orientation, presence of a headache, pupillary response, and muscle strength and coordination. Notify physician of change in neurological status. See Altered Consciousness for further details on assessment and intervention.	A change in neurological status should be considered as a possible reason for the patient's agitated behavior.
Assess patient factors which could contribute to an agitated outburst (pain, hunger, need to urinate or defecate, frustration, inability to communicate need, visual/noise disturbance, fear, depression, confusion).	Assessment will help in preventing triggers to an agitated outburst and in recognizing what may precipitate an outburst.
Assess environmental factors which could contribute to an agitated outburst (noisy, busy, unfamiliar personnel, too dark, too light, lack of privacy).	
Observe for signs of agitation: clenched fist; facial expressions; throwing objects or kicking at objects; threatening verbalizations; continuous complaints, requests, demands; hallucinations; increased motor activity such as pacing, pulling at tubes, and restlessness.	Knowing signs of escalating agitation will allow implementation of prearranged plan for managing behavior as soon as possible.

Nursing Interventions	Rationales
Document behavior on a flowsheet. State time, describe behaviors, identify the antecedents or triggers to the behavior if possible, and explain the consequence of the behavior after the nursing intervention was implemented.	Flowsheet allows patterns of behaviors, triggers, and effective interventions to be observed. Patterns will facilitate consistency among staff and will be useful when setting up an individualized behavior modification plan for the patient.
Manipulate the environment by: 1. providing for private or semiprivate room 2. decreasing noise and activity (avoid placing patient in the middle of the hallway to be observed) 3. removing hazards such as scissors, sharps boxes, long ropes, or strings 4. providing for structure and predictability by doing the same activities in the same way at the same time of the day and using consistent personnel when possible	The patient may not be cognitively able to participate in managing his or her behavior. A calm environment will help decrease stimulation that the patient cannot interpret and a structured environment will enable the patient to feel in control.
Utilize a confident, nonthreatening nursing approach: 1. Approach the patient calmly and nonhurriedly. 2. Speak slowly and with a quiet voice. 3. Avoid sudden movements. 4. Describe actions in short, simple sentences. 5. Hide anxiety.	A confident, nonthreatening approach communicates that the situation is under control and that the nurse will help the patient maintain control of himself or herself.
Utilize aids to provide safety: 1. door alarms 2. floor beds 3. bed alarms 4. time-out room (padded room where a patient can stay during an agitated outburst) 5. wheelchair with vertical bars that will prevent patient from going through doorways	Environmental aids allow the patient a way to move about with limited restriction and allow staff to observe the patient at a distance.

Nursing Interventions	Rationales
Limit visitors to one or two at a time.	Limited visitors will decrease the amount of stimulation. Family members may prefer that only family and close friends visit to prevent embarrassment of the pattient because of bizarre behaviors displayed at this time.
Employ sitters or ask family members to sit with the patient.	A sitter allows one-to-one close supervision so that the patient can freely move without being restrained. Restraints increased agitation and are potentially harmful because of their restriction. Patients may also feel more secure with someone in their room at all times or during stressful times.
Offer the patient limited choices.	Limited choices will give the patient a sense of control without being overwhelmed.
Involve the patient in high-energy-expenditure activities such as walking, wheeling chair, or punching a bag.	Moving about will wear off pent-up energy and help decrease agitation.
Promote one to two short (½–1 hr in length) naps.	Short naps will prevent the patient from being overtired and less able to process stimuli but also will prevent the patient from not being able to sleep at night.
Provide for therapies on unit in a quiet area or in patient's room.	Providing therapies away from a busy, noisy gym will decrease stimulation.

Nursing Interventions	Rationales
Administer prescribed medications and monitor for for side-effects: 1. beta blockers (propranolol) 2. benzodiazepines (lorazepam) 3. antiepileptics (carbamazepine) 4. psychotropics (Haldol, lithium)	Medications (chemical restraints) should only be used on a scheduled or as-needed basis when other interventions have not been successful in managing the aggressive, impulsive patient who is at great risk for injuring himself or herself or others. Chronic use of these medications may delay recovery because they cloud cognition and interfere with new learning.
Institute a prearranged plan for managing behavior when patient's agitation escalates: 1. Seek help from one to three or more other personnel. 2. Move patient to a place away from other patients. 3. Remain calm and communicate that you will not let patient lose control. 4. One person should speak and direct actions of other personnel. 5. Use distraction if appropriate.	A prearranged plan will allow for immediate implementation when needed. One spokesperson will decrease confusion. Distraction may be appropriate if the patient is wandering away and is congnitively able to attend to another topic.
Consult rehabilitation psychology, if available, to assist in implementing a behavior modification plan when the patient is able to participate.	Behavior modification is used when the patient's agitation is primarily from external stimuli rather than from internal stimuli.

▼

NURSING DIAGNOSIS: ALTERED ROLE PERFORMANCE

Related To injury or disability of a family member

Defining Characteristics

Change in self-perception of role
Change in others' perception of role
Denial of change in role
Change in physical/mental capacity to resume role

Change in usual patterns of responsibility
Role overload

Patient/Family Outcomes

- The patient and family will acknowledge that a change in family roles has occurred because of the injury/disability.
- The patient will maintain a sense of family worth despite fewer or less important family responsibilities.
- The family members will avoid role overload.

Nursing Interventions	Rationales
Assess the family system, including previous and current roles and relationships, significant others, cultural and religious values, economic status, past coping patterns, and family strengths and limitations.	Baseline family information gives insight into how the injury will impact on family roles and relationships.
Consult social work and rehabilitation psychology, if available, to collaborate with evaluation of family systems, plan for interventions, and family counseling.	A team approach is needed to meet the complex needs of patients and families following a TBI.
Counsel the patient and family that many role changes have and will occur since the injury/disability. Point out concrete examples, for example, the wife is now cooking instead of the disabled husband, the husband now has full responsibility for the children and caring for his cognitively impaired wife as well as working full time, or a brother may now be mowing the lawn.	Family members often assume new roles without any awareness that they have done so. Or family members may have assumed new roles with reluctance, and patients may not be aware of the multiple roles others are playing. Conflicts in families can arise because tension, anger, and jealousy exist about roles.

Nursing Interventions	Rationales
Discuss the caregiving role with the primary caregiver: 1. Remind the caregiver that it is natural to feel frustration and fear. 2. Counsel the caregiver that it is also important to care for oneself and to have understanding people to turn to for support. 3. Coach the caregiver on how to deal with specific behavior problems. 4. Provide the caregiver with a list of community agencies that may offer some type of respite or counseling.	Caregivers enable patients to stay out of institutions, but they may also feel burden, anger, and frustration about their role. Caregivers often experience role overload because they have assumed the caregiving role in addition to several other roles. Caregivers need support, guidance, and sometimes respite to continue doing what they are doing.
Counsel the family regarding realistic expectations for the recovery and function of the disabled/injured patient.	If family expectations are too low, the patient may be overprotected and not given the independence and responsibilities needed to reach full recovery. If expectations are too high, family members will add to the patient's frustration or place the patient in situations that could be harmful.
Develop a plan with the patient and family to deal with role changes: 1. The plan should include some roles and responsibilities for the injured patient. 2. The plan should avoid role overload for one family member. 3. Help family to consider giving up noncritical responsibilities and roles during periods of stress/crisis.	A plan will allow the patient and family to confront role changes and help them deal with the changes in a concrete way. It is important to the injured patient's self-esteem and recovery that he or she still has some responsibility that is important to the family. Giving up noncritical responsibilities will help decrease frustration and will lower the potential for role overload.
Practice solving problems about role conflicts that may arise among family members.	Practice in the hospital setting will enable the patient and family to work through problems as they arise at home.

Nursing Interventions	Rationales
Encourage patient and family to attend in hospital or community support groups if available.	Support groups allow patients and family members to realize that they are not alone. Other support group members give helpful advice as well as empathy.

▼

NURSING DIAGNOSIS: KNOWLEDGE DEFICIT—DIAGNOSIS AND HOME CARE

Related To family members' lack of exposure to TBI

Defining Characteristics

Verbalization of not understanding what to expect
Anxiety
Many questions
Few questions
Inappropriate or exaggerated behaviors
Inappropriate interaction with the patient

Family Outcomes

- Family members will verbalize an understanding of what has happened and what is being done for the patient.
- Family members will demonstrate skills necessary to care for the patient at home.
- Family members will interact with the patient appropriately during behavioral outbursts.

Nursing Interventions	Rationales
Assess the family members' current knowledge about brain injuries and their reaction to injury.	Allows for clearing up misconceptions that may have already occurred
Describe what a brain injury is, the type of injury the patient has, what treatment is being given to the patient, and what the rehabilitation phase is all about.	Helps decrease anxiety about the unknown and instills trust in health care team that a plan is in place.

Nursing Interventions	Rationales
Schedule periodic family conferences with the health care team to allow the patient and family to ask questions and to allow the health care team to give consistent messages to the family.	Enables fuller participation in the recovery process by the patient and family.
Teach behavior management skills.	Necessary for family members to interact effectively with a patient who has a behavioral impairment.
Teach caregivers the skills necessary to care for the patient at home (e.g., medication administration, bowel program, bladder program, tube feedings, swallowing recommendations, communication system, positioning, transfers, dressing, behavior management skills, etc.). 1. Prioritize teaching by beginning with critical skills and skills that the caregiver wants to learn. 2. Allow for the caregivers to return to demonstrate the skills. 3. Discuss common problems and ways to solve them.	
Provide written and audiovisual materials when possible.	
Plan day or weekend passes for the patient to go home before discharge.	Allows for integration of learning in the home setting before discharge.

▼

DISCHARGE PLANNING/CONTINUITY OF CARE

- Refer patient to a rehabilitation facility if further inpatient rehabilitation is necessary.
- Assure understanding by caregiver of patient home management plan.
- Arrange for home equipment from vendor if necessary (e.g., wheelchair, cushion, tube feeding pump).
- Refer to a home health care agency if continued nursing care,

occupational therapy, speech therapy, physical therapy, or home health aide assistance is needed.

- Arrange follow-up with physician for continued management postdischarge.
- Provide patient and family with the phone number of a nurse or physician to call if problems arise.
- Assist in obtaining prescriptions and medical supplies and in establishing a plan for refilling prescriptions and medical supplies when needed.
- Provide patient and family with information or brain injury support groups of educational programs in the area.
- Refer to the local chapter of the National Head Injury Foundation for further information.

REFERENCES

Cammermeyer, M. & Appeldorn, C. (Eds.). (1990). *Core curriculum for neuroscience nursing*. Chicago, IL: American Association of Neuroscience Nurses.

Hanak, M. (1992). *Rehabilitation nursing for the neurological patient.* New York: Springer.

Hickey, J. V. (1992). *The clinical practice of neurological and neurosurgical nursing* (3rd ed). Philadelphia: Lippincott.

Mumma, C. M. (Ed.). (1987). *Rehabilitation nursing: Concepts and practice: A core curriculum* (2nd ed). Skokie, IL: Rehabilitation Nursing Foundation.

Patterson, T. S. (1990). Behavioral management of the agitated head trauma client. *Rehabilitation Nursing, 15*(5), 248–249.

Common Renal and Urological Conditions and Procedures

Hemodialysis

Lynn Schoengrund, RN, MS

Hemodialysis is one form of renal replacement therapy for patients with acute and chronic renal failure. It is the passing of blood over a semipermeable membrane to remove the excess fluids, electrolytes, and metabolites that accumulate in all body tissues when renal failure occurs. Three components must be present to perform hemodialysis. One is an access to a large blood supply that will allow blood flow up to 500 mL/min. The second component is the dialyzer, or artificial kidney, which is the semipermeable membrane over which blood is passed. Excess solutes are removed from the blood by the processes of diffusion and fluid movement and solute drag. Fluid is removed by ultrafiltration, the movement of fluid under pressure. The third component is a fluid called dialysate, which is circulated on the other side of the semipermeable membrane. Dialysate mimics normal serum, containing normal or slightly less than normal quantities of sodium, chloride, potassium, bicarbonate, and calcium. Dialysate can be altered or prescribed to add or delete electrolytes for specific patient conditions.

ETIOLOGIES

- Diabetes
- Glomerulonephritis
- Chronic hypertension
- Polycystic kidneys
- Autoimmune disorders, for example, lupus or Goodpasture's
- Progression of acute renal failure to chronic renal failure
- Chronic acetaminophen use or abuse
- Heroin use

CLINICAL MANIFESTATIONS

- Severe fatigue
- Anorexia, nausea, vomiting

- Pallor
- Signs of fluid overload

CLINICAL/DIAGNOSTIC FINDINGS

See Renal Failure.

OTHER PLANS OF CARE TO REFERENCE

- Renal Failure
- Peritoneal Dialysis

▼

NURSING DIAGNOSIS: HIGH RISK FOR INFECTION

Risk Factors

- Frequent invasive procedure
- Exposure of blood and body fluids to extracorporeal equipment
- Exposure to blood-borne pathogens, for example, hepatitis and human immunodeficiency virus (HIV)
- Chronic illness

Patient Outcomes

Patient is free from infection.

Nursing Interventions	Rationales
Discuss the need for vaccinating against hepatitis B infection with the patient and family and administer the vaccine as prescribed prior to or as the patient begins chronic dialysis.	High-risk groups should be immunized against hepatitis. During the 1970s hepatitis was epidemic in dialysis units. Generally patient's infections are benign, but spread to family members or staff is common.

Nursing Interventions	Rationales
Use Universal Precautions and follow OSHA guidelines to prevent the spread of blood-borne infections to self or others.	Spread of blood-borne infections is well documented in epidemiological studies of dialysis patients. Despite immunization against hepatitis B, hepatitis C and HIV remain risks as well as other unknown viral agents. The mode of transmission of hepatitis B and C and HIV requires blood-to-blood or mucous-membrane-blood contact. This mode encompasses the ingestion of the virus from contaminated surfaces, sexual activity, and blood contact with open cuts or sores.
Inspect the fistula or graft (Figures 45.1 and 45.2) daily for signs of infection, especially at needle insertion sites. Look for redness; palpate for heat. Inspect for purulent drainage or whitened areas at needle sites. Regular needle insertion into the fistula or graft increases the risk of infection.	Early diagnosis and treatment may prevent the development of septicemia. Grafts may need to be surgically removed to prevent life threatening-infection.

▼

NURSING DIAGNOSIS: FLUID VOLUME DEFICIT

Related To excessive ultrafiltration of fluid during dialysis.

Defining Characteristics

Hypotension, orthostatic hypotension
Excessive fatigue, weakness, or dizziness
Rapid or thready pulse
Decreased weight

Patient Outcomes

- Weight, blood pressure, and pulse are stable.
- The patient does not report increased fatigue, weakness, or dizziness.

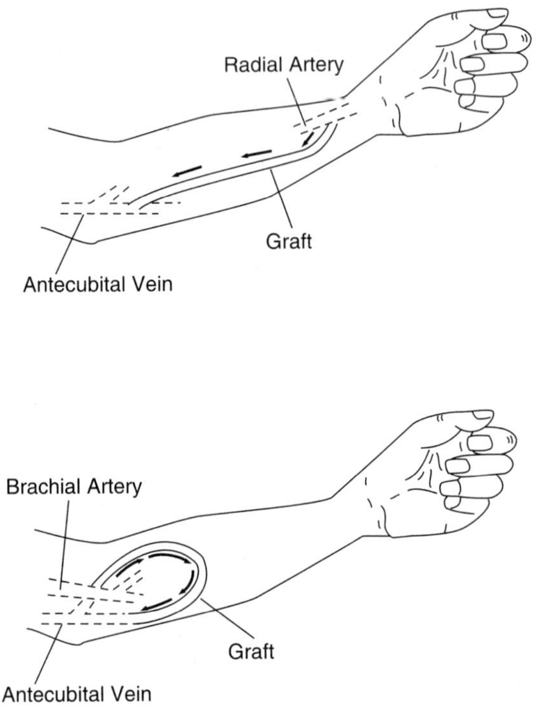

Figure 45.1 Placement of straight and curved grafts between arteries and veins. Arrows indicate the flow of blood through the grafts. From *Renal Problems in Critical Care* (p. 79) by Schoengrund and Balzer, 1985, Albany, NY: Delmar. Copyright 1985 by Delmar Publishers. Reprinted by permission.

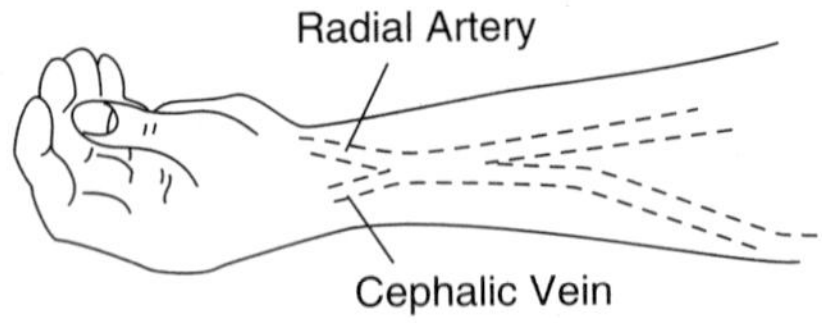

Figure 45.2 Atrioventricular fistula. The radial artery is shown in a side-to-side anastomosis with the cephalic vein. After maturation, needles are placed in the vein for hemodialysis. From *Renal Problems in Critical Care* (p. 77) by Schoengrund and Balzer, 1985, Albany, NY: Delmar. Copyright 1985 by Delmar Publishers. Reprinted by permission.

Nursing Interventions	Rationales
Assess the fluid status after dialysis: 1. Compare the predialysis weight to postdialysis weight. 2. Compare blood pressure values pre- and postdialysis. 3. Assess the jugular vein with the patient lying flat; the vein should be filled. Assess for symptoms of dizziness, increased fatigue, and weakness. Assess the patient's ability to stand and ambulate.	Hemodialysis removes fluid from vascular space. Fluid moves into the vascular space from the interstitial space and finally from the cellular space. There is a time lag in the movement of fluid from the cellular level to the vascular level; therefore patients may demonstrate hypotension while continuing to demonstrate excess total body fluids with symptoms such as edema. Control of fluid volume is based on human calculations of fluid balance and machine settings to remove fluid during dialysis. The calculations cannot always be precise. Excessive removal results in fluid volume deficit. Inadequate removal results in fluid volume excess. Therefore, assessment of fluid status after dialysis is of paramount importance.
Administer oral salt solutions (broth) for symptoms of hypotension, rapid pulse, and dizziness.	Salt solutions will move fluids quickly into the vascular space to offset hypovolemia.
Administer intravenous saline if patient is unable to drink or if hypotension is life threatening.	Severe hypotension must be treated immediately despite long-range goals of fluid removal.
Teach patients to recognize and report early symptoms of hypotension to prevent its progression.	Patients experience early symptoms of hypotension that vary by the individual. Examples may include nausea, ringing in the ears, slight apprehension, or nervous sensations.

Nursing Interventions	Rationales
Prevent need for excessive fluid removal during dialysis by assisting patients in learning their individual fluid needs. Review intake, symptoms, and dialysis treatments and assist the patients in drawing correlations.	

▼

NURSING DIAGNOSIS: HIGH RISK FOR INJURY

Risk Factors

- Increased clotting potential of diverted or artificial vessels
- Bleeding from needle sites after dialysis
- Heparinization during dialysis with overlap effect
- Diverted circulation from distal or anatomy on affected limb
- Presence of 100–1200 mL blood supply in fistula or graft

Patient Outcomes

- Dialysis access will be patent.
- No bleeding will occur from access site.

Nursing Interventions	Rationales
Regularly assess the patency of the fistula graft by palpating for a thrill or auscultating for a bruit.	The presence of arterial blood in the vein or graft produces a bruit or thrill. Absence of these signs indicates decreased flow.
Assess needle site dressings after dialysis and review amount of heparin used during dialysis.	
Teach patients to avoid constricting flow through the access by avoiding pressure of clothing or postures. Do not take blood pressure, draw blood, or place tourniquets on limb with access.	Flow through the access must be maintained at all times.
Communicate fistula/graft care and need to avoid constricting flow to all caregivers including lab technicians.	

NURSING DIAGNOSIS: BODY IMAGE DISTURBANCE

Related To

- Presence of atrioventricular (AV) graft or fistula
- Changed physical appearance (pallor, yellowing of skin)
- Dependence on technology for continued life

Defining Characteristics

Neglect of hygiene
Avoidance of fistula or graft
Focus on previous strengths
Function or appearance
Fear of rejection by others
Feelings of helplessness or hopelessness
Preoccupation with change or loss
Extension of body boundary to include components of dialysis
Refusal to acknowledge changes

Patient Outcomes

The patient will demonstrate acceptance of body image changes, as evidenced by discussing feelings and planning clothing selections.

Nursing Interventions	Rationales
Empower the patient to discuss feelings by validating rather than denying patient perceptions.	Patients will not discuss feelings if they are not in a safe environment. Denial of feelings perpetuates and accelerates the patient's negative emotions.
Assist the patient in exploring altered self-image by verbalizing fears and exploring reality.	Patients need to incorporate physical changes into their self-definition.
Assist patient in selecting clothing to cover access site and grooming to enhance appearance.	
Refer patients to psychotherapists if symptoms are severe or continued.	

▼

NURSING DIAGNOSIS: INEFFECTIVE MANAGEMENT OF THERAPEUTIC REGIMEN

Related To
- Complex treatment regimes
- Difficult required changes in life-style and habits

Defining Characteristics

Verbalization of desire to manage the treatment of illness
Verbalization of difficulty with regulation or integration of any of the regimens needed to maintain health on hemodialysis.
Verbalization of no action to make changes previously.

Patient Outcomes

The patient will
- demonstrate understanding of components of treatment plan.
- set realistic priorities to meet selected components of the plan.
- identify factors which inhibit following treatment plan.

Nursing Interventions	Rationales
Provide educational resources through literature, slides, or video tapes.	
Assist the patient in talking through perceived need for behavioral changes. Help the patient set priorities. Individualize plans by reviewing the patient's life-style.	
Provide validation for patient efforts. For example, demonstrate changes in laboratory results as dietary habits change.	
Refer patients to appropriate experts (dietitian, exercise physiologist, nephrology nurses, and physicians) for assistance in individualizing treatment regimen.	

▼

DISCHARGE PLANNING/CONTINUITY OF CARE

- Schedule outpatient dialysis treatments and provide detailed report to the dialysis caregivers.
- Assure understanding of self-management plan, especially any additional regimens added during hospitalization.
- Review symptoms that would require immediate reporting to the nephrologist.
-

REFERENCES

Lewis, S. M. & Collier, I. C. (1992). *Medical surgical nursing.* St. Louis, MO: Mosby.

Liebairt, A. (1991). Nursing management of continuous arteriovenous hemodialysis. *Heart & Lung, 20*(2), 152–160.

Patrick, M. L., Woods, S. J., Crawer, R. F., Rokoshy, J. S., & Boraine, P. (1991). *Medical surgical nursing pathophysiological concepts.* Philadelphia, PA: Lippincott.

Porth, C. M. (1990). *Pathophysiology—Concepts of altered health states.* Philadelphia, PA: Lippincott.

▼

NEPHROSTOMY

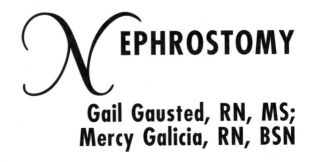

Gail Gausted, RN, MS; Mercy Galicia, RN, BSN

A nephrostomy tube insertion is performed to provide temporary or permanent renal system decompression. It is also used for external urinary diversion from the bladder or an operative site or for therapeutic medication administration to the renal collecting system.

ETIOLOGIES (INDICATIONS)

- Sepsis secondary to urethral obstruction
- Impassable ureteral obstruction related to stone, tumor, or stricture
- Diagnostic purposes: pressure perfusion studies
- Medication administration

CLINICAL MANIFESTATIONS

- flank pain
- nausea, vomiting, fever, chills
- burning on micturation
- visible hematuria
- cloudy urine

CLINICAL/DIAGNOSTIC FINDINGS

- Low hemoglobin and hematocrit
- Leukocytosis
- Visible radiopaque calculi on kidney x-ray
- Positive intravenous urogram
- Positive Whitaker test or Pfister test

▼

NURSING DIAGNOSIS: HIGH RISK FOR INJURY

Risk Factors

- Inadvertent severance of blood vessel(s) during placement of nephrostomy tube
- Surgical procedure on a highly vascular organ

Patient Outcomes

Patient will not develop hemorrhage, as evidenced by

- stable vital signs
- warm skin with usual color
- palpable peripheral pulses
- urine output of at least 30 mL/hr

Nursing Interventions	Rationales
Check vital signs, dressing, and nephrostomy tube every 2–4 hr for 48 hr, then every shift thereafter, if normal. Check dressing under patient's back.	Expect to observe bloody drainage initially. The color should change to a light pink within 48 hr. Drainage will flow with gravity.
Assess for hematuria.	Small amount of hematuria that ceases spontaneously within 6–36 hr is expected after insertion of nephrostomy tube.
Notify physician of persistent bright red drainage.	Persistent bright red drainage is indicative of abnormal bleeding.
Assess for swelling or bruising in the affected flank. Report changes to physician immediately.	Suggestive of internal bleeding.
Ensure the nephrostomy tube is securely taped to the patient's side.	Do not attempt to reposition a displaced tube.

▼

NURSING DIAGNOSIS: RISK FOR INFECTION

Risk Factors

- Presence of nephrostomy tube and urethral catheter
- Noncompliance with urinary tract and wound infection precautions
- Decreased resistance to infection

Patient Outcomes

Patient will not demonstrate signs and symptoms of local or systemic infection.

Nursing Interventions	Rationales
Monitor for postprocedural infection and prevent and/or initiate management, as appropriate.	Infection is a common postnephrostomy complication.
Obtain urine or wound culture if infection is suspected.	Facilitates organism identification, so that appropriate treatment can be instituted quickly.
Prevent interruption of closed drainage system. Do not disconnect the tubing unless absolutely necessary. Avoid contamination if tubing must be disconnected.	Nephrostomy tubes go directly into the renal collecting system and pose risk of pyelonephritis, unless precautions are maintained. Once the system is open, it is potentially contaminated.
Assess tubing for kinks. If a persistent leak exists, notify physician. Change dressings when wet; do not reinforce. Cleanse area around tube with betadine solution or hydrogen peroxide.	If urine has leaked under the dressing, it acts as a wick, enabling the microorganisms to move toward the incision. It is a good medium for bacterial growth.
Encourage fluid intake to at least 8–10 glasses/day, unless contraindicated, including 3 glasses of cranberry juice.	Rapid flow of urine through the urinary tract discourages multiplication of bacteria. It also produces a good mechanical flushing and dilutes urinary particles that cause calculus formation. Cranberry juice aids in keeping urine clear and acidic, thus inhibiting bacterial growth and preventing tube encrustation by urinary sediment.
Keep collection bags below kidney level and tubing free from kinks.	Prevents reflux, promotes urine flow, and eliminates obstruction.
Do not clamp nephrostomy tube unless ordered.	Clamping will precipitate acute pyelonephritis unless the urinary tract is proven patent.
Preform catheter/meatal care twice daily or as needed.	Prevents accumulation of mucus around the meatus.

▼

NURSING DIAGNOSIS: HIGH RISK FOR IMPAIRED SKIN INTEGRITY

Risk Factors

- Presence of nephrostomy tube
- Excessive leakage of drainage around nephrostomy tube site
- Lack of skin barrier
- Prolonged contact of skin with wet dressing.

Patient Outcomes

Patient will maintain skin integrity around the nephrostomy tube, as evidenced by absence of redness, irritation, and breakdown.

Nursing Interventions	Rationales
Keep the tube securely taped to the patient's flank. If extension tubing is used to connect the nephrostomy tube to collection device, it should be coiled and taped to abdomen as a "safety loop" or coiled and secured to bed if connected to bedside drainage.	Prevents accidental pulling or tugging of tube that may cause dislodging.
If the nephrostomy tube becomes dislodged, facilitate immediate replacement.	Dislodgement of the tube is considered an emergency. If the tube is not reinserted within 1–2 hr, the nephrostomy opening will contract, and it may be impossible to reinsert the tube through the same tract.
Report sudden onset or increase in pain in affected kidney area.	Can indicate perforation of an organ by the tube.
Report persistent gross hematuria (bright red urine, possibly with clots).	Transient hematuria can be expected for 24–48 hr after tube insertion.
Notify physician of leakage around tube and sudden decrease in urine output which can occur with blockage and/or obstruction.	Leakage should stop in about 10 days. A sudden decrease in output is a sign of tube dislodgment.

Nursing Interventions	Rationales
Hand irrigate the nephrostomy as needed as indicated with no more than 5 mL of specified irrigant using strict sterile technique.	Normal kidney pelvis holds 2–5mL of fluid; more than this amount can cause mechanical damage to the kidney or infection from pyelorenal backflow.
Inspect skin areas that are in contact with wound drainage for signs of irritation and breakdown. Protect skin from moisture or drainage around the tube. Apply skin barrier of ostomy appliance around wound where there is prolonged or copious drainage. Change dressing when wet as soon as possible. Do not reinforce.	Drainage with urine is highly irritating to skin and can easily cause breakdown of skin integrity.

▼

NURSING DIAGNOSIS: ALTERED URINARY ELIMINATION

Related To

- Presence of nephrostomy/urethral indwelling catheter
- Urinary retention.

Defining Characteristics

Disruption of urine flow through nephrostomy tube or urethral catheter
Inability of patient to void
Flank pain
Suprapubic distention and/or discomfort
Decreased urine output

Patient Outcomes

Patient will establish a normal pattern of urinary elimination after nephrostomy/urinary catheter removal (voidings > 100 mL.

Nursing Interventions	Rationales
Measure nephrostomy and urethral catheter outputs every hour for first 24–48 hr, then every 4–8 hr, and report any changes.	A sudden decrease could mean obstruction or loss of kidney function. An increase of more than 2000 mL/8 hr could indicate postobstructive diuresis, which can cause fluid and electrolyte imbalance.

Nursing Interventions	Rationales
Assess for signs of reobstruction after the nephrostomy tube is clamped and removed, that is, leakage around the nephrostomy tube site, flank pain, and fever.	The nephrostomy tube remains in place until obstruction of the urinary tract is removed. Removal occurs if clamping regimen is tolerated. Expect drainage from site for up to 12 hr after removal. The tract should close completely in 2 days, leaving a small scar.
Maintain accurate record of intake and output.	

▼

NURSING DIAGNOSIS: KNOWLEDGE DEFICIT—REGARDING FOLLOW-UP CARE

Related To
- Lack of exposure to information
- New procedure

Defining Characteristics
Inability to describe treatment plan
Inability to perform desired skills
Verbalizes deficiency of knowledge or skill of information
Expresses inaccurate interpretations of information
Repeated questions/requests for information

Patient Outcomes
Patient and significant other will
- verbalize understanding of treatment plan after discharge.
- demonstrate necessary procedures correctly.
- relate what signs and symptoms to report.
- state measures to prevent recurrent stone formation.
- demonstrate independent maintenance of nephrostomy tube.

Nursing Interventions	Rationales
Assess the patient's/significant other's ability to care for themselves/be cared for others at home in the initial hospitalization. Plan teaching sessions to include family members/significant others.	Because of the nephrostomy tube location, someone will have to help patient with dressing changes and tube management.

Nursing Interventions	Rationales
Stress importance of good hand washing before handling equipment or dressing. Review dressing removal and site cleansing using an outward circular approach. Remind not to touch the side of the dressing that touches the tube. The preferred cleansing solution preference is soap and water or antiseptic solution with an antibacterial ointment.	
Review cleansing of the bedside drainage collector and leg bag after each use and replace these bags weekly. Cleanse bags with a phosphoric acid detergent, rinse with clear water, followed by final rinse of vinegar solution (1 oz vinegar to 1 qt water). Do not use hot water.	This practice controls odor. Hot water causes odor retention.
Remind patient to keep tube taped to the flank and attached to a drainage bag. Instruct to empty the leg bag when it is two thirds full and to cleanse bag tubing tips with an alcohol or betadine solution with bag changes.	
Instruct to call if the nephrostomy tube has moved even 2–3 inches out of tract. Repositioning of the tube should never be attempted by the patient.	
Review signs and symptoms of infection. Instruct to call if redness, warmth, or drainage at the site, fever, flank pain, and bloody, cloudy, or foul-smelling urine are noticed.	Assess current knowledge regarding stone formation. Refer patient to a dietitian for prescribed diet as needed. Reinforce the importance of adequate fluid intake of at least 8–10 glasses/day.
Review activity level: 1. Exercise, lifting or straining should be avoided until permitted by physician. Walking can be done without fear of tube dislodgement.	Active, strenous physical activities can dislodge the nephrostomy tube.

Nursing Interventions	Rationales
2. Sexual activities are discouraged while the nephrostomy tube is still in place, but concerns should be discussed with physician.	
3. Sleeping on the same side as nephrostomy tube should be avoided.	This can disrupt the flow of nephrostomy tube drainage.

▼

DISCHARGE PLANNING/CONTINUITY OF CARE

- Assure patient/family understand and can perform self-care at home.
- Refer to a home care agency if continued care, teaching, or assistance with self-care management is needed.
- Arrange for follow-up with physician.
- Assist with obtaining prescriptions and supplies and establishing a plan for refilling as needed.

REFERENCES

Barr, J. E. (1988). Standards of care for the patient with a percutaneous nephrostomy tube. *Journal of Enterostoma Therapy, 15*, 147–153.

Brunner, L. & Suddarth, D. (1988). *Textbook of medical-surgical nursing*. Philadelphia, PA: Lippincott.

Ghiotto, D. (1988). A full range of care for nephrostomy patient. *RN*, April, pp. 72–74.

Guidos, B. (1988). Preparing the patient for home care of the percutaneous nephrostomy tube. *Journal of Enterostoma Therapy, 15*, 187–190.

Sage, S. J. (1992). Nephrostomy dressing procedure. *Ostomy and Wound Management Journal, 32*, 32–36.

▼

RENAL FAILURE

Lynn Schoengrund, RN, MS

Renal failure is a progressive loss of nephrons that results in loss of renal function. The initial cause of nephron loss varies, while resulting symptomatology is uniform regardless of the cause of the disease. As many as 90% of nephrons are destroyed before signs and symptoms appear, and 95% nephron loss is demonstrated before renal replacement therapy is necessary. Renal insufficiency is the term used to define the phase between symptom appearance and the need for replacement therapy. Renal insufficiency can be managed in the short term by restricting dietary protein and controlling symptoms with medications. Renal failure requires replacement therapy in the form of dialysis or renal transplant.

Clinical Clip

Functions of the Kidney

Excretory
Excretion of the end products of metabolism.

Homeostatic
Regulation of fluid and electrolyte balance.

Hormone Production
Renin-angiotensin conversion, vitamin D production, erythropoietin production.

ETIOLOGIES

- Diabetes
- Glomerulonephritis
- Chronic hypertension
- Polycystic kidneys
- Autoimmune disorders, for example, lupus or Goodpasture's
- Progression of acute renal failure to chronic renal failure

- Chronic acetaminophen use or abuse
- Heroin use

CLINICAL MANIFESTATIONS

- Severe fatigue
- Anorexia, nausea vomiting
- Pallor
- Signs of fluid overload

CLINICAL/DIAGNOSTIC FINDINGS

- Increased creatinine, blood urea nitrogen (BUN), (as high as 10 times normal)
- Decreased creatinine clearance to 5–10% of normal
- Decreased hemoglobin and hematocrit
- Altered serum electrolytes, especially elevated potassium
- Abnormally small or sclerosed kidneys possibly visualized on IVP or other radiographic film

OTHER PLANS OF CARE TO REFERENCE

- Hemodialysis
- Peritoneal Dialysis
- Hypertension

▼

NURSING DIAGNOSIS: FLUID VOLUME EXCESS

Related To

- Noncompliance with fluid restriction
- Inadequate fluid removal in dialysis
- Accumulation of fluid prior to introduction of dialysis

Defining Characteristics

Vascular distention
Systolic hypertension
Edema
Increased body weight in daily weight comparisons
Subjective reports of "heaviness"
Orthopnea, shortness of breath, rales
Exertional fatigue
Increased central venous or pulmonary artery pressures
Fluid on chest x-ray

Patient Outcomes

- Blood pressure and weight are stable.
- The patient has no shortness of breath.
- The patient does not exhibit signs of fluid overload.

Nursing Interventions	Rationales
Assess fluid status at regular intervals: 1. Measure and compare systolic blood pressure and note changes. 2. Weigh daily with similar circumstances at each weight. 3. Position the patient flat and examine the jugular veins for distention. 4. Assess the patient for edema, noting dependent areas. 5. Auscultate the lungs, listening for rales, especially at the bases.	Fluid accumulates first in the vascular space, then in the interstitial space, and lastly at the cellular level. A person of average height and weight can accumulate 5–10 lb of fluid before demonstrating edema. The immediate life-threatening mechanism of fluid excess occurs when the left ventricle cannot handle the load presented and fluid accumulates in the lungs, interfering with gas exchange. However, chronic fluid volume excess chronically strains the heart muscle and compromises the heart over time.
Develop a plan with the patient and the physician to intervene before fluid accumulation is life threatening.	
Prevent fluid overload due to excessive intake by assisting the patient in learning his or her own fluid tolerance levels by monitoring intake and correlating levels with signs and symptoms.	Individual tolerance for fluid accumulation is dependent on muscle distribution and body size.
Assist patients in controlling thirst by using other forms of oral satisfaction and scheduling fluid intake at regular intervals.	

▼

NURSING DIAGNOSIS: HIGH RISK FOR INFECTION

Risk Factors

- Chronic disease
- Decreased hemoglobin
- Decreased leukocyte effectiveness

- Increased exposure to invasive procedures
- Increased exposure to other ill individuals

Patient Outcomes
The patient is free from infection.

Nursing Interventions	Rationales
Use aseptic technique and universal precautions in all procedures (see Hemodialysis and Peritoneal Dialysis).	The frequent invasive procedures required for treatment may introduce bacterial or viral agents.
Instruct patients on universal precautions and the rationale for hospital policies and procedures which decrease the rate of nosocomial infections.	
Teach prevention of infections by avoiding circumstances that may include exposure to individuals with infections.	Understanding their own risk of infection will aid in avoiding exposure.

▼

NURSING DIAGNOSIS: ALTERED ORAL MUCOUS MEMBRANE

Related To presence of ammonia in mouth causing irritation and breakdown

Defining Characteristics
Uremic breath odor
Stomatitis
Oral lesions or ulcers
Gum ulceration or bleeding

Patient Outcomes
The patient will
- be free from bleeding and mucous membrane breakdown.
- be able to eat and drink as usual.

Nursing Interventions	Rationales
Provide for oral hygiene with a soft toothbrush at regular intervals.	

Nursing Interventions	Rationales
Teach principles of oral hygiene technique and refer to regular dental care.	
Encourage the use of vinegar mouthwash if taste or smell of ammonia is strong or disturbs the patient.	Vinegar neutralizes ammonia.

NURSING DIAGNOSIS: HIGH RISK FOR IMPAIRED SKIN INTEGRITY

Risk Factors
- Dryness and flaking of skin
- Itching and scratching
- Deposition of uremic salts in skin

Patient Outcomes
- The patient's skin is intact.

Nursing Interventions	Rationales
Inspect skin completely, daily, for pressure areas, breakdown, and edema.	Breaks in skin may appear in unusual areas due to the deposition of uremic salts.
Avoid use of tape, dressings, or linen that may cause irritation.	
Assess for complaints of itching. Provide emotional support by avoiding minimizing these symptoms.	
Use skin moisturizers and other treatments to decrease itching, for example, therapeutic baths (oatmeal) and showers. Consult skin care specialist, if available.	
If above means do not work or if itching becomes intolerable, discuss use of medications with physician.	

NURSING DIAGNOSIS: HIGH RISK FOR ACTIVITY INTOLERANCE

Risk Factors

- Decreased red blood cell (RBC) production in renal failure
- Chronic cardiac muscle fatigue due to chronic fluid overload

Patient Outcomes

- Patient is able to perform desired activities.

Nursing Interventions	Rationales
Assess the patient daily for activity tolerance by asking the patient to rate fatigue on a scale of 1–10 with activity, monitoring pulse rate with activity and observing the patient for diaphoresis.	
Monitor hematocrit and administer prescribed erythropoietin.	The hormone erythropoietin has been synthesized and is available for intravenous or subcutaneous replacement. Its dosage is titrated to maintain a hematocrit of 30–35%. The drug is well tolerated with very few side effects.
Plan activities with the patient and build activities to increase tolerance gradually.	
Refer patients to exercise specialists for a progressive exercise prescription.	Abrupt exercise can be life threatening to patients with compromised cardiac status.
Encourage to start and maintain prescribed exercise program.	Studies show renal failure patients who exercise have decreased morbidity and mortality.
During illness maintain patient activity tolerance by 1. spacing activities 2. providing short but frequent activities such as walking 3. referring to physical therapy for strengthening and stretching exercises	Acute illnesses increase the patient's risk of activity tolerance.

▼

NURSING DIAGNOSIS: ALTERED NUTRITION—LESS THAN BODY REQUIREMENTS

Related To

- Oral stomatitis
- Anorexia
- Fatigue
- Rigid dietary requirements

Defining Characteristics

Altered taste
Lack of appetite or interest in food
Loss of body weight

Patient Outcomes

- Weight is maintained.
- Caloric intake equals requirements.

Nursing Interventions	Rationales
Monitor daily weight, intake and output, and calorie count, comparing weight and intake daily.	Loss of body weight may not be readily apparent because fluid may replace lost body weight.
Monitor the patient's nitrogen balance by monitoring BUN-creatinine ratio. Report to the physician if greater than 10 : 1.	Negative nitrogen balance exists when cells are broken down to provide for energy requirements. Cell breakdown causes a rapidly rising BUN, out of proportion with increased creatinine in renal failure. Cell breakdown is an early sign of starvation which can be reversed with oral or parenteral nutritional supplements.
Involve patient in food selection. Try to meet preferences with dietary restrictions.	

NURSING DIAGNOSIS: ALTERED THOUGHT PROCESSES

Related To disturbance in neurological function due to uremia

Defining Characteristics

Inaccurate interpretation of the environment
Distractibility
Memory deficits/problems
Decreased attention span
Inappropriate non-reality-based thinking

Patient Outcomes

The patient will

- meet learning objectives.
- interpret events and the environment accurately.
- be free from anxiety or fears based on inaccurate thinking.

Nursing Interventions	Rationales
Assess patient perceptions and interpretation of information. Check level of retention of information provided at regular intervals.	Information provided does not always result in information learned. Neurological disturbances may alter patient's interpretation of events. A detailed assessment of the patient's level of understanding must be performed before developing an individualized teaching plan.
Decrease environmental crowding and limit environmental stimuli.	A quiet environment decreases the opportunities for inaccurate patient interpretations and decreases patient stress.
Space teaching sessions to allow the patient to absorb information.	
Teach patient and family the physiological basis of symptoms.	Patients and families may fear other disease processes or emotional responses.
Validate accurate patient perceptions and correct misperceptions.	Ineffective coping and noncompliance can be based on inaccurate interpretation of information by the patient.

▼

NURSING DIAGNOSIS: KNOWLEDGE DEFICIT—RENAL FAILURE AND TREATMENT OPTIONS

Related To
- New information
- Misunderstanding of previous information

Defining Characteristics
Requests for information
Verbalization of inaccurate information
Difficulty making treatment choices
Noncompliance
Inappropriate behaviors

Patient Outcomes
The patient will
- describe renal failure and recommended treatment.
- list long-term replacement therapy options and begin selection process.

Nursing Interventions	Rationales
Assess the knowledge base of renal disease, medical management, and replacement therapy options.	
Teach about the effects of renal failure. Relate each effect to symptoms the patient is experiencing. Relate treatments and medications to effects of renal failure and control of symptoms. Assist the patient in developing strategies to control symptoms and to make treatments palatable.	
Refer to the dietitian for complex diet teaching. Reinforce information provided, reviewing protein, sodium, potassium, and fluid restriction.	
Discuss importance of controlling hypertension by taking antihypertensive medication as prescribed (see Hypertension, p. 123.).	

Nursing Interventions	Rationales
Provide information on renal replacement therapy options if medical therapy is no longer effective, including hemodialysis, peritoneal dialysis, and kidney transplantation (see Hemodialysis, p. 515, and Peritoneal Dialysis, p. 543).	Transplantation options include use of a matched cadaver kidney or one donated by a relative. Extensive tests are required of patient and potential donor to determine a match. Dialysis may be needed until transplantation can be done.
Refer to dialysis, transplant staff, or physician for evaluation and specific questions and issues. Consider introducing to successful patients using each option.	
Assist the patient in weighing advantages and disadvantages of each treatment option as they impact the patient's life-style.	

▼

DISCHARGE PLANNING/CONTINUITY OF CARE

- Assure understanding of renal failure treatment, including diet, medication regimen, and replacement treatment options.
- Arrange follow-up with nephrologist for continued medical management.
- Refer to a home health agency if ongoing care is needed.
- Be sure the patient is able to contact the physician managing renal failure and is aware of symptoms that require immediate reporting, including signs of fluid overload, severe or disabling fatigue, anorexia, or nausea.
- If the patient is on or beginning dialysis, coordinate dialysis appointments and provide a detailed report to outpatient dialysis nurse.
- Refer the patient to the local Kidney Foundation chapter for information or support.

REFERENCES

Lewis, S. M. & Collier, I. C. (1992). *Medical surgical nursing*. St. Louis, MO: Mosby.

Patrick, M. L., Woods, S. J., Crawer, R. F., Rokoshy, J. S., & Boraine, P. (1991). *Medical surgical nursing pathophysiological concepts.* Philadelphia, PA: Lippincott.

Porth, C. M. (1990). *Pathophysiology—Concepts of altered health stakes.* Philadelphia, PA: Lippincott.

Toto, L. (1992). Acute renal failure: A question of location. *American Journal of Nursing, 92*(11), 44–53.

▼

PERITONEAL DIALYSIS

Lynn Schoengrund, RN, MS

Peritoneal dialysis is a form of renal replacement therapy for patients with acute and chronic renal failure. It is an intracorporeal process that utilizes the highly vascular peritoneal membrane in the abdomen as the semipermeable membrane. A soft, silastic, multilumen catheter is surgically placed in the peritoneal cavity as the access for use of the peritoneum. The peritoneal dialysis procedure is performed by the patient at home (see Tables 48.1 and 48.2). When the patient is hospitalized, it is generally performed by the bedside nurse.

ETIOLOGIES

- Diabetes
- Glomerulonephritis
- Chronic hypertension
- Polycystic kidneys
- Autoimmune disorders, for example, lupus or Goodpasture's
- Progression of acute renal failure to chronic renal failure
- Chronic acetaminophen use or abuse
- Heroin use

CLINICAL MANIFESTATIONS

- Severe fatigue
- Anorexia, nausea vomiting
- Pallor
- Signs of fluid overload

CLINICAL/DIAGNOSTIC FINDINGS

See Renal Failure, p. 532.

Table 48.1 • Steps in Peritoneal Dialysis

Inflow: Dialysate is introduced into the abdominal cavity via the dialysis catheter.

Dwell: Dialysate remains in the abdominal cavity and fluid and electrolytes are drawn in.

Outflow: Fluid is drained via the dialysis catheter.

Exchange: The preceding three steps combined. Exchanges are varied based on patient needs.

Table 48.2 • Forms of Peritoneal Dialysis

CAPD (continuous ambulatory peritoneal dialysis): Patients manually perform three or four exchanges with long dwell times at 4–6 hr. The procedure is continuous.

CCPD (continuous cycling peritoneal dialysis): Automated exchanges are performed by a machine while the patient sleeps. Six to eight exchanges are performed at home.

IPD (intermittent peritoneal dialysis): Automated exchanges are performed in a dialysis center.

OTHER PLANS OF CARE TO REFERENCE

- Renal Failure
- Hemodialysis

NURSING DIAGNOSIS: HIGH RISK FOR INFECTION

Risk Factors

- Dialysis catheter
- A foreign object which communicates to the external environment
- High dextrose concentration in dialysate
- Warm, moist environment of the peritoneal cavity
- Chronic illness

Patient Outcomes

The patient will

- not have signs and symptoms of peritonitis.
- not have signs and symptoms of catheter exit site infections.

Nursing Interventions	Rationales
Prevent introduction of bacteria during exchanges by wearing masks, washing hands well, and following manufacturers' recommendations for using supplies.	Although peritonitis may occur despite perfect technique, some occurrences may be preventable if procedures are followed with painstaking care.
Assess for peritonitis at each exchange. The earliest sign is cloudy outflow. Inspect each outflow; manufacturers' print should be visible from the other side of the bag if the outflow is not cloudy. Draw samples from outflow for culture and gram stain as indicated by protocol or medical order.	Early detection can prevent rapid spread of bacteria and prevent complications. Unchecked peritonitis may scar the peritoneum and decrease its effectiveness as a semipermeable membrane.
Report the results of cultures to physicians and add antibiotics to dialysate as prescribed using aseptic technique.	Intraperitoneal antibiotics are an effective route for treatment of peritonitis and require no placement of additional venous access.
Assess the catheter exit site for signs of infection, including redness, inflammation, purulent drainage, and crust formation at exit.	The catheter exit site or tunnel may become sites of bacterial infection.
Use aseptic technique to set up and perform all exchanges.	

▼

NURSING DIAGNOSIS: FLUID VOLUME DEFICIT

Related To

- Excessive ultrafiltration of fluid during dialysis
- Inadequate intake

Defining Characteristics

Hypotension, orthostatic hypotension
Rapid or thready pulse
Weakness, dizziness
Dry mucous membranes

Patient Outcomes

- Vital signs are within normal limits of patient.
- Mucous membranes are moist.

- Intake and output are balanced.
- Weight is stable.

Nursing Interventions	Rationales
Assess fluid balance at least daily: 1. Weigh the patient at the same point in the exchange to compare weights (after drain, before inflow); when the patient is empty is recommended. 2. Compare weights over several exchanges and several days. 3. Calculate ultrafiltration by measuring or weighing outflow. 4. Assess the patient for signs and symptoms of fluid deficit.	Removal of fluid in peritoneal dialysis is based on selection of one of three concentrations of dextrose in dialysate (1.5, 2.5, or 4.25%). Some patients will ultrafiltrate significant amounts of fluid with the lowest concentration and need to drink fluids to maintain fluid balance. Calculation of the amount of fluid that needs to be removed is not as simple as it appears since it also varies with changes in body weight, accessibility of fluid to the semipermeable membrane, and variable responses with each exchange. Responses to fluid removal vary from individual to individual and in the individual by circumstances. Illness and hospitalization affect patient routines and may increase the potential for poor oral fluid intake. Peritonitis often interferes with ultrafiltration of fluid.
Adjust schedule of dextrose concentrations in exchanges and patient intake as prescribed and indicated by assessment.	Each exchange provides an opportunity to adjust patient fluid balance.
Administer oral salt solutions (broth) if the patient is symptomatic. If symptoms are severe, administer prescribed intravenous saline solutions.	Symptoms indicate a deficit in the vascular space that needs to be corrected to maintain circulation. Saline solutions pull fluid rapidly back into the vascular space.

Nursing Interventions	Rationales
Assist patients in learning about their responses to dialysis and fluid intake by reviewing the data collected in assessment.	Patients must learn to balance their life-style and treatment by trial and error. Examples are helpful in demonstrating both techniques for decision making and results. Patients who previously were on hemodialysis have to learn new routines.

▼

NURSING DIAGNOSIS: FLUID VOLUME EXCESS

Related To inadequate ultrafiltration in peritoneal dialysis

Defining Characteristics

Hypertension
Jugular distention
Increased weight
Edema
Pulmonary congestion, rales

Patient Outcomes

- Patient will not complain of shortness of breath.
- Weight will be stable.
- Breath sounds will be normal.

Nursing Interventions	Rationales
Assess the capability of the peritoneum to ultrafiltrate fluid: 1. Measure or weigh outflow fluid. 2. Time outflow of fluid. 3. Compare ultrafiltration outflow to intake, and note concentration of dextrose.	The cause of patients' fluid balance problems must be discovered so that treatment is appropriate. Loss of ultrafiltration fluid in peritoneal dialysis is associated temporarily with peritonitis. Other patients may not regularly ultrafiltrate fluid due to scarring of the peritoneum or for unknown reasons.
Assess regularly for signs of pulmonary edema and promptly report.	Patients may need temporary or permanent hemodialysis to prevent life-threatening fluid excess.

▼

NURSING DIAGNOSIS: BODY IMAGE DISTURBANCE

Related To to presence of permanent external peritoneal dialysis catheter

Defining Characteristics

Neglect of hygiene
Avoidance of catheter or catheter care
Focus on previous functions or appearances
Fear of rejection by others
Feelings of helplessness or hopelessness
Preoccupation with changes or loss
Extension of body boundary to include components of dialysis

Patient Outcomes

The patient will

- discuss feelings and concerns about image changes.
- demonstrate acceptance of changes with effective coping mechanisms.

Nursing Interventions	Rationales
Empower the patient to discuss feelings by validating rather than denying patient perceptions.	Denial of feelings perpetuates and accelerates the patient's negative feelings. Patient's can discuss these emotions if in a safe environment.
Assist in verbalizing fears and exploring reality.	Patients will need to incorporate physical changes into their self-definition.
Assist with clothing selection that minimizes appearance of catheter.	
Refer patients to psychotherapist if symptoms are severe or continued.	

▼

NURSING DIAGNOSIS: ALTERED NUTRITION—LESS THAN BODY REQUIREMENTS

Related To

- Loss of protein across the peritoneal membrane
- Decreased appetite due to feelings of fullness of dialysate dwell

Defining Characteristics

Body weight loss
Negative nitrogen balance
Blood urea nitrogen (BUN) >15 mg/100 mL
Inadequate food intake
Muscle tone or mass loss
Weakness
Complaints of fullness

Patient Outcomes

The patient will
- maintain weight.
- eat adequate diet.

Nursing Interventions	Rationales
Assess food intake, serum BUN, creatinine, and protein as well as weight comparisons.	Simple measurements such as weight changes are masked by fluid volume changes in dialysis patients. Responding to early cues may prevent severe malnutrition.
Consult dietitian to assess nutritional status.	Plan a protein intake for the patient that offsets protein loss in peritoneal dialysis.
Work with the patient to discover foods and serving sizes that are tolerated.	Ideal methods for obtaining adequate nutrition must be discovered through trial and error.
Encourage family involvement.	

▼

NURSING DIAGNOSIS: INEFFECTIVE MANAGEMENT OF THERAPEUTIC REGIMEN

Related To
- Complexity of regimen
- Lack of knowledge
- Frustration with chronic illness

Defining Characteristics

Verbalizes desire to manage the treatment of illness
Verbalizes difficulty with regulation or integration of any of the regimens needed to maintain health on dialysis
Verbalization of no action to make changes previously

Patient Outcomes

The patient will

- demonstrate understanding of components of treatment plan.
- set realistic priorities to meet selected components of the plan.
- identify factors which inhibit following treatment plan.

Nursing Interventions	Rationales
Provide educational resources through literature slides or video tapes.	
Assist the patient in talking through perceived need for behavioral changes. Help the patient set priorities. Individualize plans by reviewing the patient's life-style.	
Provide validation for patient efforts. For example, demonstrate changes in laboratory results as dietary habits change.	
Refer patients to appropriate experts (dietitian, exercise physiologist, nephrology nurses, and physicians) for assistance in individualizing treatment regimen.	

▼

DISCHARGE PLANNING/CONTINUITY OF CARE

- Assure that patient has sufficient supplies for treatment at home.
- Provide detailed report of hospitalization to dialysis caregivers.
- Assure understanding of self-management plan and any additional care regimens due to hospitalization.
- Review symptoms that require immediate reporting to the nephrologist.

REFERENCES

Covalesky, R. (1990). Myths and facts about peritoneal dialysis. *Nursing, 20*(4), 91.

Lewis, S. M. & Collier, I. C. (1992). *Medical surgical nursing*. St. Louis, MO: Mosby.

Patrick, M. L., Woods, S. J., Crawer, R. F., Rokoshy, J. S. & Boraine, P. (1991). *Medical surgical nursing pathophysiological concepts.* Philadelphia, PA: Lippincott.

Porth, C. M. (1990). *Pathophysiology—Concepts of altered health states.* Philadelphia, PA: Lippincott.

▼

Common Infectious Disease and Skin Conditions

ACQUIRED IMMUNODEFICIENCY SYNDROME: OPPORTUNISTIC INFECTIONS, SECONDARY CANCERS AND NEUROLOGICAL DISEASE

LuAnn Greiner, RN, BSN

A healthy immune system is required in order for the body to defend itself against infection. Individuals with the human immunodeficiency virus (HIV) experience a depletion of T4 (CD4, T-helper) lymphocytes, which in turn predisposes them to opportunistic infections, secondary cancers, and neurological disease indicative of the progression of HIV to acquired immunodeficiency syndrome (AIDS), a chronic, life-threatening illness. Regardless of the particular AIDS-defining illness (Table 49.1) the individual presents with, the plan of care must incorporate the physical, psychosocial and cognitive manifestations of the development and progression of AIDS.

ETIOLOGIES

- Presence of the HIV
- Depletion of T4 (CD4, T-helper) lymphocytes leading to immunodeficiency predisposing to opportunistic infections, secondary cancers, and neurological disease

CLINICAL MANIFESTATIONS

- Nausea and vomiting
- Persistent diarrhea
- Persistent fever
- Anorexia
- Dysphagia
- Involuntary weight loss

- Night sweats
- Abdominal pain
- Peripheral neuropathy
- Headache
- Persistent cough
- Dyspnea on exertion
- Mental status changes
- Chest pain
- Fatigue
- Anemia
- Skin lesions/rash
- Vision changes
- Cytopenias
- Hypotension
- Dehydration
- Recurrent yeast infections

Table 49.1 • AIDS-Defining Illnesses

AIDS dementia
Bacterial infections (2 or more within 2 years)
Candidiasis (esophageal, pulmonary)
Coccidioidomycosis
Cryptococcal meningitis
Cryptosporidiosis
Cytomegalovirus (CMV)
Herpes simplex virus (HSV)
Herpes varicella-zoster virus (HZV)
Histoplasmosis
Invasive cervical cancer
Isosporiasis
Kaposi's sarcoma (KS)
Lymphoid interstitial pneumonia (LIP)
Mycobacterium avium complex (MAC)
Mycobacterium kansasii
Non-Hodgkin's lymphoma
Nonpulmonary tuberculosis
Pneumocystis carinii pneumonia (PCP)
Primary lymphoma of the brain
Pulmonary tuberculosis
Progressive multifocal leukoencephalopathy (PML)
Recurrent bacterial pneumonia (2 or more in 12-month period)
Salmonellosis
Toxoplasmosis
Wasting syndrome

Note: From Centers for Disease Control, January 1 1993.

▼

CLINICAL/DIAGNOSTIC FINDINGS

- Total T4 lymphocyte count <200
- Abnormal chest x-ray consistent with pulmonary involvement
- Cultures (blood, wound, spinal fluid, stool, sputum) and/or tissue

biopsy positive for organisms indicative of opportunistic infection or secondary cancer
- Central nervous system lesion on head magnetic resonance imaging (MRI) indicative of opportunistic infection or tumor growth
- Abnormal ambulatory oxygen desaturation study consistent with *Pneumocystis carinii* pneumonia (PCP)
- Ophthalmologic changes consistent with cytomegaloviral retinitis

OTHER PLANS OF CARE TO REFERENCE

- Pain Management: Patient-Controlled Analgesia
- Nutrition/Support: Total Parenteral Nutrition
- Pneumonia
- Long-Term Venous Access
- Hepatitis
- Lumbar Puncture
- Alterations in Conciousness
- Prevention and Care of Pressure Ulcers

▼

NURSING DIAGNOSIS: HIGH RISK FOR SOCIAL ISOLATION

Risk Factors
- Activity intolerance associated with acute illness and progression of disease
- Presence, and associated stigma, of a communicable disease
- Long-term hospitalization
- Financial instability
- Loss of established relationships
- Unemployment or underemployment
- Loss of usual means of transportation
- Homosexual or bisexual identity
- Relocation secondary to long-term care needs
- History of intravenous (IV) drug use and associated stigma
- Lack of adequate child care

Patient Outcomes
The patient will
- convey that feelings of isolation are validated by others.
- identify risk factors contributing to social isolation.
- identify and utilize resources available to reduce or eliminate risk factors.

Nursing Interventions	Rationales
Assess for risk factors contributing to social isolation and feelings of loneliness.	
Validate the patient's feelings of social isolation and provide emotional support.	Validation of the subjective feeling of social isolation is imperative to collaboration with the patient in reducing or eliminating risk factors.
In collaboration with patient, identify existing support systems and their effectiveness.	
Reduce or eliminate risk factors contributing to social isolation: 1. Initiate physical therapy: muscle-strengthening exercises to promote maximum activity tolerance and sense of well-being. 2. Contact hospital social worker for assistance with financial concerns and establishment of community-based support. 3. Assist with referral to local AIDS service organization and/or local support groups available to persons with HIV/AIDS, if desired. 4. Identify and encourage participation in diversional activities that contribute to feelings of productivity and promote interaction with others. 5. Identify alternative means of transportation. 6. Assist with arrangements for provision of child care, if needed. 7. Provide supportive counseling to assist patient in exploring feelings associated with sexual identity, current illness, and presence of communicable disease. 8. Assist with referral to drug treatment program, if desired.	

Nursing Interventions	Rationales
Assist significant others in understanding the implications of chronic, life-threatening illness on one's self-image and identifying ways to provide support.	

▼

NURSING DIAGNOSIS: PAIN

Related To

- Neuropathy
- Malignancy
- Immobility
- Diagnostic procedures
- Tissue ischemia
- Fear
- Anxiety

Defining Characteristics

Reports or demonstrates pain
Necessity of diagnostic tests/invasive procedures
Fear and anxiety associated with pain experience
Inability to concentrate
Insomnia

Patient Outcomes

The patient will

- convey that others validate the pain experience.
- identify the location and intensity of the pain.
- identify precipitating factors that increase the pain experience.
- identify side effects of pain-relieving measures and ways to manage them.
- attain optimal pain relief with improved comfort, rest, and mobility.

Nursing Interventions	Rationales
Assess subjective and objective data to illicit character and intensity of pain experience.	Complete information regarding the patient's pain experience will contribute to optimal pain relief measures.
Validate the patient's feeling of pain.	Validation of the pain experience will decrease associated fear and anxiety.

Nursing Interventions	Rationales
Identify aggravating factors which contribute to the pain experience, for example, fear of pain, activity, and oral intake.	
Identify measures currently used to relieve pain, including prescribed medications, recreational drug use, and nonpharmacological pain-relieving measures.	Discussion of current use of pain-relieving measures will illicit further information regarding the patient's pain experience and coping mechanisms.
Differentiate between chronic (greater than 6 months) and acute pain and administer analgesics accordingly.	Differentiation of chronic and acute pain will assist in identifying the most effective treatment modalities. Analgesics provide the most consistent pain relief when administered on a scheduled rather than an as-needed basis.
Instruct patient on management of common side effects of pain-relieving medications, specifically constipation, nausea, vomiting, and sedation.	Common side effects must be managed appropriately to maintain optimal pain relief.
Offer alternative pain-relieving therapies as indicated based on patient interest and ability to participate, for example, guided imagery, massage, music, and art therapy.	
Assess response to pain-relieving measures and consult with physician if optimal pain relief has not been achieved.	Multiple factors will influence the response to pain-relieving measures, necessitating ongoing evaluation and adjustment.

▼

NURSING DIAGNOSIS: KNOWLEDGE DEFICIT—TREATMENT AND PROGRESSION

Related To

- New diagnosis
- Lack of exposure to information

Defining Characteristics

First admission to inpatient setting for AIDS-defining illness
Anxiety associated with progression of life-threatening illness

Inability of patient/significant other to verbalize understanding of diagnosis, treatment, and long-term therapies
Initiation of long-term IV therapies
Denial of presence or progression of disease

Patient Outcomes

The patient will

- verbalize understanding of diagnosis, treatment, and long-term therapies associated with acute/chronic illness.
- demonstrate correct technique for administration of IV therapies.
- perform proper infection control techniques and verbalize understanding of their role in prevention of disease transmission.
- define a plan for ongoing health care and identify and utilize available health care resources.

Nursing Interventions	Rationales
Assess for current knowledge of HIV infection and progression of disease and provide necessary information based on patient readiness to learn and physical and cognitive status.	Patients will present with extreme variations in the level of understanding of HIV infection and disease progression. Teaching will range from basic concepts of HIV infection to detailed information about specific AIDS-defining illness.
Instruct patient and significant other regarding specific presenting illness including signs and symptoms, treatment options, side effects of medications, and proper infection control techniques.	An understanding of the treatment plan is vital to quality of life and self-empowerment in the midst of chronic, life-threatening illness.
Utilize available resources, including written materials, videos, and consultation with HIV clinical nurse specialist, if available.	Written materials and videos will reinforce verbal instruction. The HIV clinical nurse specialists are experts in HIV education/ management.
Contact home infusion services to provide instruction and coordination of supplies for home IV therapies, if applicable.	Short- or long-term home IV therapy will require detailed instruction and ongoing support after discharge.
If home IV therapy is indicated, instruct patient and/or significant other on care and maintenance of venous access devices.	Self-care activities promote independence. Meticulous IV line and site care decreases risk of phlebitis and line contamination.

Nursing Interventions	Rationales
Initiate referral to visiting nurse for reinforcement and monitoring of treatment plan, if indicated.	Patient and/or significant other will likely need ongoing nursing support and teaching following acute illness.
Initiate referral to local AIDS service organization (ASO).	Individuals who avail themselves of ASO services gain significant knowledge regarding disease process and treatment modalities.

▼

NURSING DIAGNOSIS: HIGH RISK FOR INFECTION—NOSOCOMIAL

Risk Factors

- Weakened immune system related to presence of HIV
- Multiple invasive procedures
- Skin breakdown secondary to immobility and infection
- Bone marrow suppression as a side effect of immunosuppressive medications
- Long-term IV therapy/presence of venous access device

Patient Outcomes

The patient will

- identify risk factors for nosocomial infections.
- remain free of nosocomial infection throughout hospitalization.
- describe measures to maintain skin integrity.

Nursing Interventions	Rationales
Assess for risk factors associated with nosocomial infection: 1. baseline assessment of skin 2. baseline neutrophil count 3. use of bone marrow–suppressing agents 4. invasive procedures 5. indications for presence of long-term venous access device	
Monitor neutrophil count and initiate neutropenic precautions if count drops below 500.	Transient neutropenia can occur secondary to the use of bone marrow–suppressing agents, further placing the patient at risk for nosocomial infection.

Nursing Interventions	Rationales
Adhere to universal precautions and body substance isolation at all times.	To reduce the risk of transmission of pathogens.
Follow strict aseptic technique when performing treatments and invasive procedures.	
Promote optimal skin integrity. 1. Perform site care to all venous lines every 72 hr. 2. Reposition immobilized patients every 2 hr. 3. Maintain adequate nutrition and fluid intake. 4. Follow strict aseptic technique with all dressing changes. 5. Maximize activity for patients restricted to bed. 6. Provide air mattress for bed, foam, or gel pad for chairs. 7. Assess skin thoroughly every 8 hr and prn. 8. Administer antidiarrheals as indicated. 9. If patient is incontinent of urine, provide perianal care every 2 hr and prn. Consider use of condom or indwelling catheter to prevent excoriation of skin. 10. Apply emollients to dry areas of skin.	The effects of immobility, the wasting syndrome and the altered nutritional status associated with AIDS, and the presence of excretions and secretions as the result of fevers, incontinence, and wound drainage each contribute to skin breakdown and, in turn, increased risk for nosocomial infection.
Instruct visitors on proper handwashing techniques and other safety measures to prevent transmission of infections to which patient is susceptible, for example, upper respiratory infections and herpes simplex virus.	

Nursing Interventions	Rationales
Consult with physician to consider long-term venous access device if IV therapy is indicated for longer than 2 weeks.	The frequency with which short-term venous access devices must be changed and the patient's susceptibility to infection negate the use of these devices if IV therapy is indicated for longer than 2 weeks.

NURSING DIAGNOSIS: GRIEVING

Related To
- Loss of financial and physical independence
- Loss of social supports
- Changes in life-style secondary to progression of AIDS.

Defining Characteristics
Reports an actual or perceived loss
Anger
Depression
Withdrawal
Denial of need for assistance from others

Patient Outcomes
Patient will
- convey feelings of grief and loss.
- identify and utilize appropriate coping mechanisms for working through grief.
- identify and utilize available resources for counseling and support.

Nursing Interventions	Rationales
Establish a safe, trusting relationship that encourages expression of feelings.	
Provide supportive counseling that acknowledges patient's grief experience and associated feelings.	
Encourage to make choices in plan of care to increase feelings of control.	

Nursing Interventions	Rationales
Provide realistic, straightforward prognostic information when resolution of acute illness or progression of disease is not indicated.	
In collaboration with patient, identify effective coping mechanisms for working through grief.	
Identify and encourage participation in hospital and community-based support programs, for example, inpatient support group, local AIDS service organization.	

▼

NURSING DIAGNOSIS: HIGH RISK FOR IMPAIRED PHYSICAL MOBILITY/SELF-CARE DEFICITS

Risk Factors

- Progressive, debilitating illness
- Visual, cognitive, and sensory impairments
- Malnutrition as a result of chronic diarrhea, wasting syndrome, and inability to maintain adequate oral intake
- Pain

Patient Outcomes

Patient will

- identify and utilize adaptive techniques to perform daily activities and optimize independence.
- identify and utilize community agencies to assist with self-care needs and ongoing support.

Nursing Interventions	Rationales
Obtain baseline and ongoing data of functional abilities and limitations using established functional assessment tools.	Early detection and ongoing monitoring of physical limitations allow initiation of therapies that promote optimal function and independence.

Nursing Interventions	Rationales
Identify factors which place patient at risk and institute interventions to minimize risks: 1. Monitor fluid losses and maintain adequate hydration. 2. Consult registered dietitian to assist in optimizing nutritional status. 3. Consult physical and occupational therapy for instruction on muscle-strengthening exercises and energy expenditure modifications. 4. Teach active and/or passive range-of-motion exercises as indicated. 5. Initiate pain-relieving measures and administer analgesics as prescribed to maximize activity tolerance.	Contributing factors must be identified and corrected to maximize activity tolerance.
Facilitate use of assistive devices as indicated.	
Initiate referral to a home care agency for functional assessment and initiation of ongoing physical and occupational therapies.	

▼

NURSING DIAGNOSIS: HIGH RISK FOR INJURY

Risk Factors

- Weakness and fatigue
- Visual, cognitive, and sensory deficits
- Sedation associated with analgesics
- Hypotension associated with anemia, dehydration

Patient Outcomes

Patient will

- remain free from injury.
- identify potential hazards in the environment.
- describe general safety measures.
- obtain necessary adaptive equipment to promote safety.

Nursing Interventions	Rationales
Identify potential hazards in the hospital and home environment.	
Obtain baseline data regarding visual, cognitive, and sensory and physical limitations/deficits.	This information will direct the type of interventions and adaptive equipment needed.
Provide for orientation to the hospital environment.	
Initiate safety measures when patient is identified to be at risk for falls: 1. frequent reorientation 2. use of siderails 3. 24-hr sitter or attendant care 4. bed alarm 5. condom or indwelling catheter 6. close proximity to unit desk 7. assistance with activities 8. call light in reach at all times 9. use of soft wrist or chest restraint if other safety measures fail	
Discuss general safety measures in the home and provide necessary adaptive equipment.	
Initiate home care referral to perform functional assessment and initiate safety measures as indicated.	

▼

DISCHARGE PLANNING/CONTINUITY OF CARE

- Initiate a discharge planning meeting that includes the patient, significant others, and representatives from all involved disciplines and referral agencies.
- Provide with necessary home care supplies and prescriptions and establish a plan for refilling prescriptions.
- Review and finalize home care plan, ensuring that adequate support services are available to the patient.
- Initiate referral to a home health care agency for ongoing nursing, therapy, and attendant care.

- Initiate referral to local AIDS service organization or other counseling agency for ongoing psychosocial support.
- Arrange for follow-up appointments with primary physician.
- Provide telephone numbers in case of questions or emergencies.
- Identify avenues for caregiver support and respite.

REFERENCES

Aranda-Naranjo, B. (1993). The effect of HIV on the family: Implications for care. *AIDS Patient Care, 7*(1), 27–29.

Bartlett, J. G. & Finkbeiner, A. K. (1991). *The guide to living with HIV Infection.* Baltimore, MD: Johns Hopkins University Press.

Kelly, F., & Holman, S. (1993). The new faces of AIDS. *American Journal of Nursing, 93*(2), 26–34.

Lewis, A. (Ed.). (1988). *Nursing care of the person with AIDS/ARC.* Rockville, MD: Aspen.

Wolfe, L. (1992). Grief, AIDS and the gay community. *AIDS Patient Care, 6*(4), 194–197.

▼

HEPATITIS

Lynn Schoengrund, RN, MS

Hepatitis is widespread inflammation of liver tissue which may interrupt bile flow resulting in cholestasis. Complete recovery is the most common result of hepatitis; however, complications can include chronic persistent hepatitis, chronic active hepatitis, fulminant hepatitis, and cirrhosis of the liver. Chronic persistent hepatitis is a delayed convalescent period, characterized by fatigue and hepatomegaly. Chronic active hepatitis is distinguished from chronic persistent hepatitis by the ongoing process of liver necrosis. This process usually results in cirrhosis. Fulminant hepatitis is severe liver impairment and liver cell necrosis that may result in liver failure. This type of complication may be seen with toxic reactions to drugs.

ETIOLOGIES

Viral hepatitis types include
- A
- B
- non-A, non-B
- C
- drugs
- poisons

CLINICAL MANIFESTATIONS

- Anorexia, nausea, vomiting
- Right upper quadrant pain
- Decreased sense of smell and taste
- Malaise, headache, fever, arthralgias, fatigue
- Urticaria, jaundice

CLINICAL/DIAGNOSTIC FINDINGS

- Hepatitis A: presence of immunoglobulin M (IgM) antibody in serum or hepatitis A virus in stool
- Hepatitis B: presence of hepatitis antigen in serum
- All types:
  - elevated serum glutamic oxaloacetic/pyruvic transaminases (SGOT, SGPT)
  - elevated serum bilirubin
  - elevated urine bilirubin

▼

NURSING DIAGNOSIS: ALTERED NUTRITION—LESS THAN BODY REQUIREMENTS

Related To
- Anorexia
- Nausea
- Vomiting
- Malaise
- Fatigue

Defining Characteristics
Weight loss
Poor dietary intake
Loss of muscle mass or tone
Pale mucous membranes

Patient Outcomes
- Weight is maintained.
- The patient does not experience nausea and vomiting.

Nursing Interventions	Rationales
Assess nutritional status. Include daily record of calories consumed. Record daily weight.	Prevention of catabolism and increasing patient weakness are possible if measures to provide nutrition are instituted.
Provide high-calorie snacks and small, frequent meals. Meet individual requests.	Maintaining patient diet is preferred method for maintaining nutritional status.

Nursing Interventions	Rationales
If weight loss is persistent or if the patient shows continuing signs of malnutrition, discuss with physician and refer to the dietitian or nutritional support team if available for enteral supplements or parenteral nutrition.	
Administer enteral or parenteral feedings as prescribed and frequently reassess the patient's nutritional status. See Total Parenteral Nutrition or Enteral Nutrition.	

▼

NURSING DIAGNOSIS: ACTIVITY INTOLERANCE/SELF-CARE DEFICIT—BATHING/HYGIENE

Related To

- Fatigue
- Malaise
- Arthralgia
- Weakness

Defining Characteristics

Verbal report and/or demonstrated inability to perform activities
Complaints of weakness, fatigue, or pain with activities

Patient Outcomes

The patient will

- gradually increase activity without symptoms.
- begin to participate in activities of daily living.

Nursing Interventions	Rationales
Assess patient's response to activity (dyspnea, tachycardia, fatigue).	
Plan a daily schedule which balances activity with rest. Inform all other care providers of rest schedule.	

Nursing Interventions	Rationales
Assist with bathing, hygiene, and other activities of daily living until able to resume.	
Instruct patient on passive range-of-motion (ROM) exercises to be done while in bed.	Range-of-motion exercises increase joint flexibility and stretch muscles.
Provide regular ambulation for short distances.	Muscle wasting may occur if the patient is totally inactive. Protein breakdown from muscle wasting will contribute to poor nutritional status.
Consult occupational/physical therapy for muscle-strengthening exercises and strategies for conserving energy.	

▼

NURSING DIAGNOSIS: PAIN—PRURITIS

Related To bile salt accumulation

Risk Factors

- Inactivity or bedrest
- Deposition of bilirubin in the skin
- Dry, itchy skin

Patient Outcomes

Skin is intact; patient comfort is maintained.

Nursing Interventions	Rationales
Wash skin frequently with mild soap. Apply lotion to prevent dryness.	Deposition of bilirubin may cause skin dryness and itching.
Discourage scratching of skin. Use commonsense strategies to decrease itching, for example, lotion application, use of unbleached linen, and frequent gown/linen changes.	

▼

NURSING DIAGNOSIS: KNOWLEDGE DEFICIT—HEPATITIS TRANSMISSION

Related To
- No previous exposure to information
- Inappropriate behavior

Defining Characteristics
Verbalizes lack of knowledge about disease acquisition
No correlation between previous activity and disease

Patient Outcomes
The patient will
- state methods of disease transmission.
- describe ways to prevent transmission.
- identify a personal plan to prevent transmission of hepatitis.

Nursing Interventions	Rationales
Educate patient regarding disease transmission (see Table 50.1.)	
Refer patient to community resources specific for the mode of transmission of disease for that patient. For example, develop lists of resources for clean needles and syringes; refer to clinics or resources for condoms.	
Teach safe sex techniques.	
Teach proper hygiene, especially washing of hands and washing of food prior to eating.	
Report home environments without sanitary facilities to the proper authorities.	
Inform patient that the Center for Disease Control recommends human immunodeficiency virus (HIV) testing for people exposed to other sexually transmitted diseases.	

Table 50.1 • Transmissions Of Hepatitis Viruses

Virus	Mode Of Transmission	Source Of Infection/Spread Disease	Serological Monitor
Hepatatis A (HA)	Fecal, oral, i.e., fecal contamination and oral ingestion	Crowded conditions, poor personal hygiene, contaminated food, persons with subclinical infection	HA Ag
Hepatatis B (HB)	Percutaneous and permucosal infected blood and body fluids at birth, sexual contact	Contaminated needles and syringes, contaminated blood products, at-risk sexual behaviors, i.e., homosexual activity, multiple partners, contact with asymptomatic carriers	HB Ag
Non-A, non-B hepatitis (includes hepatitis C)	Percutaneous and parenteral	Blood and blood products, needles and syringes	Hepatitis C virus

▼

DISCHARGE PLANNING/CONTINUITY OF CARE

- Assure understanding of self-management plan, including building activity tolerance slowly and maintaining an adequate diet.
- Refer to a home health agency if continued nursing care or assistance is needed.
- Arrange follow-up with a physician to provide continuing care.
- Assure understanding of the mode of transmission of the disease, especially through sexual contacts, to prevent spread of the disease.

REFERENCES

Lewis, S. M. & Collier, I. C. (1992). *Medical surgical nursing.* St. Louis, MO: Mosby.

Maddrey, W. C. (1989). Viral hepatitis today. *Emergency Medicine, 21*(16), 124–136.

Patrick, M. L., Woods, S. J., Crawer, R. F., Rokoshy, J. S., & Boraine, P. (1991). *Medical surgical nursing pathophysiological concepts.* Philadelphia, PA: Lippincott.

Porth, C. M. (1990). *Pathophysiology—Concepts of altered health states.* Philadelphia, PA: Lippincott.

▼

PREVENTION AND CARE OF PRESSURE ULCERS

Barbara King, RN, RN-C;
Susan Murray, RN, MS

Pressure ulcers are defined as an area of localized tissue damage caused by ischemia due to pressure. The most frequently identified pressure ulcer sites are over bony prominences, which include scapula, elbows, iliac crest, sacrum, trochanters, and heels.

ETIOLOGIES

- Intrinsic factors
  - compromised nutritional status
  - advanced age
  - elevated glucose levels
  - decreased circulation
  - decreased sensation
  - decreased immune status
  - decreased skin turgor
- Extrinsic factors
  - excessive pressure
  - excessive shearing
  - excessive friction
  - excessive moisture

CLINICAL MANIFESTATIONS

Stage I
- Nonblanchable erythema
- Epidermis intact

Stage II
- Loss of epidermis
- Painful
- Free of necrotic tissue

Stage III
- Loss of dermis to subcutaneous tissue
- Usually not painful
- May include
  - necrotic tissue
  - sinus tract formation/undermining (tunneling or track formation under the skin
  - exudate
  - infection

Stage IV
- Deep tissue destruction extending to fascia, muscle, or bone usually not painful
- May include
  - necrotic tissue
  - sinus tract formation/undermining
  - exudate
  - infection

CLINICAL/DIAGNOSTIC FINDINGS

- Altered nutritional state
  - hypoalbunemia
  - weight loss
  - hypocholesterolemia
  - decreased total lymphocyte count
  - negative nitrogen balance
  - protein deficiency
  - anemia
  - hyperglycemia
  - decreased serum transferrin
- Altered circulatory state
  - dehydration
  - low diastolic blood pressure
  - edema
  - decreased hematocrit/hemoglobin
- Infected pressure ulcers
  - elevated white blood cell (WBC) count
  - positive wound culture
  - osteomyelitis
  - fever

▼

NURSING DIAGNOSIS: HIGH RISK FOR IMPAIRED SKIN INTEGRITY

Risk Factors

- Intrinsic factors: decreased serum albumin, obesity, emaciation, low diastolic blood pressure, peripheral neuropathy, elderly, poor skin

turgor, immunocompromised, hyperglycemia, medications, dehydration, edema
- Extrinsic factors: incontinence, diaphoresis, immobility, decreased activity, mechanical factors (shearing, friction, pressure), hypothermia

Patient Outcomes

Patient/caregiver will
- maintain intact skin.
- state necessary measures to reduce pressure/shearing/friction/moisture.
- state importance of adequate nutrition and fluid to maintain skin integrity.

Nursing Interventions	Rationales
Establish a position change schedule.	Frequency must be tailored to individual patient needs. The schedule should include major position changes and minor weight shifts at least every 2 hr.
Utilize pressure reduction/relief device in conjunction with position change schedule. (See Table 51.1)	Capillary closing pressure is 25–32 mmHg. Pressure-reducing devices lower pressure as compared to a standard hospital mattress or chair surface but do not reduce pressure below 32 mmHg. Therefore, the device must be used in conjunction with a turning schedule. Pressure relief devices (low air loss bed and air-fluidized bed) lower capillary closing pressure below 32 mmHg.
Assist with ambulation as tolerated.	
Utilize measures to decrease shearing and friction:	Shearing of skin layers occurs when patients slide down in bed.
1. Place head of bed less than 30° when not contraindicated.	
2. Use turning sheet, trapeze, lifts, and transfer boards.	Reduce surface cling and friction.
3. Use powder or cornstarch on surfaces contacting the skin.	Absorbs moisture; reduces friction.
4. Apply transparent dressing to high-risk areas.	Reduces surface friction.

Nursing Interventions	Rationales
Utilize measures to reduce excessive moisture: 1. Utilize pressure relief/reduction device which provides aeration (e.g., vented air mattress, low air loss beds, air-fluidized beds). 2. Apply moisture barrier creme to contacting skin. 3. Change gowns and linens when wet, as needed.	Excessive moisture and/or contact with urine or stool causes maceration and/or chemical erosion to the skin.
Monitor patient's nutritional and hydration status by assessing 1. intake and output 2. daily weight 3. calorie count 4. dietary consult 5. vital signs 6. BUN, creatine, cholesterol, albumin	Tissue hydration and positive nitrogen balance are critical for wound healing. Adequate fluid intake is necessary to maintain intact skin.
Provide education to patient/family/caregiver which includes 1. effects of and measures to decrease pressure/shearing/moisture/friction to the skin 2. Effects of medical problems on circulation and skin integrity 3. routine skin care and inspection of skin for signs of impending skin breakdown. 4. importance of adequate fluid and nutritional intake	

▼

NURSING DIAGNOSIS: IMPAIRED SKIN INTEGRITY

Related To pressure

Defining Characteristics

Nonblanchable erythema
Disruption of skin surface and layers

Patient Outcomes

Patient will

- not develop further pressure ulcer formation.

- have adequate nutritional and fluid intake.
- verbalize signs and symptoms of infected wound.
- demonstrate activities and treatments which will promote wound healing.
- show signs of progressive wound healing.

Table 51.1 • Pressure-Reducing/Relieving Devices

Devices	Indications for Use
Waffle/egg crate foam mattress overlay: no pressure reduction/relief	Comfort only, does not provide pressure reduction/relief
Static air mattress: pressure reduction only	High-risk patient; presence of stage I or II pressure ulcer; presence of stage III or IV pressure ulcer and awaiting surgical consult
Low airloss bed: pressure relief provided	Limited mobility with one other factor: • Anasarca • Drainage and/or body fluids contained in pouching device • Presence of stage III or IV pressure ulcer • Postoperative myocutaneous flap • Pain management
Air-fluidized bed: pressure relief provided	Immobility with one other factor: • Drainage and/or body fluids not contained in pouching device. • Presence of stage III or IV pressure ulcer • Postoperative myocutaneous flap • Pain management • Hypothermia/hyperthermia

▼

Nursing Interventions	Rationales
Identify stage of pressure ulcer.	See Clinical Manifestations.

Nursing Interventions	Rationales
Assess pressure ulcer for: 1. size 2. location 3. undermining/sinus formation 4. necrotic tissue 5. local infection (erythema, induration, purulent drainage, malodorous drainage, crepitus) 6. characteristics of exudate 7. pain to the wound and surrounding tissues	
Measure the depth or undermining of a pressure ulcer using the following technique: 1. With a gloved hand, insert a 6-inch cotton-tipped applicator into the deepest portion of the wound. 2. Grasp the fully inserted applicator with the thumb and forefinger at the point where the applicator meets the wound surface. 3. Carefully remove the applicator while maintaining the marking point. Measure from the tip of the applicator to the grasp point. This will indicate the wound depth.	Accurate measurement of wound size is necessary in order to evaluate the healing process.
Monitor patient for signs and symptoms of systemic infection, including 1. fever 2. leukocytosis 3. confusion 4. tachycardia 5. hypotension 6. malaise	

Nursing Interventions	Rationales
Monitor fluid and nutritional status: 1. intake and output 2. daily weight 3. calorie count 4. dietary consult 5. vital signs 6. BUN, creatinine cholesterol, albumin	
Institute measures to reduce pressure, shearing, friction, and moisture.	
Debride necrotic tissue, if present:	Presence of necrotic tissue hinders wound healing.
1. use of enzymatic debridement agents (Elase, Travase)	Enzymatic agents chemically break down necrotic tissue; ineffective unless moist environment is present.
2. physiological debridement using transparent dressings	Transparent dressings increase leukocyte migration and autolysis of necrotic tissue; cannot be used when clinical infection is present.
3. mechanical debridement with wet/dry gauze dressings	Wet/dry dressings provide nonselective debridement. Granulation tissue as well as necrotic tissue will be removed.
4. surgical consult for sharp debridement	Sharp debridement provides quick and effective removal of necrotic tissue.
Clean wound with appropriate cleanser at each dressing change. (See Table 51.2)	Wound cleansing promotes removal of wound debris and bacteria from wound surface.
Apply dressing as indicated by wound stage. Dressings may include gauze, hydrocolloid, hydrogels, calcium alginate, and transparent and polymeric foam. (See Table 51.3.)	Wound dressings absorb excess exudate, obliterate dead space, and keep the wound surface moist. Dead space hinders wound healing and predisposes the tissue to abscess formation. A moist wound surface enhances cellular migration and wound healing.

Nursing Interventions	Rationales
Implement teaching plan which includes preventative measures, instructions in wound care, and signs and symptoms of infection.	The patient/caregiver needs to be educated regarding the process of skin breakdown and preventative measures. Wound healing requires correct use of cleansing solution and dressing application.

▼

DISCHARGE PLANNING/CONTINUITY OF CARE

- Observe patient/family/caregiver performing wound care.
- Provide with the necessary supplies and equipment prior to discharge and review plan for obtaining additional supplies.
- Arrange follow-up with local physician
- Consult a home health agency if continued nursing care or additional support services are needed.

Table 51.2 • Wound Cleansers

Cleanser	Use	Considerations
Normal saline	Cleanser recommended for all wounds	
Povidone-iodine	Effective in controlling bacterial growth in wounds	Inhibits and destroys macrophages and fibroblasts
Hydrogen peroxide	Provides mechanical cleansing via effervescent action	Destroys fibroblasts
Dankin's solution	Controls odor; is useful for staphylococcal and streptococcal infections; liquefies necrotic tissue	Destroys fibroblasts unless properly diluted
Acetic acid	Appropriate for *Pseudomonas* infections	Destroys fibroblasts when properly diluted

▼

Table 51.3 • Wound Dressings

Dressing	Indications	Features
Gauze		
Impregnated • Aquaphor, Vaseline, Xerofoam	Most wound sites	Protects wounds
Not impregnated • Adaptic, Kling, Telfa	Most wound sites	Protects wounds
Transparent (film) • Acuderm, OpSite, Tegaderm	Superficial abrasions, blisters, minor burns, donor sites, stage I or II pressure ulcers	Maintains physiological environment, provides bacterial barrier, transparent, conforms to wound, waterproof, provides autolytic debridement
Hydrogel • Spenco, Vilgilon, Elastogel	Stage I, II, or III dermal ulcers, donor sites, second-degree burns, abrasions, blisters, lacerations	Maintains physiological environment when dressing is moist, relieves pain, translucent, provides debridement
Polymeric (foam) • Epi-lock, Lyofoam, Allevyn	Stage I, II, or III pressure ulcers, dermal ulcers, donor sites, second-degree burns, abrasions, blisters, lacerations	Maintains physiological environment, reduces pain, provides autolytic debridement if dressing stays moist
Hydrocolloid • DuoDerm, Restore, Comfeel	Stage I, II, or III pressure ulcers, dermal ulcers, donor sites, second-degree burns, abrasion, blisters	Provides moist environment for wound healing, bacterial barrier, enhances autolytic debridement, waterproof, reduces pain
Calcium Alginate • Kaltostat, Sorbsan	Moderate to heavy exudating wounds, control of minor bleeding, can be used in infected wounds, stage I, II, III, or IV pressure ulcers, venous stasis ulcers, diabetic ulcers, arterial ulcers, donor sites, dermal ulcers	Dressing absorbs exudate and forms a gel plug, creating a moist environment for wound healing, conforms to wound, provides autolytic debridement, painless to remove, provides hemostasis

Note: The dressing brands listed are only a sampling of the many products available. We do not endorse the use of any particular product.

▼

REFERENCES

Braden, B. & Bergstrom N. (1989). Clinical utility of the Braden Scale for predicting pressure sore risk. *Decubitus, 2*(3), 44–51.

International Association of Enterostomal Therapy (IAET). (1989). Standards of care dermal wounds: pressure sores. IAET.

Krasner, D. (1990). *Chronic wound care—A clinical source book for health care professionals.* King of Prussia, PA: Health Management Publications.

Mertz, M. (1990). Intervention: Dressing effects on wound healing. In *New directions in wound healing.* ConvaTec, NJ: Squibb and Sons.

Pressure ulcers in adults: Prediction and prevention. (1992). Rockville, MD: U.S. Department of Health and Human Services, Public Health Service Agency for Health Care Policy and Research.

▼

VENOUS STASIS ULCER

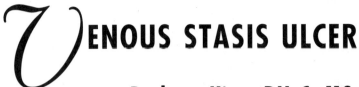

Barbara King, RN-C, MS;
Susan Murray, RN, MS

Venous stasis ulcers are a result of prolonged venous hypertension, usually in the lower calf. Skin layers affected by venous ulcer formation are epidermis, dermis, and subcutaneous tissue. Location of ulcers are typically just above the medial malleolus of the ankle.

ETIOLOGIES

- Deep-vein thrombosis
- Thrombophlebitis
- Obesity
- Valvular incompetence
- Varicosities

CLINICAL MANIFESTATIONS

- Edema
- Pigmentation changes
- Varicose veins
- Pain
- Cutaneous changes

CLINICAL/DIAGNOSTIC FINDINGS

- Doppler ultrasonagraphy revealing absence of venous reflux or obstruction

OTHER PLANS OF CARE TO REFERENCE

- Prevention and Care of Pressure Ulcers

▼

NURSING DIAGNOSIS: ALTERED PERIPHERAL TISSUE PERFUSION

Related To venous stasis

Defining Characteristics

Assessment of the lower extremities will find:
Edema which increases with prolonged standing
Dilated tortuous superficial veins
Erythema followed by a deep brown skin discoloration
Loss of hair growth
Chronic dryness and scaling
Pain relieved with elevation or walking
Presence of ulcers just above the medial malleolus
Irregularly shaped ulcers with welldefined boarders

Patient Outcomes

The patient will
- attain intact skin.
- demonstrate improved peripheral circulation.

Nursing Interventions	Rationales
Assess lower extremities for presence or absence of edema, pigmentation changes, and presence or absence or diluted/tortuous superficial veins.	
Monitor peripheral pulses frequently.	
Ongoing assessment of ulcer should include the following: 1. location 2. size 3. ulcer stage 4. demarcation 5. color 6. condition of surrounding tissue 7. presence of necrosis 8. presence of infection	

Nursing Interventions	Rationales
Implement measures to optimize venous return:	Elimination of venous stasis is necessary to promote ulcer healing and maintain tissue integrity.
1. Keep legs elevated higher than heart when lying down.	
2. Encourage patient to avoid sitting with legs crossed.	Acute angulation of vessels decreases venous return.
3. Encourage patient to avoid prolonged standing.	Prolonged standing increases hydrostatic pressure and venous distention, thus increasing venous stasis.
4. Ambulate as tolerated.	Ambulating improves venous return through activation of the muscle pump.
5. Encourage to avoid use of constrictive clothing.	
6. Correctly fit and apply lower extremity support devices (e.g., Ace wraps, pressure gradient support stockings, zinc-impregnated gauze wrap, intermittent compression device).	Support devices provide an appropriate pressure gradient to enhance venous return.
Implement measures to reduce pressure/shearing/friction/moisture, as needed, to enhance ulcer healing (see Prevention and Care of Pressure Ulcers, see p. 576).	
Debride necrotic issue if present using	Presence of necrotic tissue hinders wound healing.
1. enzymatice debridement agents (Elase, Travase)	Enzymatic agents chemically break down necrotic tissue and keep wound clear of pyrogenic crusting. Ineffective unless moist environment is present.
2. physiological debridement using transparent dressings	Transparent dressings increase leukocyte migration and autolysis of necrotic tissue. Transparent dressings cannot be used when clinical infection is present. Transparent dressings may not be effective over heavy exudating wounds.

Nursing Interventions	Rationales
3. mechanical debridement with wet/dry gauze dressings	Wet/dry dressings provide nonselective debridement. Granulation tissue as well as necrotic tissue will be removed.
Clean ulcer with appropriate cleanser with each dressing change. (See Table 51.2.)	
Apply dressing as indicated by ulcer stage. Examples of dressing include Hydracolloid, Hydrogel, calcium alginate, moist gauze, and zinc-impregnated gauze wrap (Unna boot). (See Table 51.3.)	

▼

NURSING DIAGNOSIS: PAIN—LOWER EXTREMITIES

Related To chronic venous insufficiency

Defining Characteristics

Early disease stage: verbalization of leg pain which improves with ambulating and elevation

Later disease stage: verbalization of leg pain which is severe and may necessitate analgesic use

Guarded movement

Patient Outcomes

Patient will describe increased comfort.

Nursing Interventions	Rationales
Assess pain for the following factors: 1. location 2. duration 3. intensity 4. precipitation and alleviating factors	
Implement measure to provide pain relief: 1. Administer analgesics as prescribed.	

Nursing Interventions	Rationales
2. Apply lower extremity support devices.	
3. Elevate lower extremities.	
4. Encourage ambulation as tolerated.	

▼

NURSING DIAGNOSIS: KNOWLEDGE DEFICIT—DISEASE PROCESS, TREATMENT PLAN, AND PREVENTION

Related To
- Misinterpretation
- Lack of exposure to information

Defining Characteristics
Verbalization of problem
Inaccurate perception of underlying disease process
Inaccurate performance of wound care
Inaccurate knowledge of preventative treatments

Patient Outcomes
The patient will
- verbalize understanding of disease process and plan of treatment.
- correctly demonstrate ulcer care.
- verbalize understanding of preventive strategies.

Nursing Interventions	Rationales
Discuss significance of underlying disease state (venous stasis) and its relationship to ulcer formation.	Education of the patient regarding the pathophysiology, prevention, and treatment of a venous stasis ulcer are critical elements for ulcer care.

Nursing Interventions	Rationales
Educate regarding preventive strategies, which include: 1. Keep legs elevated higher than heart level when lying down. 2. Avoid sitting with legs crossed. 3. Avoid prolonged standing. 4. Avoid use of constrictive clothing. 5. Correct application of lower extremity vascular support device. 6. Avoid tobacco use in all forms. 7. Maintain sufficient fluid intake. 8. Avoid use of devices which may produce thermal trauma (e.g., heating pads, hot water bottles, hot or cold solutions or soaks, ice packs). 9. Avoid use of solutions which may produce chemical trauma (e.g., corn and callous removal preparations, drying or irritating agents such as alcohol). 10. Wear properly fitting footwear when up ambulating, for protection of feet.	
Provide information regarding proper care of skin on legs and feet which includes: 1. Keep legs and feet clean and apply moisturizing lotion. 2. Inspect legs and feet daily for signs of irritation or ulcer formation. 3. Wear white natural fiber socks which are nonconstricting. 4. Keep toenails neatly trimmed. 5. Notify local physician if changes develop in lower extremity: sensation, temperature, color, pain, or presence of drainage.	

DISCHARGE PLANNING/CONTINUITY OF CARE

- Assure understanding of ulcer care.
- Observe patient performing ulcer care.
- Provide with the necessary supplies and equipment needed prior to discharge and review plan for obtaining additional supplies.
- Consult a home health agency if additional nursing care and/or support services are needed.
- Arrange follow-up with local physician.

REFERENCES

International Association of Enterostomal Therapy (IAET). (1989). *Standards of care of dermal wounds: Leg ulcers.* Irvine, CA: IAET.

Krasner, D. (1990). *Chronic wound care: A clinical source book for health care professionals.* King of Prussia, PA: Health Management Publications.

INDEX

Note: Page numbers followed by t indicate tables; numbers in italic indicate figures.

B

E

I

J

K

N

O

P

Q

R

T

U

X

Z